CAROTID ARTERY STENTING: THE BASICS

CONTEMPORARY CARDIOLOGY

CHRISTOPHER P. CANNON, MD

SERIES EDITOR

For further volumes:
http://www.springer.com/series/7677

CAROTID ARTERY STENTING: THE BASICS

Edited by

JACQUELINE SAW

University of British Columbia, Vancouver, BC, Canada

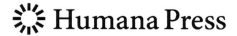 Humana Press

Editor
Jacqueline Saw, MD, FRCPC
Clinical Assistant Professor
University of British Columbia
Vancouver General Hospital
Vancouver, BC, Canada
jsaw@interchange.ubc.ca

Series Editor
Christopher P. Cannon

ISBN 978-1-60327-313-8   e-ISBN 978-1-60327-314-5
DOI 10.1007/978-1-60327-314-5

Library of Congress Control Number: 2009921124

Cover illustration: Figure 17D in Chapter 11

Printed on acid-free paper

springer.com

To my family for their love, support, and understanding: my parents Juliana and Nicholas, my husband David, and our son and daughter, Evan and Kate. And to the members of the Division of Cardiology at Vancouver General Hospital, for their enduring guidance and mentorship.

PREFACE

Carotid artery stenting has evolved remarkably over the past three decades to become a promising alternative to carotid endarterectomy, especially for patients deemed to have high surgical risks. Several crucial developments have enabled carotid stenting to be performed safely and achieve durable effectiveness in stroke prevention. The key advancements comprise technological innovations, improvement in operator skills and experience, and optimization of patient selection. Modern-day carotid stenting is performed with dedicated carotid self-expanding stents and emboli protection devices, with several FDA-approved platforms that are currently available for use. Nevertheless, despite utilizing the best equipment, carotid stenting can be challenging in unsuitable complex patients with difficult anatomy, and may result in catastrophic cerebral complications. Thus, the vital roles of the interventionist as a gatekeeper in patient selection, and as a meticulous skilled proceduralist entrusted to execute the procedure safely, cannot be underestimated.

This textbook serves as a learning resource on the multifaceted management of patients with carotid artery stenosis, with the key focus on extracranial carotid artery stenting. Details on contemporary aspects of carotid stenting are discussed, including review of supporting studies and guidelines, technical perspectives, and peri-procedural management. This textbook is intended to complement the "hands-on" experience of interventional trainees and established interventionists.

Jacqueline Saw, MD, FRCPC

CONTENTS

CONTRIBUTORS

ALEX ABOU-CHEBL, MD - *Department of Neurology, University of Louisville School of Medicine, Louisville, KY*

ADIL AL-RIYAMI, MD - *Interventional Cardiology, Vancouver General Hospital, Vancouver, BC, Canada*

FAISAL ALQUOOFI, MD, FRCPC - *Interventional Cardiology, University of Calgary and Foothills Hospital, Calgary, AB, Canada*

DEEPAK L. BHATT, MD, FACC - *Integrated Interventional Cardiovascular Program at Brigham and Women's Hospital and the VA Boston Healthcare System, TIMI Group, Boston, MA*

ROBERT H. BOONE, MD - *Interventional Cardiology, St Paul's Hospital, Vancouver, BC, Canada*

ANTHONY Y. FUNG, MBBS - *Interventional Cardiology, Division of Cardiology, Vancouver General Hospital, Vancouver, BC, Canada*

MARLENE GRENON, MD, FRCSC - *Division of Vascular Surgery, University of British Columbia, St. Paul's Hospital, Vancouver, BC, Canada*

PERCY P. JOKHI, MBBS, PhD - *Interventional Cardiology, Vancouver General Hospital, Vancouver, BC, Canada*

RONAK S. KANANI, MD, FRCP - *Interventional Cardiology, University of Calgary, Foothills Hospital, Calgary, AB, Canada*

JUHANA KARHA, MD - *Cleveland Clinic Foundation, Cleveland, OH*

USMAN KHAN, MD - *Department of Neurology, University of Louisville School of Medicine, Louisville, KY*

ROHIT KHURANA, MD - *Interventional Cardiology, Vancouver General Hospital, Vancouver, BC, Canada*

JONATHON LEIPSIC, MD - *Department of Radiology, St Paul's Hospital, Vancouver, BC, Canada*

PETER RUCHIN, MD - *Interventional Cardiologist, Wagga Wagga Base Hospital and Calvary Health Care Riverina, Wagga Wagga, New South Wales, Australia*

RAVISH SACHAR, MD - *Interventional Cardiologist, Wake Heart and Vascular, Raleigh, NC*

JACQUELINE SAW, MD, FRCPC - *Interventional Cardiology, Division of Cardiology, Vancouver General Hospital, University of British Columbia, Vancouver, BC, Canada*

RAVI S. SIDHU, MD, MEd, FRCSC, FACS - *Division of Vascular Surgery, St. Paul's Hospital, University of British Columbia, Vancouver, BC, Canada*

ANDREW STAROVOYTOV, MD - *Interventional Cardiology Research, Vancouver General Hospital, Vancouver, BC, Canada*

PHILIP TEAL, MD - *Department of Neurology, Vancouver General Hospital, University of British Columbia, Vancouver, BC, Canada*

SIMON WALSH, MD - *Interventional Cardiology, Southern Health and Social Care Trust, Portadown, Northern Ireland*

DAVID A. WOOD, MD - *Interventional Cardiology, Vancouver General Hospital, Vancouver, BC, Canada*

I CAROTID ARTERY STENOSIS AND MANAGEMENT

1 Carotid Artery Stenosis Prevalence and Medical Therapy

Rohit Khurana, BMBCH, PhD and Philip Teal, MD

CONTENTS

ABSTRACT

Stroke is a leading cause of disability and mortality worldwide, with the burden projected to increase. A substantial proportion of ischemic stroke syndromes are secondary to occlusive carotid disease. Established cerebrovascular disease is a marker of disease in other vascular territories and predicts future global athero-thrombotic events. A number of landmark trials have established an evidence base supporting medical intervention strategies to prevent recurrent vascular events. In addition to lifestyle modification, antiplatelet therapy, statins, and anti-hypertensive agents should be routinely administered to stroke patients.

Keywords: Carotid bruit; Carotid stenosis; Stroke; Cerebrovascular disease; Stroke syndrome; Secondary prevention; Antiplatelet therapy; Statin; ACE inhibitor

PREVALENCE OF CAROTID ARTERY STENOSIS (EXTRACRANIAL AND INTRACRANIAL)

Incidence and Economic Burden

Stroke ranks as the third leading cause of death, after ischemic heart disease and cancer. There are >700,000 incident strokes in the United States each year, resulting in >160,000 deaths annually. In 2004, the economic burden was estimated at $53.6

From: *Contemporary Cardiology: Carotid Artery Stenting: The Basics*
Edited by: J. Saw, DOI 10.1007/978-1-60327-314-5_1,
© Humana Press, a part of Springer Science+Business Media, LLC 2009

billion in direct and indirect costs. It is also the most important cause of disability, with 20% of survivors requiring institutional care after 3 months and 15–30% becoming permanently disabled. The burden is projected to worsen over the next 20 years, in part due to an ageing population, especially in developing countries.

Etiology

Strokes are either ischemic or hemorrhagic in origin, with the majority (80%) being ischemic. The management of these subtypes is very different, so the clinical distinction between the two is essential and facilitated by the use of CT and/or MR imaging. Three quarters of ischemic strokes involve the anterior circulation and the remaining quarter involves the posterior vertebrobasilar system. Approximately 25% of these ischemic events are related to occlusive disease of the cervical internal carotid artery and 8–10% are secondary to intracranial arterial stenosis. Figure 1 shows the potential sites of thromboembolic origin.

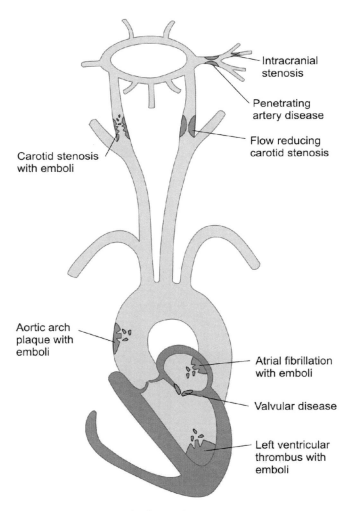

Fig. 1. Potential sources of thromboembolic strokes.

Epidemiologic studies have also shown ethnicity to affect stroke incidence. The Northern Manhattan Stroke Study revealed that Hispanics and blacks had a higher incidence and significantly greater proportion of intracranial atherosclerotic strokes than whites (P=0.003 and 0.023, respectively) *(1)*. The proportions of lacunar, extracranial atherosclerotic, and cryptogenic stroke were not significantly different among the three race–ethnic groups, although blacks (21%) and Hispanics (22%) had a slightly greater proportion of lacunar strokes than whites (16%).

Prevalence of Concomitant Coronary Artery Disease

The Reduction of Atherothrombosis for Continued Health (REACH) Registry collected data on atherosclerosis risk factors and treatment on >68,000 stable patients (44 countries) between 2003 and 2004, of whom nearly 19,000 patients had established cerebrovascular disease (CVD). Stroke patients are at high risk of recurrent stroke but also other vascular events. From this cohort, 40% had symptomatic atherothrombotic disease in ≥1 additional vascular beds: 36% coronary artery disease, 10% peripheral arterial disease, and 6% both *(2)*. Multiple disease locations predict a greater cardiovascular (CV) event rate after 1 year. The incidence of the end point of CV death, MI, or stroke or of hospitalization for atherothrombotic events was 14.5% for patients with established CVD after 1 year. These event rates increased with the number of symptomatic arterial disease locations, ranging from 12.6% for patients with one, 21.1% for patients with two, and 26.3% for patients with three symptomatic arterial disease locations (P<0.001 for trend) *(3)*. In addition, angiographically documented CAD has been identified as an important predictor of progression of extracranial carotid atherosclerosis *(4)*.

Risk of Stroke with Coronary Artery Bypass Surgery

High-grade asymptomatic carotid artery stenosis (>80%) occurs in roughly 8–12% of patients scheduled for coronary artery bypass surgery, with the incidence of perioperative stroke dependent upon stenosis severity, being <2% for mild stenosis (<50% severity), increasing to 10% for moderate lesions (50–80% severity), and 11–19% for severe lesions (>80% severity) *(5)*. Patients with bilateral high-grade stenosis or occlusion have up to a 25% incidence of perioperative stroke. Therefore, screening for concurrent carotid disease prior to cardiac surgery is important and routinely performed to allow a more accurate estimation of perioperative risk. Issues regarding necessity, timing, and mode for treating any detected carotid stenosis are an ongoing controversy in the surgical literature.

CORRELATION OF CAROTID STENOSIS TO STROKES

The risk of stroke is highly dependent on the severity of carotid stenosis and symptom status. In the NASCET (North American Symptomatic Carotid Endarterectomy Trial) study *(6)*, the risk of ipsilateral strokes at 5 years for patients with mild (<50%) stenosis on angiography was 18.7 and 7.8% for those with and without symptoms, respectively. For those with more severe (75–94%) stenosis, the rates were higher with a risk of 27.1 and 18.5% in the symptomatic and asymptomatic cohorts, respectively. These results were supported by the European Carotid Surgery Trial (ECST) which randomized 3,024 patients with carotid stenosis, who within the previous 6 months had experienced at least one transient or mild symptomatic ischemic vascular event in the distribution of one or both carotid arteries *(7)*. The stroke incidence at 3 years was 20.6% in patients with severe stenosis (>80% ECST criteria, which correlates to >60% using NASCET-derived angiographic criteria).

For asymptomatic carotid stenosis, the risk is lower than that associated with symptomatic disease. In observational studies, the rate of ipsilateral stroke was 1–3% per year among patients with asymptomatic stenosis >50% *(8)*, and the risk in NASCET was 3.2% per year for asymptomatic stenosis of 60–99% *(6)*. The manifestation of symptoms will depend on the severity and progression of the stenosis, the adequacy of collateral vessels, the character of the atherosclerotic plaque, and the presence or absence of other risk factors for stroke. Figure 2 from Moore et al. shows the relationship between stenosis severity and annual incidence of ipsilateral stroke in asymptomatic patients from multiple studies performed in the 1980s and 1990s *(9)*. The annual stroke risk is much higher with stenosis >80% severity that is medically treated, and thus this is a commonly accepted threshold for revascularization in asymptomatic patients.

Significance of a Carotid Bruit

The detection of a carotid bruit is poorly specific (<20%) for severe carotid stenosis *(10)*. Coupled with the complex management of asymptomatic stenosis, this led the United Preventive Services Task Force to recommend against routine neck auscultation for carotid bruits *(11)*. The prognostic implications of a bruit have therefore focused on the subsequent incidence of cerebrovascular and cardiovascular events. A carotid bruit weakly predicts cerebrovascular events in patients who are otherwise asymptomatic for cerebrovascular conditions *(12)*, but for patients with symptomatic carotid bruits (e.g., non-disabling strokes and transient ischemia in the ipsilateral carotid distribution), prognosis depends more on the severity of stenosis than on the presence of the bruit *(13)*. A recent meta-analysis estimated that people with carotid bruits have twice the risk of myocardial infarction and cardiovascular death compared with people who do not *(14)*.

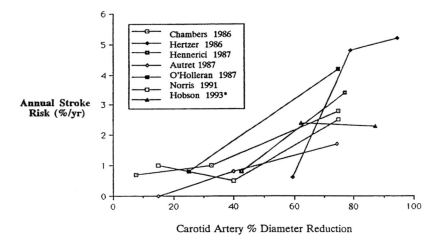

Fig. 2. Asymptomatic carotid artery stenosis severity and annual ipsilateral stroke risk, reproduced with permission from Moore et al. *(9)*.

TYPICAL STROKE SYNDROMES ASSOCIATED WITH EXTRACRANIAL CAROTID STENOSIS

Stroke manifests as a spectrum of symptoms and signs that correlate with the area of the brain supplied by the affected blood vessel. Anatomical mapping of the primary motor and sensory cortex is often visually depicted as a homunculus (Fig. 3). The anterior cerebral circulation comprises the internal carotid artery and its branches (anterior choroidal, anterior cerebral, and middle cerebral arteries) and supplies most of the cerebral cortex and subcortical white matter, basal ganglia, and internal capsule. Anterior circulation strokes are commonly associated with symptoms and signs that indicate hemispheric dysfunction (Table 1), such as aphasia, apraxia, and agnosia. They also produce hemiparesis, hemisensory disturbances, and visual field defects, but these can also occur with posterior circulation strokes. The posterior cerebral circulation consists of the paired vertebral arteries, the basilar arteries, and their branches. Strokes in this territory are characterized by brainstem dysfunction (Table 1), including drop attacks, coma, vertigo, nausea and vomiting, cranial nerve palsies, ataxia, and crossed sensorimotor deficits that affect the face on one side of the body and the limbs on the other. An algorithm to assist with the management of patients with extracranial carotid stenosis is summarized in Fig. 4.

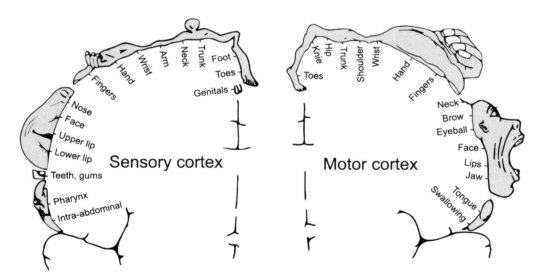

Fig. 3. Cortical homunculus: a coronal view depicting the relationship between the anterior circulation to the primary motor and sensory cortex.

EVIDENCE-BASED MEDICAL THERAPY FOR PATIENTS WITH CAROTID STENOSIS

Two main strategies exist for the treatment of carotid stenosis. First, risk factor modifying therapy can be used to stabilize or halt progression of the carotid plaque. The second approach is revascularization of carotid stenosis by surgical

Table 1
Symptoms and Signs of Anterior and Posterior Circulation Ischemia

Symptom or sign	*Incidence**	
	Anterior (%)	*Posterior (%)*
Headache	25	3
Altered consciousness	5	16
Aphasia †	20	0
Visual field defect	14	22
Diplopia †	0	7
Vertigo †	0	48
Dysarthria	3	11
Drop attacks †	0	16
Hemi- or monoparesis	38	12
Hemisensory deficit	33	9

* Most patients have multiple symptoms or signs.
† Most useful distinguishing features.
Modified from Simon RP, Aminoff MJ, Greenberg DA: Clinical Neurology, 1999.

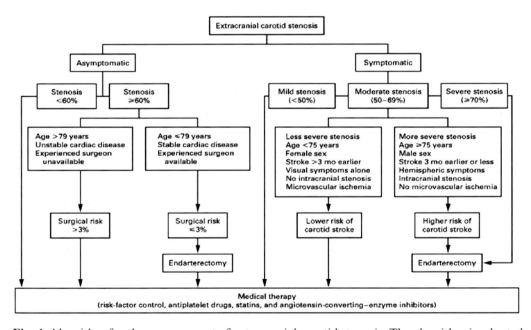

Fig. 4. Algorithm for the management of extracranial carotid stenosis. The algorithm is adapted from the Guidelines of the American Heart Association and the National Stroke Association.

(endarterectomy) or percutaneous intervention (angioplasty and stenting), to reduce the high early risk of recurrent events and long-term vascular events. This section will focus on the evidence underlying medical interventions that diminish the risk from carotid stenosis and its clinical sequelae. The chronology of progress for established secondary prevention for carotid stenosis is summarized in Fig. 5. Most patients qualify for at least one and many for up to three or more interventions at hospital discharge.

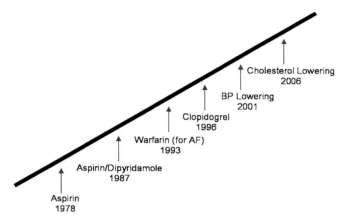

Fig. 5. Chronology of evidence base supporting secondary prevention measures for ischemic stroke.

Primary Prevention of Traditional Cardiovascular Risk Factors

Traditional cardiovascular risk factors correlate with carotid artery stenosis *(15)*. Markers of hemostatic function such as von Willebrand factor, factor VIIIc, fibrinogen, and white blood cell count are also associated with ischemic stroke incidence *(16)*, but the steadily reducing mortality from stroke is largely attributable to improved control of the modifiable risk factors, primarily hypertension *(17)*, but also LDL cholesterol with statins *(18)*, smoking cessation, and more widespread use of antiplatelet agents.

ANTIPLATELET THERAPIES

Aspirin

Low cost, patient accessibility, and low toxicity have led to early and widespread use of aspirin in both primary and secondary stroke prevention. The Physician's Health Study was the largest randomized clinical trial in 22,071 healthy men evaluating the effect of low-dose aspirin for primary prevention of cardiovascular mortality *(19)*. There was a 44% relative risk reduction (RRR) of MI (95% CI 0.45–0.70, $p < 0.00001$). A non-significant but slightly increased risk of stroke was seen, primarily of hemorrhagic stroke, and no reduction in cardiovascular mortality was observed. Subgroup analysis revealed that the benefit was predominantly in patients >50 years old. There was no increase in the incidence of gastrointestinal bleeds caused by aspirin (95% CI 0.98–1.53, $p = 0.08$).

The Women's Health Study randomized 39,876 asymptomatic women ≥45 years of age to receive 100 mg aspirin or placebo on alternate days and followed them for 10 years. This landmark trial was the first primary prevention study of aspirin therapy in women alone. In contrast to trials recruiting predominantly men, aspirin was shown to decrease the risk of stroke without affecting the risk of MI or vascular death *(20)*, with the most consistent benefit being for women ≥65 years of age, with a 30% RRR in ischemic stroke.

Table 2
Design of Trials Included in the Meta-analysis

Trial	No. of patients	Trial participant characteristics	Female (%)	Aspirin dose	Mean follow-up (years)
Physician's Health Study (19)	2,2071	Healthy male physicians	0	325 mg every other day	5
British Doctor's trial (50)	5,139	Healthy male physicians	0	500 mg/day	6
Thrombosis Prevention trial (51)	5,085	Men at high risk for IHD	0	75 mg/day	6.4
Hypertension Optimal Treatment trial (52)	18,790	Men and women with hypertension	47	75 mg/day	4
Primary Prevention Project (53)	4,495	Men and women with >1 CV risk factor	58	100 mg/day	3.6
Women's Health Study (20)	39,876	Healthy female health care professionals	100	100 mg/day	10.1

Adapted from Berger et al. (3).

A sex-specific meta-analysis of 6 trials, incorporating 95,456 individuals, of aspirin therapy for the primary prevention of cardiovascular events, addressed this differential gender effect of aspirin (3) (Table 2). This confirmed the beneficial effect of aspirin on the risk of stroke for women and on the risk of MI for men. However, there were relatively small numbers of MI among women and strokes among men, which emphasizes the need for further evidence before definitively concluding that men and women differ in their cardiovascular response to aspirin.

With respect to *secondary prevention*, the Antiplatelet and Antithrombotic Trialists' Collaboration examined all trials of antiplatelet drugs among patients at high risk for vascular events. Aspirin was the most commonly used antiplatelet agent in 21 trials enrolling patients (n=23,020) with a prior ischemic stroke or TIA. Random assignment to the antiplatelet therapy arm compared with placebo resulted in a 22% risk reduction for long-term secondary prevention (29 month mean duration of follow-up) (21), which equates to the prevention of 36 events in 2 years for every 1,000 patients treated. No relationship was apparent between aspirin dosage and efficacy. A second meta-analysis, which pooled the data from 11 randomized trials (n=9,469) of long-term aspirin versus control with prior ischemic stroke or TIA, showed that aspirin reduced the risk of adverse vascular events by nearly 15% (22), with the benefit uniform across all doses from 50 to 1,500 mg/day. Currently available clinical data do not support the routine, long-term use of aspirin dosages greater than 75–81 mg/day in the setting of cardiovascular disease prevention *(23)*. Higher dosages are associated with increased risks of gastrointestinal bleeding.

Aspirin and Acute Stroke

Evidence from about 40,000 randomized patients (International Stroke Trial and Chinese Acute Stroke Trial) showed that aspirin administration within 48 hours of ischemic stroke onset reduced 14-day morbidity and mortality *(24, 25)*. Overall, the benefit within this short time frame is small, with an absolute reduction of death or non-fatal stroke for 9 patients per 1,000 treated. There was also a small increase in extracranial bleeding.

Dipyridamole

Dipyridamole alone and in combination with aspirin has been extensively evaluated for secondary stroke prevention. The second European Stroke Prevention Study (ESPS-2) that recruited 6,602 patients demonstrated a 16% reduction in recurrent stroke risk ($P=0.039$) and a 15% risk reduction in stroke or death ($P=0.015$) in the dipyridamole-only arm (200 mg twice daily, extended-release formulation) compared to placebo *(26)*. Combination with 25 mg once-daily aspirin more than doubled the benefit with a resultant 37% reduction in recurrent stroke incidence ($P<0.001$) and a 24% reduction in stroke or death ($P<0.001$). However, there was no significant impact on mortality alone. Patients treated with dipyridamole experienced a higher incidence of headaches leading to an 8% discontinuation rate. A meta-analysis of 6 trials ($n=7,795$ patients) with background aspirin showed that random assignment to the combination of aspirin/dipyridamole was associated with an 18% risk reduction in serious vascular events compared to aspirin alone, with no additional bleeding risk *(27)*. This finding has been confirmed in a recently reported meta-analysis which concluded a statistically significant 18% risk reduction in the prevention of major vascular events *(28)*. The latter analysis revealed the benefit to be greater for extended-release dipyridamole, versus immediate release preparations, which may reflect a true pharmacological effect or lack of statistical power in studies using immediate release dipyridamole. Aspirin with extended-release dipyridamole is therefore accepted as first-line therapy in treating patients to prevent recurrent stroke.

Clopidogrel

Clopidogrel monotherapy for *secondary prevention* in high-risk patients was shown to be more beneficial than aspirin in the Clopidogrel versus Aspirin in Patients at Risk of Ischemic Events (CAPRIE) trial, which randomized 19,185 individuals with a recent MI, ischemic stroke, or symptomatic peripheral vascular disease (PVD) to either clopidogrel 75 mg or aspirin 325 mg once daily *(29)*. Patients were followed for 1–3 years. For the ischemic stroke group, mean time from stroke onset to randomization was 53 days; 59% of qualifying events were atherothrombotic and 40% lacunar. However, the beneficial effect of clopidogrel was primarily driven by the PVD cohort, who achieved a relative risk reduction (RRR) of 23.8%. In contrast, in those patients for whom ischemic stroke was the qualifying event, the difference was much smaller (RRR, 7.3%) and not statistically significant.

The value of aspirin/clopidogrel combination therapy is less clear. The MATCH trial assigned 7,599 patients with recent ischemic stroke or TIA already on clopidogrel 75 mg once daily to additional 75 mg aspirin or placebo *(26)*. After 18 months of follow-up, combination therapy did not significantly affect the primary end point, a composite of ischemic stroke, MI, vascular death, or hospitalization for acute ischemia ($P = 0.36$). The dual antiplatelet regimen incurred a significantly greater and cumulative risk of life-threatening gastrointestinal and intracranial hemorrhage. Post hoc sub-analysis of the CHARISMA trial, for patients with a history of atrial fibrillation, confirmed the observations from the MATCH trial *(30)*. Combination therapy is not currently recommended unless there is another indication for the addition of clopidogrel such as a recent acute coronary syndrome or percutaneous intervention (particularly if a drug-eluting stent is used).

The direct comparison of clopidogrel and a combination aspirin/dipyridamole formulation in secondary stroke prevention was recently reported in the Prevention Regimen for Effectively avoiding Second Strokes (PRoFESS) trial *(31)*. There were 20,332 patients with non-cardioembolic stroke randomly assigned to 25 mg of aspirin plus 200 mg of extended-release dipyridamole twice daily or 75 mg of clopidogrel daily. The patients were followed for a mean of 2.5 years. There was no difference between the two groups with respect to either the primary outcome measure of recurrent stroke or the secondary outcome of stroke, MI, or vascular death.

Summary of Antiplatelet Agents

Determination of the optimal, evidence-based regimen for secondary stroke prevention is challenging because trials of antiplatelet agents have involved patients with heterogeneous vascular risk profiles and because composite end points have been used in the placebo-controlled and comparative studies. The effects of each antiplatelet regimen for chronic secondary prevention of adverse vascular events are summarized in Table 3. The current recommendations for secondary stroke prevention are summarized in Table 4.

Table 3
Summary of the Effects of Varying Antiplatelet Regimens on the Composite Outcome of Stroke, MI, or Vascular Death (Serious Vascular Events) Among Patients with TIA and Ischemic Stroke for Chronic Secondary Prevention

Antiplatelet	*Comparator*	*No. of trials*	*n*	*Follow-up (months)*	*Serious vascular event rate reduction (95% CI)*
Aspirin	Placebo	11	9,649	17–50	RR 0.87 (0.81–0.94) *(55)*
Dipyridamole	Placebo	1	3,303	24	OR 0.81 (0.67–0.99) *(26)*
Clopidogrel	Aspirin	1	6,431	22	RR 0.93 (0.81–1.06) *(29)**
Clopidogrel + aspirin	Aspirin	1	3,245	28 †	RR 0.78 (0.62–0.98) *(3)**
Dipyridamole + aspirin	Aspirin	6	7,795	15–36	RR 0.82 (0.74–0.91) *(56)*
Clopidogrel + aspirin	Clopidogrel	1	7,599	18	RR 0.94 (0.84–1.05) *(26)*
Dipyridamole + aspirin	Clopidogrel	1	20,332	30 †	HR 1.01 (0.92–1.11) *(31)*

† Median duration.
* Subgroup analysis of stroke population within larger clinical trial.
Adapted from O'Donnell et al. *(54)*.
RR, risk ratio; OR, odds ratio; and HR, hazard ratio.

Table 4
Recommendations for Oral Antiplatelet Therapy

Class I recommendations

1. For patients with non-cardioembolic ischemic stroke or TIA, antiplatelet agents rather than oral anticoagulation are recommended to reduce the risk of recurrent stroke and other cardiovascular events *(Level of Evidence: A)*
2. Aspirin (50–325 mg/day) monotherapy, the combination of aspirin and extended-release dipyridamole, or clopidogrel monotherapy are all acceptable options for initial therapy *(Level of Evidence: A)*
3. The combination of aspirin and extended-release dipyridamole is recommended over aspirin alone *(Level of Evidence: A)*

Class II recommendations

1. Clopidogrel may be considered over aspirin alone on the basis of direct comparison trials *(Level of Evidence: B)*
2. For patients allergic to aspirin, clopidogrel is reasonable *(Level of Evidence: B)*

Class III recommendation

The addition of aspirin to clopidogrel increases the risk of hemorrhage. Combination therapy of aspirin and clopidogrel is not routinely recommended for ischemic stroke or TIA patients unless they have a specific indication for this therapy (i.e., coronary stent, acute coronary syndrome)

Modified from the 2008 update to the AHA/ASA guidelines update for secondary stroke prevention *(57)*.

STATINS

The association of ischemic stroke with atherosclerosis and by implication, elevated low-density lipoprotein (LDL) cholesterol, is intuitive. However, observational studies from 10 to 20 years ago exploring this relationship reported conflicting results *(32)*. More recently, the subject was analyzed in the Women's Health Study which reported a strong positive correlation between the risk of ischemic stroke and both total cholesterol ($P<0.001$) and LDL cholesterol ($P<0.003$) levels *(33)*. However, the most compelling evidence attributing statin therapy and reduction of stroke incidence is derived from primary prevention trials in coronary artery disease (CAD) patients such as the Heart Protection Study (HPS) *(34)*. This study randomized 20,536 patients with established or at risk of CAD to simvastatin 40 mg or placebo. Notably, the majority (84%) had no history of cerebrovascular disease. During the 4.8 years of follow-up, simvastatin reduced the risk of first stroke in the overall population by 25% versus placebo (95% CI 15–34%; $P<0.0001$), driven largely by the 28% reduction in ischemic stroke (95% CI 19–37%; $P<0.0001$). There was no apparent difference between the groups in the incidence of hemorrhagic stroke ($P=0.8$). Of the 20,536 patients randomized, 13,386 (65%) had diagnosed CAD; when the analysis was confined to these patients, there was a 25% proportional reduction in the rate of stroke (95% CI 12–36%; $P=0.0005$). This reduction was associated with an absolute difference in LDL cholesterol of 39 mg/dL between the treatment groups. A similar ischemic stroke incidence reduction was observed with the much older 4S and CARE primary prevention CAD trials, which evaluated 20–40 mg simvastatin and 40 mg pravastatin, respectively *(35, 36)*.

More aggressive statin treatment also reduced stroke risk. The Treating to New Targets (TNT) trial randomized 10,001 patients to standard lipid lowering with atorvastatin 10 mg or to intensive lipid lowering with atorvastatin 80 mg, with a median follow-up of 4.9 years *(37)*. The higher dose group experienced a greater reduction in LDL cholesterol lowering, 77 versus 101 mg/dL, and a 25% reduction in the risk of fatal or non-fatal stroke ($P=0.021$). Among patients with no history of stroke (95% of randomized patients), there were fewer cerebrovascular events in the atorvastatin 80 mg group than in the 10 mg group ($P=0.032$) and also a trend toward fewer second strokes, although the latter did not reach statistical significance ($P=0.07$).

One exception to the favorable effects of statins on stroke risk in patients with CAD emerged from a post hoc analysis of the PROspective Study of Pravastatin in the Elderly at Risk (PROSPER) trial *(38)*. PROSPER randomized 5,804 older patients (70–82 years) with established cardiovascular disease (CVD) (44% had a history of CVD and 11% had a history of stroke) or at high cardiovascular risk to pravastatin 40 mg or placebo. Pravastatin treatment reduced LDL cholesterol by 34% from a baseline mean of 147 to 95 mg/dL, but did not significantly impact the incidence of stroke versus placebo (95% CI 0.81–1.31; $P=0.81$). One possible explanation for this differing result may be that in contrast to the trials mentioned above, PROSPER included patients with prior stroke.

Secondary Stroke Prevention

The HPS also analyzed secondary stroke prevention in patients without CAD. Of the total enrollment, 3,280 had a history of cerebrovascular disease and 55% (1,804) of these patients had no history of clinical CAD. In this subgroup analysis, simvastatin did not show a significant effect on stroke recurrence (169 simvastatin patients and 170 placebo patients had a stroke during follow-up; HR 0.98; 95% CI 0.79–1.22) despite a significant impact on LDL cholesterol lowering. The reason for this lack of benefit is unclear. Notably, patients who had a stroke within 6 months were excluded, and on average the cerebrovascular event occurred 4.3 years before enrollment.

More than 120,000 patients now have participated in randomized trials evaluating statin therapy for stroke prevention *(39)*. Most clinical trials evaluating statin effectiveness are primary prevention trials. With the exception of atorvastatin use in the Stroke Prevention by Aggressive Reduction in Cholesterol Levels (SPARCL) trial, the precise role and mechanism for statin-derived benefit in secondary prevention remain ill-defined. The SPARCL study randomized 4,731 patients with a prior stroke or TIA, but no evidence of CAD, to either atorvastatin 80 mg or placebo *(40)*. Unlike in the HPS, patients with cerebral hemorrhage were not excluded and comprised 2% of patients, whereas ischemic stroke accounted for 67% of patients and TIA 31% of patients. During the median 4.9 years of follow-up, the atorvastatin cohort experienced significantly lower rates of strokes (RR 0.85, $P=0.03$) and strokes or TIAs (RR 0.77, $P<0.001$) than placebo-treated patients. This study did, however, find an increased risk of hemorrhagic strokes (RR 1.25, 95% CI 1.06–1.47), the reason for which is unclear.

The discordant findings between SPARCL and HPS on the impact of stroke recurrence, as shown in Fig. 6, may have several explanations *(41)*. The risk of stroke recurrence is higher during the first year. This is where early statin use may exert most benefit, by helping to stabilize atherosclerotic plaques, whether

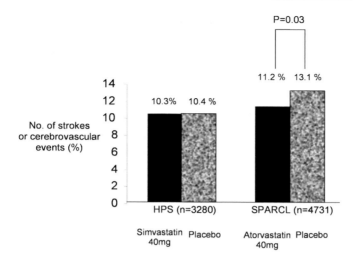

Fig. 6. The incidence of recurrent stroke in patients without CAD for the Heart Protection SPARCL studies. Modified from Nassief et al. *(41)*.

contributing to the incident stroke or at other sites. In SPARCL, the mean time between the index event and enrollment was 3 months, whereas in the HPS it was 4.3 years. Second, greater LDL cholesterol reduction was achieved with atorvastatin 80 mg over simvastatin 40 mg and preliminary analyses do support this being a contributing factor. The LDL cholesterol level after 1 month on treatment was associated with stroke risk reduction, with each 10% reduction in LDL cholesterol during the first month of treatment associated with a 4% reduction in stroke risk ($P = 0.005$). Table 5 summarizes the current guidelines with respect to statin use for secondary stroke prevention.

Table 5
Recommendations for Lipid Management

Class I recommendations
1. Ischemic stroke or TIA patients with elevated cholesterol, comorbid coronary artery disease, or evidence of an atherosclerotic origin should be managed according to NCEP III guidelines, which include lifestyle modification, dietary guidelines, and medication recommendations *(Level of Evidence: A)*
2. Statin agents are recommended, and the target goal for cholesterol lowering for those with CHD or symptomatic atherosclerotic disease is an LDL-C level <100 mg/dL. An LDL-C level <70 mg/dL is recommended for very high-risk persons with multiple risk factors *(Level of Evidence: A)*
3. On the basis of SPARCL trial, administration of statin therapy with intensive lipid-lowering effects is recommended for patients with atherosclerotic ischemic stroke or TIA and without known CHD to reduce the risk of stroke and cardiovascular events *(Level of Evidence: B)*

Class II recommendation
1. Ischemic stroke or TIA patients with low HDL cholesterol may be considered for treatment with niacin or gemfibrozil *(Level of Evidence: B)*

Modified from the 2008 update to the AHA/ASA guidelines update for secondary stroke prevention *(57)*.

ACE INHIBITORS

Systolic and diastolic hypertension has long been recognized as an important modifiable risk factor for stroke prevention. Outcome trials have demonstrated that a persistent reduction in blood pressure reduces the risk of stroke, with the value of anti-hypertensive therapy in primary stroke prevention unequivocal. A 17 trial meta-analysis involving 47,667 patients treated predominantly with a diuretic and/or beta-blocker-based regimen concluded that a decrease of 5–6 mmHg in diastolic pressure or 10–12 mmHg in systolic pressure conferred a 38% reduction in primary stroke (both fatal and non-fatal) incidence after 2–3 years of treatment *(42)*. The Blood Pressure Lowering Treatment Trialists' Collaboration reported that ACE inhibitors yielded a comparable cardiovascular event risk reduction to combined diuretics and BB versus a placebo regimen, with a slightly lesser reduction in blood pressure *(43)*. This suggests that ancillary blood pressure-independent effects of ACE inhibitors may influence outcome as proven in the HOPE trial.

The Heart Outcomes Prevention Evaluation (HOPE) trial revealed that the benefits of ACE inhibitor-mediated blood pressure lowering also extended to normotensive patients *(34)*. This study randomized >9,000 patients at high risk for major vascular events to either ramipril 10 mg once daily or placebo for a mean of 5 years. High risk was defined as documented coronary or peripheral arterial disease, or the presence of diabetes plus greater than or equal to one additional risk factor (dyslipidemia, hypertension, microalbuminuria, smoking). There were 47.6% hypertensive patients. Compared with placebo, ramipril caused a 32% reduction in stroke risk, with benefits apparent by the end of the first year.

Secondary Stroke Prevention

In patients with a history of stroke, blood pressure continues to be an important risk factor. The Perindopril Protection Against Recurrent Stroke Study (PRO-GRESS) was a randomized study of 6,105 patients with a history of stroke or TIA within 5 years, evaluating perindopril against placebo *(44)*. The entry criteria did not specify a blood pressure value, but treatment with agents other than ACE inhibitor was recommended for patients with uncontrolled hypertension before they entered the trial. Physicians retained the option to add indapamide to perindopril to improve blood pressure control. The treatment arm (amalgamated data from the perindopril alone and perindopril plus indapamide regimen) reduced blood pressure by 9/4 mmHg, with a 28 and 26% reduction in stroke and major cardiovascular event rate, respectively, over 3.9 years. Notably, perindopril *alone* did not yield any measurable impact on outcome. A major limitation of this trial was the failure to include a group randomized to indapamide alone. Several other large trials have provided evidence that for most cardiovascular outcomes, it is the absolute value of blood pressure reduction, rather than the particular regimen used, that determines the benefits of treatment *(43, 45, 46)*. This emphasizes the need for more than one agent to achieve the necessary target, and should include an ACE inhibitor.

ANTICOAGULANTS

Warfarin is an effective secondary prevention strategy for patients with atrial fibrillation and reduces the RR of recurrent stroke in patients with TIA or minor stroke by ~70% (hazard ratio 0·34, 95% CI 0·20–0·57) *(47)*. This effect of warfarin is partly offset by a small risk of major bleeding, especially intracerebral hemorrhage (0·3–0·6% per year), which rises with age, high blood pressure, use of warfarin in combination with antiplatelet agents, and increasing intensity of anticoagulation. Evidence suggests that the combination of warfarin and aspirin might also be associated with an increased risk of bleeding without evidence of benefit *(48)*. In patients without atrial fibrillation, presenting with TIA, or minor stroke, warfarin is not better than aspirin as a secondary prevention agent *(49)*. Possible exceptions are patients with thrombus in the carotid artery, critical carotid stenosis awaiting surgery, and carotid dissection.

CONCLUSIONS

Carotid stenosis is an important cause of stroke and its disabling sequelae. Symptomatic patients with severe carotid artery stenosis are at much greater risk for future cerebrovascular events than are asymptomatic patients. The presence of carotid disease also predicts future coronary and peripheral vascular events *(3)*. Accordingly, secondary prevention for stroke has evolved over recent years with a robust evidence base supporting modifying risk factors to reduce global atherothrombotic risk. In addition to smoking cessation, routine therapy to reduce fatal and non-fatal stroke now includes antiplatelet therapy, statins, and ACE inhibitors, with the latter two agents having neuroprotective attributes beyond LDL cholesterol and blood pressure lowering, respectively. In terms of future direction, safer anti-thrombotic alternatives to warfarin, such as direct thrombin inhibitors and Factor Xa inhibitors, are being assessed in trials to add to the increasing scope of therapeutic intervention.

REFERENCES

1. White H, Boden-Albala B, Wang C, et al. Ischemic stroke subtype incidence among whites, blacks, and Hispanics: the Northern Manhattan Study. Circulation 2005;111:1327–1331.
2. Rother J, Alberts MJ, Touze E, et al. Risk factor profile and management of cerebrovascular patients in the REACH Registry. Cerebrovasc Dis 2008;25:366–374.
3. Bhatt DL, Fox KA, Hacke W, et al. Clopidogrel and aspirin versus aspirin alone for the prevention of atherothrombotic events. N Engl J Med 2006;354:1706–1717.
4. Byington RP, Furberg CD, Crouse JR, 3rd, Espeland MA, Bond MG, Pravastatin, Lipids, and Atherosclerosis in the Carotid Arteries (PLAC-II). Am J Cardiol 1995;76:54C–59C.
5. Bittl JA, Hirsch AT, Concomitant peripheral arterial disease and coronary artery disease: therapeutic opportunities. Circulation 2004;109:3136–3144.
6. Inzitari D, Eliasziw M, Gates P, et al. The causes and risk of stroke in patients with asymptomatic internal-carotid-artery stenosis. North American Symptomatic Carotid Endarterectomy Trial Collaborators. N Engl J Med 2000;342:1693–1700.
7. MacMahon S, Sharpe N, Gamble G, et al. Effects of lowering average of below-average cholesterol levels on the progression of carotid atherosclerosis: results of the LIPID Atherosclerosis Substudy. LIPID Trial Research Group. Circulation 1998;97:1784–1790.
8. Norris JW, Zhu CZ, Bornstein NM, Chambers BR, Vascular risks of asymptomatic carotid stenosis. Stroke 1991;22:1485–1490.
9. Moore WS, Barnett HJ, Beebe HG, et al. Guidelines for carotid endarterectomy. A multidisciplinary consensus statement from the Ad Hoc Committee, American Heart Association. Circulation 1995;91:566–579.
10. Chambers BR, Norris JW, Outcome in patients with asymptomatic neck bruits. N Engl J Med 1986;315:860–865.
11. Wolff T, Guirguis-Blake J, Miller T, Gillespie M, Harris R, Screening for carotid artery stenosis: an update of the evidence for the U.S. Preventive Services Task Force. Ann Intern Med 2007;147:860–870.
12. Heyman A, Wilkinson WE, Heyden S, et al. Risk of stroke in asymptomatic persons with cervical arterial bruits: a population study in Evans County, Georgia. N Engl J Med 1980;302:838–841.

13. Rothwell PM, Eliasziw M, Gutnikov SA, et al. Analysis of pooled data from the randomised controlled trials of endarterectomy for symptomatic carotid stenosis. Lancet 2003;361:107–116.
14. Pickett CA, Jackson JL, Hemann BA, Atwood JE, Carotid bruits as a prognostic indicator of cardiovascular death and myocardial infarction: a meta-analysis. Lancet 2008;371:1587–1594.
15. Davis BR, Vogt T, Frost PH, et al. Risk factors for stroke and type of stroke in persons with isolated systolic hypertension. Systolic Hypertension in the Elderly Program Cooperative Research Group. Stroke 1998;29:1333–1340.
16. Folsom AR, Rosamond WD, Shahar E, et al. Prospective study of markers of hemostatic function with risk of ischemic stroke. The Atherosclerosis Risk in Communities (ARIC) Study Investigators. Circulation 1999;100:736–742.
17. Lawes CM, Bennett DA, Feigin VL, Rodgers A, Blood pressure and stroke: an overview of published reviews. Stroke 2004;35:1024.
18. Amarenco P, Labreuche J, Lavallee P, Touboul PJ, Statins in stroke prevention and carotid atherosclerosis: systematic review and up-to-date meta-analysis. Stroke 2004;35: 2902–2909.
19. Final report on the aspirin component of the ongoing Physicians' Health Study. Steering Committee of the Physicians' Health Study Research Group. N Engl J Med 1989;321:129–135.
20. Ridker PM, Cook NR, Lee IM, et al. A randomized trial of low-dose aspirin in the primary prevention of cardiovascular disease in women. N Engl J Med 2005;352:1293–1304.
21. Corti R, Fuster V, Fayad ZA, et al. Lipid lowering by simvastatin induces regression of human atherosclerotic lesions: two years' follow-up by high-resolution noninvasive magnetic resonance imaging. Circulation 2002;106:2884–2887.
22. O'Holleran LW, Kennelly MM, McClurken M, Johnson JM, Natural history of asymptomatic carotid plaque. Five year follow-up study. Am J Surg 1987;154:659–662.
23. Campbell CL, Smyth S, Montalescot G, Steinhubl SR, Aspirin dose for the prevention of cardiovascular disease: a systematic review. JAMA 2007;297:2018–2024.
24. The International Stroke Trial (IST): a randomised trial of aspirin, subcutaneous heparin, both, or neither among 19435 patients with acute ischaemic stroke. International Stroke Trial Collaborative Group. Lancet 1997;349:1569–1581.
25. CAST: randomised placebo-controlled trial of early aspirin use in 20,000 patients with acute ischaemic stroke. CAST (Chinese Acute Stroke Trial) Collaborative Group. Lancet 1997;349:1641–1649.
26. Diener HC, Bogousslavsky J, Brass LM, et al. Aspirin and clopidogrel compared with clopidogrel alone after recent ischaemic stroke or transient ischaemic attack in high-risk patients (MATCH): randomised, double-blind, placebo-controlled trial. Lancet 2004;364:331–337.
27. Leonardi-Bee J, Bath PM, Bousser MG, et al. Dipyridamole for preventing recurrent ischemic stroke and other vascular events: a meta-analysis of individual patient data from randomized controlled trials. Stroke 2005;36:162–168.
28. Verro P, Gorelick PB, Nguyen D, Aspirin plus dipyridamole versus aspirin for prevention of vascular events after stroke or TIA: a meta-analysis. Stroke 2008;39:1358–1363.
29. A randomised, blinded, trial of clopidogrel versus aspirin in patients at risk of ischaemic events (CAPRIE). CAPRIE Steering Committee. Lancet 1996;348:1329–1339.
30. Hart RG, Bhatt DL, Hacke W, et al. Clopidogrel and aspirin versus aspirin alone for the prevention of stroke in patients with a history of atrial fibrillation: subgroup analysis of the CHARISMA randomized trial. Cerebrovasc Dis 2008;25:344–347.
31. Sacco RL, Diener HC, Yusuf S, et al. Aspirin and extended-release dipyridamole versus clopidogrel for recurrent stroke. N Engl J Med 2008;359(12):1238–1251.
32. Cholesterol, diastolic blood pressure, and stroke: 13,000 strokes in 450,000 people in 45 prospective cohorts. Prospective studies collaboration. Lancet 1995;346:1647–1653.
33. Kurth T, Everett BM, Buring JE, Kase CS, Ridker PM, Gaziano JM, Lipid levels and the risk of ischemic stroke in women. Neurology 2007;68:556–562.
34. Yusuf S, Zhao F, Mehta SR, Chrolavicius S, Tognoni G, Fox KK, Effects of clopidogrel in addition to aspirin in patients with acute coronary syndromes without ST-segment elevation. N Engl J Med 2001;345:494–502.
35. Plehn JF, Davis BR, Sacks FM, et al. Reduction of stroke incidence after myocardial infarction with pravastatin: the Cholesterol and Recurrent Events (CARE) study. The Care Investigators. Circulation 1999;99:216–223.
36. Randomised trial of cholesterol lowering in 4444 patients with coronary heart disease: the Scandinavian Simvastatin Survival Study (4S). Lancet 1994;344:1383–1389.

37. Waters DD, LaRosa JC, Barter P, et al. Effects of high-dose atorvastatin on cerebrovascular events in patients with stable coronary disease in the TNT (treating to new targets) study. J Am Coll Cardiol 2006;48:1793–1799.

38. Shepherd J, Blauw GJ, Murphy MB, et al. Pravastatin in elderly individuals at risk of vascular disease (PROSPER): a randomised controlled trial. Lancet 2002;360:1623–1630.

39. O'Regan C, Wu P, Arora P, Perri D, Mills EJ, Statin therapy in stroke prevention: a meta-analysis involving 121,000 patients. Am J Med 2008;121:24–33.

40. Amarenco P, Goldstein LB, Szarek M, et al. Effects of intense low-density lipoprotein cholesterol reduction in patients with stroke or transient ischemic attack: the Stroke Prevention by Aggressive Reduction in Cholesterol Levels (SPARCL) trial. Stroke 2007;38:3198–204.

41. Nassief A, Marsh JD, Statin therapy for stroke prevention. Stroke 2008;39:1042–1048.

42. Chalmers J, Trials on blood pressure-lowering and secondary stroke prevention. Am J Cardiol 2003;91:3G–8G.

43. Turnbull F, Effects of different blood-pressure-lowering regimens on major cardiovascular events: results of prospectively-designed overviews of randomised trials. Lancet 2003;362:1527–1535.

44. Randomised trial of a perindopril-based blood-pressure-lowering regimen among 6,105 individuals with previous stroke or transient ischaemic attack. Lancet 2001;358:1033–1041.

45. Staessen JA, Wang JG, Thijs L, Cardiovascular protection and blood pressure reduction: a meta-analysis. Lancet 2001;358:1305–1315.

46. Neal B, MacMahon S, Chapman N, Effects of ACE inhibitors, calcium antagonists, and other blood-pressure-lowering drugs: results of prospectively designed overviews of randomised trials. Blood Pressure Lowering Treatment Trialists' Collaboration. Lancet 2000;356:1955–1964.

47. Secondary prevention in non-rheumatic atrial fibrillation after transient ischaemic attack or minor stroke. EAFT (European Atrial Fibrillation Trial) Study Group. Lancet 1993;342:1255–1262.

48. Akins PT, Feldman HA, Zoble RG, et al. Secondary stroke prevention with ximelagatran versus warfarin in patients with atrial fibrillation: pooled analysis of SPORTIF III and V clinical trials. Stroke 2007;38:874–880.

49. Mohr JP, Thompson JL, Lazar RM, et al. A comparison of warfarin and aspirin for the prevention of recurrent ischemic stroke. N Engl J Med 2001;345:1444–1451.

50. Halliday A, Mansfield A, Marro J, et al. Prevention of disabling and fatal strokes by successful carotid endarterectomy in patients without recent neurological symptoms: randomised controlled trial. Lancet 2004;363:1491–1502.

51. Thrombosis prevention trial: randomised trial of low-intensity oral anticoagulation with warfarin and low-dose aspirin in the primary prevention of ischaemic heart disease in men at increased risk. The Medical Research Council's General Practice Research Framework. Lancet 1998;351:233–241.

52. Hansson L, Zanchetti A, Carruthers SG, et al. Effects of intensive blood-pressure lowering and low-dose aspirin in patients with hypertension: principal results of the Hypertension Optimal Treatment (HOT) randomised trial. HOT Study Group. Lancet 1998;351:1755–1762.

53. de Gaetano G, Low-dose aspirin and vitamin E in people at cardiovascular risk: a randomised trial in general practice. Collaborative Group of the Primary Prevention Project. Lancet 2001;357:89–95.

54. O'Donnell MJ, Hankey GJ, Eikelboom JW, Antiplatelet therapy for secondary prevention of noncardioembolic ischemic stroke: a critical review. Stroke 2008;39:1638–1646.

55. Algra A, Van Gijn J, Koudstaal PJ, Secondary prevention after cerebral ischaemia of presumed arterial origin: is aspirin still the touchstone? J Neurol Neurosurg Psychiatry 1999;66:557–559.

56. De Schryver EL, Algra A, van Gijn J, Dipyridamole for preventing stroke and other vascular events in patients with vascular disease. Cochrane Database Syst Rev 2006:CD001820.

57. Adams RJ, Albers G, Alberts MJ, et al. Update to the AHA/ASA recommendations for the prevention of stroke in patients with stroke and transient ischemic attack. Stroke 2008;39:1647–1652.

2 Carotid Revascularization: Carotid Endarterectomy

Marlene Grenon, MD, FRCSC
and Ravi S. Sidhu, MD, MEd, FRCSC, FACS

CONTENTS

ABSTRACT

Carotid endarterectomy (CEA) is a procedure that has reliably decreased the risk of cerebrovascular events and death in patients with severe carotid stenosis. In this chapter, important concepts in the preoperative assessment of patients undergoing CEA will be reviewed. An overview of the clinical trials highlighting current indications will be provided, followed by a discussion of the surgical technique, complications, and controversies related to CEA.

Keywords: Carotid endarterectomy; Technique; Patch

INTRODUCTION

Stroke is the third leading cause of death in the United States, and the second leading cause of death worldwide *(1)*. It is the most common cause of death as a result of a neurological disorder. About 750,000 patients are diagnosed with this entity yearly in the United States and more than 15 million around the globe *(2)*, which corresponds to an incidence of new stroke of approximately 160 per 100,000 population per year *(3, 4)*.

From: *Contemporary Cardiology: Carotid Artery Stenting: The Basics*
Edited by: J. Saw, DOI 10.1007/978-1-60327-314-5_2,
© Humana Press, a part of Springer Science+Business Media, LLC 2009

PREOPERATIVE ASSESSMENT

The patient with carotid stenosis may be asymptomatic or symptomatic with different stroke syndromes. The stroke syndromes include transient ischemic attack (TIA), stroke (with or without recovery), stroke in evolution, crescendo TIA, and, as considered by some, progressive intellectual dysfunction. The patient suffering from a stroke syndrome will usually undergo work-up with one or more radiological modalities. The causes of stroke are generally classified as atherosclerotic (20–30%), cardioembolic (30%), or other origin (40%). Several diseases or presentations may come into play, including changes in hemodynamic parameters, hematologic diagnosis, hereditary or degenerative disorders, inflammatory diseases, infectious problems, metabolic issues, intoxications (e.g., amphetamine), and vasospasm seen with migraine, trauma, or dissection. Hence, it is essential that investigations rule out other causes for the presenting stroke syndrome. Depending on the clinical presentation, potential investigations include ECG, telemetry, carotid duplex ultrasound, echocardiography, CT scan of the head, and basic laboratory blood tests.

With respect to carotid stenosis and specifically carotid bifurcation disease, angiography and duplex ultrasound are established methods of investigation. In view of the rapidly changing radiological diagnostic tools and the emergence of computed tomography angiogram (CTA) and magnetic resonance angiogram (MRA), familiarity with interpretation, limitations, and advantages of these modalities is important. In addition to defining the presence of carotid stenosis, other anatomic details are important to guide therapeutic alternatives and approaches. For example, anatomy which is known to complicate CEA and which may warrant consideration for CAS include low lesions, high lesions (above C2), prior CEA, history of other major neck operation (radical neck, laryngectomy, tracheostomy, etc.), cervical fusion or immobility, and prior neck radiation *(5)*.

In the preoperative work-up of a patient, it is also important to consider if the patient is at "physiological" high risk for surgery, which may also warrant consideration for other alternatives such as carotid artery stenting or medical management. These factors include, but are not restricted to, advanced age, contralateral carotid occlusion, cardiac disease, and renal insufficiency *(6)*.

It is of utmost importance in the evaluation of the patient who has recently suffered a stroke and has not recovered completely to assess whether he or she is a candidate for surgery. This requires considerable experience and judgment. Likewise, the timing of surgery is another controversial topic. It has been suggested that patients should wait 4–6 weeks after the event prior to proceeding with CEA *(7, 8)*. However, the patient may be at high risk of a recurrent neurologic event during that period *(9–11)*. After an ischemic event, the 30-day risk of stroke is 4.9% in the presence of severe carotid stenosis *(12)*. On the other hand, the mortality and risk of stroke at CEA is 20% in the presence of stroke in evolution or crescendo TIA *(13)*. Hence, this remains a subject of debate.

Particular steps in the preoperative management of patients planning to undergo CEA include the appropriate antiplatelet medication. Aspirin therapy is continued in the perioperative period. Anticoagulation with heparin should be considered prior to CEA for high-grade stenosis and symptoms (acute stroke or crescendo TIA) to prevent another ischemic episode or complete arterial occlusion *(14, 15)*.

INDICATIONS FOR CEA

The objective of CEA is the prevention of strokes. Carotid artery operations should be considered for patients where surgery will improve the natural history of the disease more than the corresponding medical treatment, if it can be done in a safe manner. The section below reviews conclusions made from the randomized trials conducted to compare CEA and medical management in patients with symptomatic and asymptomatic carotid stenosis.

Symptomatic Carotid Artery Stenosis

The first study involving patients with symptomatic carotid stenosis was the Joint Study of Extracranial Arterial Occlusion *(16)*, which began in 1959. This study randomized 1,225 patients to either CEA (621 patients) or medical management (604 patients). The survival rate at 43 months follow-up was significantly different, being 80% in the surgical group and 50% in the medical group. There were also less neurological events among the surgical group. This was the first strong evidence of the advantage of CEA over medical therapy in symptomatic carotid stenosis patients.

In the 1990s, three major studies were published which furthered the evidence for CEA: the North American Symptomatic Carotid Endarterectomy Trial (NASCET), the European Carotid Surgery Trial (ECST), and the Veterans Affairs Symptomatic Trial (VAST). Several problems remain with comparison of these studies because of the diagnostic measures used. For example, ultrasound exams were not standardized and the criteria used for severity of the carotid lesion were based on different catheter angiographic criteria.

NASCET enrolled from 50 centers in North America and segregated patients according to stenosis of 30–69% and 70–99% (angiographically). To be eligible to enter the study, the centers had to demonstrate CEA combined mortality and morbidity of <5%. Patients were eligible if they had a TIA or minor stroke within 3 months of randomization. In the group with 70–99% stenosis, 328 were randomized to CEA and 331 to medical therapy (which included aspirin and control of other risk factors). The study was stopped prematurely because of the superiority of CEA over medical therapy, and patients in the medical therapy group were advised to undergo CEA. Overall, the cumulative ipsilateral stroke risk was 9% in the surgical group and 26% in the medical group at 2 years ($p<0.001$). This corresponded to an absolute risk reduction of 17% and relative risk reduction of 65%. Numbers needed to treat were six patients at 2 years *(12)*. For the group with 50–70% stenosis, there was moderate benefit of CEA over medical treatment *(17)*. This corresponded to a relative risk reduction of 39%. The study however demonstrated no definite survival benefits for women and patients with retinal symptoms over hemispheric symptoms.

The ECST trial took place over 10 years and recruited 2,518 patients from 14 countries within 6 months of a stroke, TIA, or retinal infarction *(18)*. Patients were divided into three groups, including carotid stenosis of 70–99, 30–69, and 0–29%, respectively. Randomization ratio was 1:2 for medical vs. surgical, and medical management was left to the treating physician. Patients with 70–99% stenosis had a lower risk of ipsilateral stroke (2.8% for CEA vs. 16.8% medical management) and lower risk of combined death, ipsilateral stroke, or any other stroke (12.3% CEA vs. 21.9% medical treatment) at 3 years with CEA. There was no significant advantage with CEA among the mild or moderate stenosis groups *(18, 19)*.

The VAST trial was published in 1991 and included 189 symptomatic patients with carotid stenosis >50% from 16 centers. TIA was included in the primary end point (which also consisted of death and stroke). Overall, the risk of neurological event among patients randomized to CEA was 7.7 vs. 19.4% in the medical group at 12 months ($p=0.011$) (20). A subgroup analysis of patients with greater severity of carotid stenosis >70% showed a larger proportional reduction in neurologic events with CEA. Thus, the study investigators concluded that CEA was more effective than medical management for patients with high-grade stenosis.

Asymptomatic Carotid Stenosis Trials

Overall, five randomized trials had addressed the role of CEA among patients with asymptomatic carotid stenosis. These are the Carotid Surgery versus Medical Therapy in the Asymptomatic Carotid Stenosis (CASANOVA) trial, the Mayo Clinic Asymptomatic Carotid Endarterectomy trial, the Veterans Affairs Asymptomatic Trial (VAAT), the Asymptomatic Carotid Atherosclerosis Study (ACAS), and the Asymptomatic Carotid Surgery Trial (ACST) Collaborative Study.

The CASANOVA trial randomized patients with asymptomatic carotid stenosis (50–90%) to CEA (260 patients) or medical management (204 patients) which included aspirin. One hundred and eighteen patients in the medical arm crossed over to CEA because of pre-elected criteria of treating patients with bilateral stenosis >50% or unilateral stenosis >90% surgically. The analysis, which was done in an intention-to-treat manner, demonstrated no benefit of CEA over medical management (21). The study raised several criticisms related to the trial design, and thus the results should be interpreted with caution.

The Mayo Clinic study was a small study that randomized 71 patients with asymptomatic carotid stenosis. The study was terminated early because of high number of cardiac events among patients undergoing CEA, which had been attributed to the absence of aspirin in the surgical group (22). Too few neurological events occurred in the study, which prevented any meaningful conclusions.

The VAAT study included 444 men with internal carotid stenosis >50%. Two hundred and eleven patients were randomized to surgery and 233 to medical therapy alone (23). The combined ipsilateral neurological events were 8% among surgical patients and 20.6% among medically treated patients on Kaplan–Meier analysis ($p<0.001$). The incidence of ipsilateral stroke alone was 4.7% in the surgical group and 9.4% in the medical group, with borderline significance ($p=0.056$).

The ACAS study was the first influential trial for asymptomatic carotid stenosis up until the most recent ACST trial (19). This study randomized 1,662 men and women with asymptomatic (>60%) carotid stenosis to medical or surgical management. Overall, the ipsilateral stroke rate at 5 years from Kaplan–Meier analysis was 5.1% in the surgical group and 11% in the medical group ($p=0.004$), which corresponded to a relative risk reduction of 53% and an absolute risk reduction of 1% per year.

The most recent and largest asymptomatic carotid stenosis randomized trial published is the Asymptomatic Carotid Surgery Trial (ACST) Collaborative Study (24). In this study, 3,120 asymptomatic patients with substantial carotid narrowing (>60%) were randomized between immediate CEA and indefinite deferral of any CEA. They were followed for up to 5 years. In the surgical group, the 5-year all-stroke risk was 6.4% compared to 11.8% in the deferral group ($p<0.0001$), reducing the net 5-year risk of stroke by half in the population studied.

Lesions that may cause particular surgical dilemma are bilateral carotid lesions, contralateral carotid occlusion (with ipsilateral stenosis), and tandem lesions. At the present time, if bilateral carotid stenoses are found, two options are present. The first is to repair only the symptomatic side and follow the contralateral side. The other option is to treat both (usually at 6 weeks interval), proceeding first with CEA on the side with the higher degree of stenosis. It is not considered a safe option to address both sides simultaneously because of increased mortality and morbidity, particularly in the presence of tissue swelling, airway obstruction, or possibilities of bilateral palsies of the recurrent laryngeal nerve *(25)*. In the presence of one occluded carotid artery and a contralateral carotid stenosis, the occluded side should obviously be left alone and the stenotic side addressed only if the intervention is thought to impact natural history (as the risk of surgery is increased with contralateral occlusion). Lastly, it is felt that in the presence of a tandem lesion, if the intracranial portion has a higher degree of stenosis than the extracranial portion, then it is best to treat it medically.

Ulcerated lesions are also a controversial issue. They are classified as type A if the length is <10 mm^2, type B if 10–40 mm^2, and type C if >40 mm^2 *(26)*. Type C lesions are thought to have an associated risk of stroke of 7.5%/year *(27)*. At the present time, it is thought that asymptomatic type A should be left alone. If a type C is present and the patient has acceptable risk, this may warrant prophylactic CEA. The decision for type B relies much on the surgeon's individual conviction and the experience of the operating team *(26)*. These criteria for ulcerated lesions have not been subject to the same scientific scrutiny as the criteria for symptomatic and asymptomatic stenosis; hence, considerable surgical judgment is required.

Summary of the Indications

The general indications for CEA are thus summarized in Table 1, adapted from reference *(28)*.

Table 1
Indications for CEA in Patients with Carotid Artery Stenosis

Symptomatic patients (CEA morbidity and mortality <6%)	
Proven indications	≥TIA in the last 6 months and carotid stenosis ≥70%
	Mild stroke with carotid stenosis ≥70%
Acceptable indications	TIA in the past 6 months with stenosis 50–69%
	Progressive stroke and stenosis ≥70%
	Mild or moderate stroke in the past 6 months and stenosis 50–69%
	CEA ipsilateral to TIA and stenosis ≥70%, combined with required coronary artery bypass grafting
Uncertain indications	TIA with stenosis <50%
	Mild stroke with stenosis <50%
	Symptomatic acute carotid artery thrombosis
Inappropriate indications	Moderate stroke with stenosis <50%, not receiving aspirin
	Single TIA, stenosis <50%, not receiving aspirin
	High-risk patient, mild or moderate stroke, stenosis <50%, not receiving aspirin
	Global ischemic symptoms with stenosis <50%
	Acute internal carotid dissection, asymptomatic, receiving heparin

(Continued)

Table 1
(Continued)

Asymptomatic patients (CEA morbidity and mortality <3%)

Proven indications	Stenosis ≥60%
Acceptable indications	None defined
Uncertain indications	High-risk patient or surgeon with a morbidity–mortality risk >3%
	Combined CEA and coronary artery bypass surgery
	Non-stenotic ulcerative lesions
Inappropriate indications	CEA combined stroke morbidity–mortality rate >5%

SURGICAL TECHNIQUE

Patients undergoing CEA are kept NPO after midnight the day before surgery. They are taken to the operating room where a cervical block is done if local anesthesia is planned, or alternatively, they are placed under general anesthesia (see below for "*CEA Under Local Anesthesia vs. General Anesthesia*"). The patient is positioned with the neck slightly hyperextended and the head slightly turned away from the side to be operated on. The endarterectomy site is prepped and draped from the midline, in an area encompassing the clavicle, sternal notch, and mandible. The incision can be vertical along the anterior border of the sternocleidomastoid (SCM), on an imaginary line connecting the sternoclavicular junction and the mastoid process, or an oblique incision (across the skin crease over the side of the neck). The subcutaneous tissues are divided and the anterior border of the SCM identified. The dissection continues anterior to SCM until the facial vein, a tributary of the internal jugular vein, is encountered and ligated. The internal jugular vein is then usually retracted laterally and the carotid artery is identified (Fig. 1). Proximal control is obtained at the common carotid artery (CCA) proximal to the level of disease (usually at the level of the omohyoid muscle) by surrounding it with a vessel loop. If sinus bradycardia arises, 1–2 ml of 1% lidocaine is injected in the tissues between the external carotid artery (ECA) and the internal carotid artery (ICA).

Once proximal control is obtained, dissection is continued more distally around the ECA where vascular control is gained of the external carotid artery and its first branch, the superior thyroid artery. Subsequently, control should be gained distally at the ICA. Careful attention throughout the dissection is important to minimize manipulation of the carotid artery. Extreme care must be exerted during the dissection not to injure surrounding nerves, such as the vagus or hypoglossal nerves (Fig. 2). Dissection may lead to division of the ansa cervicalis, a branch of the hypoglossal nerve, which is acceptable. Some challenges may be encountered during the case, such as high ending of the plaque in the ICA or high bifurcation. If additional exposure is needed of the ICA, the first maneuver is to extend the skin incision all the way up to the mastoid process, which will allow division of the posterior belly of the digastric muscle. If further exposure is needed, the styloid process can be divided and the mandible displaced anteriorly.

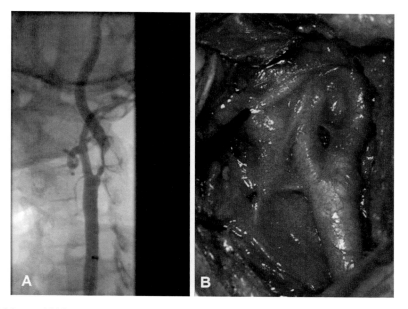

Fig. 1. (A) Normal bifurcation of the left internal carotid artery at C4 as shown on angiography and (B) surgical appearance of the carotid bifurcation after cut-down during carotid endarterectomy.

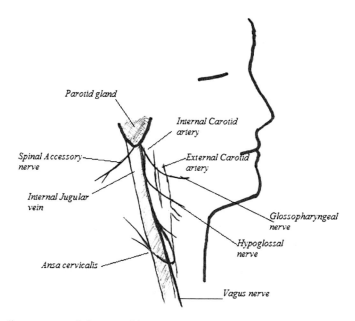

Fig. 2. Surrounding nerves of the carotid artery.

Once proximal and distal control of the vessel is obtained, heparin is given intravenously (5,000 units). If it is decided to use shunting, the type and size of shunt should be decided upon prior to clamping the vessel. The vessel is clamped and/or loops tightened proximally and distally. A longitudinal arteriotomy is made from the CCA to the ICA. The plaque is endarterectomized using a small flat surgical instrument by elevating the diseased plaque off the normal remaining arterial wall in a transmedial plane. It is critical to choose the optimal plane of dissection between the diseased intima and the circular fibers of the media. It is recommended to complete the endarterectomy proximally first (sharply), then to proceed to the distal portion of the vessel, which will often "flake away". The vessel is then closed primarily or with a patch (see below, "*Patch vs. Primary Closure*") using 6.0 polypropylene suture. Prior to unclamping, it is important to flush. The ICA is unclamped last.

Completion study may be performed as per the surgeons' preference. This may include a completion angiogram or B-mode ultrasound with waveform analysis and continuous Doppler. If a defect or intimal flap is found, it should be corrected to prevent any thromboembolic complications. Once hemostasis is achieved, a soft drain may be left in place (to be removed the day after surgery). Protamine may be given at the surgeon's discretion, keeping in mind possible hypotension and ana-phylactic reactions. The platysma is closed with a running suture and the skin is approximated with clips or a subcuticular suture.

Patients are awakened in the operating room, where the surgeon ensures that no neurological deficit is present. They are then transferred to the recovery room where they are observed for a period of approximately 6 hours. Patients are usually discharged home on the first or second postoperative day if no complication occurs. They are continued on their antiplatelet and secondary preventative therapy.

Postoperatively, a carotid duplex should be performed at 2–6 weeks after CEA. If satisfactory, another duplex should be done 6 months to 1 year later, then every year subsequently. If there is evidence of moderate contralateral disease or recurrent stenosis, scanning may be performed at 6–12 month intervals *(29)*.

Shunting or Not

No randomized trials have been conducted that demonstrate superiority of shunting *(30)*, although routine shunt insertion is known to have low perioperative death and stroke rates *(31)*. Even though some centers and surgeons recommend routine shunting, it is important to be aware that a shunt may be cumbersome during performance of the endarterectomy and closure of the vessel. Furthermore, there is a risk of plaque dislodgement and air embolization distal in the ICA. For those who do not perform routine shunting, the tolerance to cerebral clamping may be evaluated in several ways. If the operation is done under local anesthesia, 1–3 minutes after clamping is performed, the patient is asked to talk and perform a few mathematical tasks. Another approach is electroencephalographic monitoring, which has resurged recently after a period of disfavor. Lastly, others have advocated the assessment of back-bleeding, which may require considerable experience and judgment. Parameters that are evaluated include a back-bleeding pressure less than 25 mmHg *(32)*.

CEA Under Local Anesthesia vs. General Anesthesia

CEA under local anesthesia allows evaluation of cerebral tolerance to clamping; however, it does add challenges to the operation. For example, anxious patients may add to the stress of the surgical team, especially if the case is protracted. Hence, it should be reserved for patients who are felt to be able to tolerate the psychological stress of the procedure. If the local anesthesia approach is chosen, collaboration is needed between the anesthetist and the surgical team. A superficial cervical plexus block or a combination of superficial and deep cervical block may be used *(33, 34)* in combination with local anesthesia. Studies have suggested that stroke and death rates may be reduced by local anesthesia *(35, 36)*. The frequency of arrhythmias and acute myocardial infarction also appears to be reduced *(37)*. A randomized controlled trial (The General Anaesthetic versus Local Anaesthetic for Carotid Surgery Trial – GALA) is presently enrolling patients to assess this question.

In contrast, CEA under general anesthesia is felt to provide better control of the airway and ventilator mechanics. Furthermore, there may be improved cerebral blood flow and better tolerance to clamping with halogenated anesthetic agents *(38)*. Lastly, it results in less stress to the surgical team compared to an awake patient, with easier control of intra-operative complications.

Patch vs. Primary Closure

Once endarterectomy is performed, the surgeon is confronted with the choice of primary closure of the carotid artery or the use of a patch material. The traditional approach is to patch patients believed to be at high risk of recurrence, such as women and those with small carotid arteries. Several randomized controlled trials *(39–46)* and meta-analyses *(47–49)* have been conducted that evaluated the outcomes of patch closure vs. primary closure during CEA. In a meta-analysis conducted in 2,000, patching was superior to primary closure *(47)*. An update of the analysis performed by Bond in 2004 demonstrated that patching, with vein or prosthetic materials, significantly reduced the risk of ipsilateral stroke (1.6 vs. 4.5%) at 30 days *(48)*. This benefit persisted over the long term, with a lower risk of carotid restenosis (18.6 vs. 4.8%). With regard to selective or "discretionary" patching, there have been a few reports to date *(50–52)*. Pappas et al. *(50)* reported lower rates of stroke among primary closure patients but no long-term difference in restenosis. The authors concluded that selective patching was advocated. The other two studies reported no significant difference between patch closure and primary closure. These studies remain retrospective in nature. Based on these data, it appears that perhaps more evidence exists for routine patching, although it remains justifiable to use primary closure in large-caliber ICA (>6 mm diameter) *(53)*.

Type of Patch

The different materials available for patching include autologous vein graft, Dacron, ePTFE, and bovine pericardium. Surgeons may have their preference based on the malleability or other characteristics of the material. A meta-analysis of seven randomized controlled trials reported little difference between the types of patch material *(54)*. Hence, at the present moment, there is no consensus that any particular type of patch material is better than the other. A possible disadvantage of vein patch is patch disruption *(55–58)*, and that of prosthetic material is infection.

A Variant Approach: Eversion Endarterectomy

Although most surgeons perform open CEA, some prefer the eversion endarterectomy technique. This involves a similar dissection as the standard endarterectomy. However, the origin of the ICA is then transected and the ICA is "rolled" up distally while removing the diseased plaque in the transmedial plane. At the end of the diseased plaque, the artery is "rolled back" and sewn to the carotid bifurcation.

This suture line is purported to be less prone to restenosis compared to closure of a longitudinal arteriotomy as is performed in a standard CEA. A randomized study has been conducted, followed by a Cochrane database review, which suggested that eversion endarterectomy may carry equivalent death and stroke rate *(59–62)*. Downfalls of the technique are that not all patients are suitable, and the insertion of a shunt may be more difficult if it is needed. At the present time, however, it is still felt that the evidence is uncertain to firmly recommend one technique or another.

COMPLICATIONS

Complications related to CEA can be classified as early or late, and local or systemic (Table 2). Some of the most devastating complications involve the neurological system. These tend to occur early, within the first 30 days after surgery.

Early Complications

STROKE OR DEATH

Although most strokes are delayed (the patient initially wakes up postoperatively with normal neurological function), they tend to happen within the first 24 hours of surgery. These are usually due to endarterectomy site thrombosis and/or embolism. Death can also result from surgery, often in combination with a neurological event. Studies have reported a 30-day mortality of 1–3% in patients with symptomatic carotid stenosis *(20, 63, 64)* and 0.1–2% in patients with asymptomatic carotid stenosis *(64, 65)*. The combined incidence of stroke and death in the same time period is 5.5–7.0% in the symptomatic patients and 1.5–4.5% in the asymptomatic patients. Community-based surveys follow these results closely *(66–73)*.

HYPERPERFUSION/CEREBRAL HEMORRHAGE

The classic presentation of hyperperfusion and cerebral hemorrhage syndrome is unilateral headache, seizure, and cerebral hemorrhage, which peaks at postoperative

Table 2
Complications Related to CEA

Early complications	Incidence
Stroke or death	5.5–7% symptomatic patients
	1.5–4.5% asymptomatic patients
Hyperperfusion syndrome	2–3%
Cerebral hemorrhage	0.2–0.8%
Cranial nerve injury	8.6%
Hemorrhage requiring surgery	1–3%
Cardiac events	
– Cardiac death	0.4%
– Non-fatal myocardial infarction	0.8%
– Cardiac arrhythmias	1.6%
– Congestive heart failure	1.0%
– Angina	1.3%
Late complications	
Recurrent stenosis	10% at 2 years, 17% at 10 years
False aneurysm	Rare

days 2–7. The incidence of hyperperfusion is 2–3% *(74–76)*, which in 0.2–0.8% progresses to cerebral hemorrhage *(64, 77–79)*. The syndrome is thought to be secondary to changes in autoregulation in the cerebral territory of the endarterecto-mized carotid stenosis. It is critical to promptly and aggressively investigate and treat this complication.

CRANIAL NERVE INJURIES

In the NASCET trial, the incidence of cranial nerve injury was 8.6%, with the hypoglossal being injured in 3.7% of cases, the vagus in 2.5%, and the marginal mandibular branch of the facial nerve in 2.2% *(12, 80)*. Injury to the vagus nerve usually manifests as dysfunction of the recurrent laryngeal nerve and is noted by ipsilateral vocal cord paralysis with hoarseness of the voice, impaired phonation, and ineffective cough. Although the ansa cervicalis, a branch of the hypoglossal nerve, can be divided without much noticeable neurological deficit, division of the hypoglossal nerve itself will result in tongue palsy with impaired annunciation and deglutition. Injury to the marginal branch of the facial nerve will lead to drooping of the corner of the mouth and drooling.

Cranial nerve injuries that are less common include injury to the superior lar-yngeal nerve, spinal accessory nerve, glossopharyngeal nerve, and the sympathetic chain. Injury to the superior laryngeal nerve may result in voice fatigue and altera-tion, although it is mostly asymptomatic. Injury to the sympathetic chain may lead to Horner's syndrome. If the glossopharyngeal nerve is affected, impairment in swallowing and recurrent aspiration may occur. Spinal accessory injury may lead to shoulder pain and dropping and winging of the scapula. The greater auricular nerve may also be injured during the superficial part of the dissection. This will usually result in paresthesia and hyperesthesia around the ear.

HEMORRHAGE AND INFECTION

Hemorrhage requiring surgical intervention occurs in about 1–3% of patients *(64, 72, 81, 82)*. It is critical to be aware of this complication in order to avoid airway compromise. Disruption of the venous patch may happen in 0.1–0.7% of cases *(55–58)* and is usually due to poor quality of vein which leads to necrosis. Infection rarely occurs, but could lead to hemorrhage if situated in the deep tissues.

SYSTEMIC COMPLICATIONS

Hemodynamic instability may be seen after CEA. Hypotension and bradycardia are usually related to hyperactivity of the carotid baroreceptor because of restora-tion of compliance of the vessel wall. Hypertension is secondary to absent or decreased baroreceptor activity. Cardiac complications reported in the NASCET trial *(80)* include perioperative cardiac deaths (0.4%), non-fatal myocardial infarc-tions (0.8%), arrhythmias (1.6%), congestive heart failure (1.0%), or angina (1.3%).

Late Complications

RECURRENT STENOSIS

The meta-analysis by Frericks et al. demonstrated a rate of recurrence of 10% at 2 years and 17% at 10 years *(83)*. It is important to distinguish recurrent stenosis from residual stenosis in the early postoperative period. During the first 2 years post-CEA, the cause of recurrent stenosis is intimal hyperplasia, which often regresses. After several years post-CEA, progressive atherosclerosis is the usual cause.

FALSE ANEURYSM

False aneurysms at the endarterectomy sites are extremely rare. Their incidence has decreased since monofilament sutures have been used for arteriotomy closure, which decrease the risk of infection.

CONCLUSIONS

Carotid stenosis remains a major public health issue with an important burden on the population. Although CEA has demonstrated its efficacy over several decades now, a few controversies still remain with regard to the technical approaches. It will be interesting to see future long-term outcomes in comparison to carotid artery stenting. At the moment, it remains the gold standard to treat most patients with a high-grade carotid stenosis.

REFERENCES

1. World Health Organization (WHO). Surveillance in brief: Update of noncommunicable diseases and mental health surveillance activities. Issue No. 5 Geneva, WHO, 5:1–5, 2003. Available at www.who.int/entity/ncd_surveillance/media.org
2. American Heart Association. Heart and Stroke Facts Statistics-1999: Statistical Supplement. American Heart Association, Dallas, TX.
3. Kannel WB. Epidemiology of cerebrovascular disease: an epidemiologic study of cerebrovascular disease. In American Neurological Association and American Heart Association: Cerebral Vascular Diseases. Grune & Stratton, New York, 1966, pp. 53–66.
4. Kuller LH, Cook LP, Friedman GD. Survey of stroke epidemiology studies: Committee on Criteria and Methods, Council of Epidemiology, American Heart Association. Stroke 1972;3: 579–85.
5. Schneider PA, Kasirajan K. Difficult anatomy: what characteristics are critical to good outcomes of either CEA or CAS? Semin Vasc Surg 2007;20:216–25.
6. Landis GS, Faries PL. A critical look at "high-risk" in choosing the proper intervention for patients with carotid bifurcation disease. Semin Vasc Surg 2007;20:199–204.
7. Caplan LR, Skillman J, Ojemann R, Fields WS. Intracerebral hemorrhage following carotid endarterectomy: a hypertensive complication? Stroke 1978;9:457–460.
8. Giordano JM, Trout HH, 3rd, Kozloff L, DePalma RG. Timing of carotid artery endarterectomy after stroke. J Vasc Surg 1985;2:250–255.
9. Dosick SM, Whalen RC, Gale SS, Brown OW. Carotid endarterectomy in the stroke patient: computerized axial tomography to determine timing. J Vasc Surg 1985;2:214–219.
10. Khanna HL, Garg AG. 774 carotid endarterectomies for strokes and transient ischemic attacks: comparison of results of early vs. late surgery. Acta Neurochir Suppl (Wien) 1988;42:103–106.
11. Gasecki AP, Ferguson GG, Eliasziw M, Clagett GP, Fox AJ, Hachinski V, Barnett HJ. Early endarterectomy for severe carotid artery stenosis after a nondisabling stroke: results from the North American Symptomatic Carotid Endarterectomy Trial. J Vasc Surg 1994;20:288–295.
12. Beneficial effect of carotid endarterectomy in symptomatic patients with high-grade carotid stenosis. North American Symptomatic Carotid Endarterectomy Trial Collaborators. N Engl J Med 1991;325:445–453.
13. Nehler MR, Moneta GL, McConnell DB, Edwards JM, Taylor LM, Jr., Yeager RA, Porter JM. Anticoagulation followed by elective carotid surgery in patients with repetitive transient ischemic attacks and high-grade carotid stenosis. Arch Surg 1993;128:1117–1121; discussion 1121–1123.
14. Inzitari D, Eliasziw M, Gates P, Sharpe BL, Chan RK, Meldrum HE, Barnett HJ. The causes and risk of stroke in patients with asymptomatic internal-carotid-artery stenosis. North American Symptomatic Carotid Endarterectomy Trial Collaborators. N Engl J Med 2000;342:1693–1700.

15. Eckstein HH, Schumacher H, Dorfler A, Forsting M, Jansen O, Ringleb P, Allenberg JR. Carotid endarterectomy and intracranial thrombolysis: simultaneous and staged procedures in ischemic stroke. J Vasc Surg 1999;29:459–471.
16. Bauer RB, Meyer JS, Fields WS, Remington R, Macdonald MC, Callen P. Joint study of extracranial arterial occlusion. 3. Progress report of controlled study of long-term survival in patients with and without operation. JAMA 1969;208:509–518.
17. Barnett HJ, Taylor DW, Eliasziw M, Fox AJ, Ferguson GG, Haynes RB, Rankin RN, Clagett GP, Hachinski VC, Sackett DL, Thorpe KE, Meldrum HE, Spence JD. Benefit of carotid endarterectomy in patients with symptomatic moderate or severe stenosis. North American Symptomatic Carotid Endarterectomy Trial Collaborators. N Engl J Med 1998;339:1415–1425.
18. MRC European Carotid Surgery Trial: interim results for symptomatic patients with severe (70–99%) or with mild (0–29%) carotid stenosis. European Carotid Surgery Trialists' Collaborative Group. Lancet 1991;337:1235–1243.
19. Endarterectomy for asymptomatic carotid artery stenosis. Executive Committee for the Asymptomatic Carotid Atherosclerosis Study. JAMA 1995;273:1421–1428.
20. Mayberg MR, Wilson SE, Yatsu F, Weiss DG, Messina L, Hershey LA, Colling C, Eskridge J, Deykin D, Winn HR. Carotid endarterectomy and prevention of cerebral ischemia in symptomatic carotid stenosis. Veterans Affairs Cooperative Studies Program 309 Trialist Group. JAMA 1991;266:3289–3294.
21. Carotid surgery versus medical therapy in asymptomatic carotid stenosis. The CASANOVA Study Group. Stroke 1991;22:1229–1235.
22. Results of a randomized controlled trial of carotid endarterectomy for asymptomatic carotid stenosis. Mayo Asymptomatic Carotid Endarterectomy Study Group. Mayo Clin Proc 1992; 67:513–518.
23. Hobson RW, 2nd, Weiss DG, Fields WS, Goldstone J, Moore WS, Towne JB, Wright CB. Efficacy of carotid endarterectomy for asymptomatic carotid stenosis. The Veterans Affairs Cooperative Study Group. N Engl J Med 1993;328:221–227.
24. Mohammed N, Anand SS. Prevention of disabling and fatal strokes by successful carotid endarterectomy in patients without recent neurological symptoms: randomized controlled trial. MRC asymptomatic carotid surgery trial (ACST) collaborative group. Lancet 2004; 363: 1491–1502. Vasc Med 2005;10:77–78.
25. Betterman K, Toole JF. Diagnostic Evaluation of and Medical Management of Patients with Ischemic Cerebrovascular Disease. Rutherford Textbook of Vascular Surgery. 6th ed. W.B. Saunders, Philadelphia, PA; 2005, p.1906.
26. Moore WS, Boren C, Malone JM, Roon AJ, Eisenberg R, Goldstone J, Mani R. Natural history of nonstenotic, asymptomatic ulcerative lesions of the carotid artery. Arch Surg 1978;113: 1352–1359.
27. Dixon S, Pais SO, Raviola C, Gomes A, Machleder HI, Baker JD, Busuttil RW, Barker WF, Moore WS. Natural history of nonstenotic, asymptomatic ulcerative lesions of the carotid artery. A further analysis. Arch Surg 1982;117:1493–1498.
28. Moore, WS. Extracranial Cerebrovascular Disease: The Carotid Artery. Vascular and Endovascular Surgery. A Comprehensive Review. 7th ed. W.B. Saunders, Philadelphia, PA; 2006, p.634.
29. Ricotta JJ, DeWeese JA. Is routine carotid ultrasound surveillance after carotid endarterectomy worthwhile? Am J Surg 1996;172:140–142; discussion 143.
30. Counsell C, Salinas R, Naylor R, Warlow C. Routine or selective carotid artery shunting for carotid endarterectomy (and different methods of monitoring in selective shunting). Cochrane Database Syst Rev 2000:CD000190.
31. Naylor AR, Hayes PD, Allroggen H, Lennard N, Gaunt ME, Thompson MM, London NJ, Bell PR. Reducing the risk of carotid surgery: a 7-year audit of the role of monitoring and quality control assessment. J Vasc Surg 2000;32:750–759.
32. Moore WS, Hall AD. Carotid artery back pressure: a test of cerebral tolerance to temporary carotid occlusion. Arch Surg 1969;99:702–710.
33. Stoneham MD, Doyle AR, Knighton JD, Dorje P, Stanley JC. Prospective, randomized comparison of deep or superficial cervical plexus block for carotid endarterectomy surgery. Anesthesiology 1998;89:907–912.
34. Pandit JJ, Bree S, Dillon P, Elcock D, McLaren ID, Crider B. A comparison of superficial versus combined (superficial and deep) cervical plexus block for carotid endarterectomy: a prospective, randomized study. Anesth Analg 2000;91:781–786.

35. Fiorani P, Sbarigia E, Speziale F, Antonini M, Fiorani B, Rizzo L, Massucci M. General anaesthesia versus cervical block and perioperative complications in carotid artery surgery. Eur J Vasc Endovasc Surg 1997;13:37–42.

36. Tangkanakul C, Counsell C, Warlow C. Local versus general anaesthesia for carotid endarterectomy. Cochrane Database Syst Rev 2000:CD000126.

37. Allen BT, Anderson CB, Rubin BG, Thompson RW, Flye MW, Young-Beyer P, Frisella P, Sicard GA. The influence of anesthetic technique on perioperative complications after carotid endarterectomy. J Vasc Surg 1994;19:834–842; discussion 842–843.

38. Christensen MS, Hoedt-Rasmussen K, Lassen NA. Cerebral vasodilatation by halothane anaesthesia in man and its potentiation by hypotension and hypercapnia. Br J Anaesth 1967;39:927–934.

39. De Vleeschauwer P, Wirthle W, Holler L, Krause E, Horsch S. Is venous patch grafting after carotid endarterectomy able to reduce the rate of restenosis? Prospective randomized pilot study with stratification. Acta Chir Belg 1987;87:242–246.

40. Al-Rawi PG, Turner CL, Waran V, Ng I, Kirkpatrick PJ. A randomized trial of synthetic patch versus direct primary closure in carotid endarterectomy. Neurosurgery 2006;59:822–828; discussion 828–829.

41. Eikelboom BC, Ackerstaff RG, Hoeneveld H, Ludwig JW, Teeuwen C, Vermeulen FE, Welten RJ. Benefits of carotid patching: a randomized study. J Vasc Surg 1988;7:240–247.

42. Lord RS, Raj TB, Stary DL, Nash PA, Graham AR, Goh KH. Comparison of saphenous vein patch, polytetrafluoroethylene patch, and direct arteriotomy closure after carotid endarterectomy. Part I. Perioperative results. J Vasc Surg 1989;9:521–529.

43. Ranaboldo CJ, Barros D'Sa AA, Bell PR, Chant AD, Perry PM. Randomized controlled trial of patch angioplasty for carotid endarterectomy. The Joint Vascular Research Group. Br J Surg 1993;80:1528–1530.

44. Myers SI, Valentine RJ, Chervu A, Bowers BL, Clagett GP. Saphenous vein patch versus primary closure for carotid endarterectomy: long-term assessment of a randomized prospective study. J Vasc Surg 1994;19:15–22.

45. Katz D, Snyder SO, Gandhi RH, Wheeler JR, Gregory RT, Gayle RG, Parent FN, 3rd. Long-term follow-up for recurrent stenosis: a prospective randomized study of expanded polytetrafluoroethylene patch angioplasty versus primary closure after carotid endarterectomy. J Vasc Surg 1994;19:198–203; discussion 204–205.

46. AbuRahma AF, Khan JH, Robinson PA, Saiedy S, Short YS, Boland JP, White JF, Conley Y. Prospective randomized trial of carotid endarterectomy with primary closure and patch angioplasty with saphenous vein, jugular vein, and polytetrafluoroethylene: perioperative (30-day) results. J Vasc Surg 1996;24:998–1006; discussion 1006–1007.

47. Counsell C, Salinas R, Warlow C, Naylor R. Patch angioplasty versus primary closure for carotid endarterectomy. Cochrane Database Syst Rev 2000:CD000160.

48. Bond R, Rerkasem K, Naylor AR, Aburahma AF, Rothwell PM. Systematic review of randomized controlled trials of patch angioplasty versus primary closure and different types of patch materials during carotid endarterectomy. J Vasc Surg 2004;40:1126–1135.

49. Counsell CE, Salinas R, Naylor R, Warlow CP. A systematic review of the randomised trials of carotid patch angioplasty in carotid endarterectomy. Eur J Vasc Endovasc Surg 1997;13:345–354.

50. Pappas D, Hines GL, Yoonah Kim E. Selective patching in carotid endarterectomy: is patching always necessary? J Cardiovasc Surg (Torino) 1999;40:555–559.

51. Golledge J, Cuming R, Davies AH, Greenhalgh RM. Outcome of selective patching following carotid endarterectomy. Eur J Vasc Endovasc Surg 1996;11:458–463.

52. Cikrit DF, Larson DM, Sawchuk AP, Thornhill C, Shafique S, Nachreiner RD, Lalka SG, Dalsing MC. Discretionary carotid patch angioplasty leads to good results. Am J Surg 2006;192:e46–e50.

53. Byrne J, Feustel P, Darling RC, 3rd. Primary closure, routine patching, and eversion endarterectomy: what is the current state of the literature supporting use of these techniques? Semin Vasc Surg 2007;20:226–235.

54. Bond R, Rerkasem K, Naylor R, Rothwell PM. Patches of different types for carotid patch angioplasty. Cochrane Database Syst Rev 2004:CD000071.

55. Riles TS, Lamparello PJ, Giangola G, Imparato AM. Rupture of the vein patch: a rare complication of carotid endarterectomy. Surgery 1990;107:10–12.

56. Tawes RL, Jr., Treiman RL. Vein patch rupture after carotid endarterectomy: a survey of the Western Vascular Society members. Ann Vasc Surg 1991;5:71–73.

57. O'Hara PJ, Hertzer NR, Krajewski LP, Beven EG. Saphenous vein patch rupture after carotid endarterectomy. J Vasc Surg 1992;15:504–509.

58. Yamamoto Y, Piepgras DG, Marsh WR, Meyer FB. Complications resulting from saphenous vein patch graft after carotid endarterectomy. Neurosurgery 1996;39:670–675; discussion 675–676.
59. Cao P, Giordano G, De Rango P, Zannetti S, Chiesa R, Coppi G, Palombo D, Spartera C, Stancanelli V, Vecchiati E. A randomized study on eversion versus standard carotid endarterectomy: study design and preliminary results: the Everest Trial. J Vasc Surg 1998;27:595–605.
60. Cao P, Giordano G, De Rango P, Zannetti S, Chiesa R, Coppi G, Palombo D, Peinetti F, Spartera C, Stancanelli V, Vecchiati E. Eversion versus conventional carotid endarterectomy: late results of a prospective multicenter randomized trial. J Vasc Surg 2000;31:19–30.
61. Cao P, Giordano G, De Rango P, Caporali S, Lenti M, Ricci S, Moggi L. Eversion versus conventional carotid endarterectomy: a prospective study. Eur J Vasc Endovasc Surg 1997;14: 96–104.
62. Cao P, De Rango P, Zannetti S. Eversion vs conventional carotid endarterectomy: a systematic review. Eur J Vasc Endovasc Surg 2002;23:195–201.
63. Randomised trial of endarterectomy for recently symptomatic carotid stenosis: final results of the MRC European Carotid Surgery Trial (ECST). Lancet 1998;351:1379–1387.
64. Ferguson GG, Eliasziw M, Barr HW, Clagett GP, Barnes RW, Wallace MC, Taylor DW, Haynes RB, Finan JW, Hachinski VC, Barnett HJ. The North American Symptomatic Carotid Endarterectomy Trial: surgical results in 1415 patients. Stroke 1999;30:1751–1758.
65. Towne JB, Weiss DG, Hobson RW, 2nd. First phase report of cooperative Veterans Administration asymptomatic carotid stenosis study – operative morbidity and mortality. J Vasc Surg 1990;11:252–258; discussion 258–259.
66. Bratzler DW, Oehlert WH, Murray CK, Bumpus LJ, Moore LL, Piatt DS. Carotid endarterectomy in Oklahoma Medicare beneficiaries: patient characteristics and outcomes. J Okla State Med Assoc 1996;89:423–429.
67. Karp HR, Flanders WD, Shipp CC, Taylor B, Martin D. Carotid endarterectomy among Medicare beneficiaries: a statewide evaluation of appropriateness and outcome. Stroke 1998; 29:46–52.
68. Cebul RD, Snow RJ, Pine R, Hertzer NR, Norris DG. Indications, outcomes, and provider volumes for carotid endarterectomy. JAMA 1998;279:1282–1287.
69. Kucey DS, Bowyer B, Iron K, Austin P, Anderson G, Tu JV. Determinants of outcome after carotid endarterectomy. J Vasc Surg 1998;28:1051–1058.
70. Kresowik TF, Bratzler DW, Kresowik RA, Hendel ME, Grund SL, Brown KR, Nilasena DS. Multistate improvement in process and outcomes of carotid endarterectomy. J Vasc Surg 2004;39:372–380.
71. Kresowik TF, Hemann RA, Grund SL, Hendel ME, Brenton M, Wiblin RT, Adams HP, Ellerbeck EF. Improving the outcomes of carotid endarterectomy: results of a statewide quality improvement project. J Vasc Surg 2000;31:918–926.
72. Kresowik TF, Bratzler D, Karp HR, Hemann RA, Hendel ME, Grund SL, Brenton M, Ellerbeck EF, Nilasena DS. Multistate utilization, processes, and outcomes of carotid endarterectomy. J Vasc Surg 2001;33:227–234; discussion 234–235.
73. Bond R, Rerkasem K, Rothwell PM. Systematic review of the risks of carotid endarterectomy in relation to the clinical indication for and timing of surgery. Stroke 2003;34:2290–2301.
74. Ascher E, Markevich N, Schutzer RW, Kallakuri S, Jacob T, Hingorani AP. Cerebral hyperperfusion syndrome after carotid endarterectomy: predictive factors and hemodynamic changes. J Vasc Surg 2003;37:769–777.
75. Coutts SB, Hill MD, Hu WY. Hyperperfusion syndrome: toward a stricter definition. Neurosurgery 2003;53:1053–1058; discussion 1058–1060.
76. Ogasawara K, Yukawa H, Kobayashi M, Mikami C, Konno H, Terasaki K, Inoue T, Ogawa A. Prediction and monitoring of cerebral hyperperfusion after carotid endarterectomy by using single-photon emission computerized tomography scanning. J Neurosurg 2003;99:504–510.
77. Solomon RA, Loftus CM, Quest DO, Correll JW. Incidence and etiology of intracerebral hemorrhage following carotid endarterectomy. J Neurosurg 1986;64:29–34.
78. Schroeder T, Sillesen H, Boesen J, Laursen H, Sorensen P. Intracerebral haemorrhage after carotid endarterectomy. Eur J Vasc Surg 1987;1:51–60.
79. Piepgras DG, Morgan MK, Sundt TM, Jr., Yanagihara T, Mussman LM. Intracerebral hemorrhage after carotid endarterectomy. J Neurosurg 1988;68:532–536.
80. Paciaroni M, Eliasziw M, Kappelle LJ, Finan JW, Ferguson GG, Barnett HJ. Medical complications associated with carotid endarterectomy. North American Symptomatic Carotid Endarterectomy Trial (NASCET). Stroke 1999;30:1759–1763.

81. Kunkel JM, Gomez ER, Spebar MJ, Delgado RJ, Jarstfer BS, Collins GJ. Wound hematomas after carotid endarterectomy. Am J Surg 1984;148:844–847.
82. Welling RE, Ramadas HS, Gansmuller KJ. Cervical wound hematoma after carotid endarterectomy. Ann Vasc Surg 1989;3:229–231.
83. Frericks H, Kievit J, van Baalen JM, van Bockel JH. Carotid recurrent stenosis and risk of ipsilateral stroke: a systematic review of the literature. Stroke 1998;29:244–250.

3 Carotid Stenting Registries and Randomized Trials

Percy P. Jokhi, MBBS, PhD
and Jacqueline Saw, MD, FRCPC

CONTENTS

ABSTRACT

Considerable advances have been made in the development of carotid artery stenting (CAS). Increased operator experience and training have been coupled with improvements in technique and design of dedicated low-profile equipment, and the use of cerebral protection is becoming widespread. As a rival to CEA, the evidence in favor of CAS is most robust in high surgical risk patients. Results from ongoing rigorous large randomized trials are anticipated to address the utility of CAS in standard and low-risk patients.

Keywords: Carotid artery stenting; Randomized controlled trial; Registry; Case series

INTRODUCTION AND HISTORICAL BACKGROUND

Following the first reported carotid endarterectomy (CEA) by Eastcott in 1954 *(1)*, widespread uptake of this technique meant that by the early 1980s, CEA was the most frequently performed vascular surgical procedure. However,

From: *Contemporary Cardiology: Carotid Artery Stenting: The Basics*
Edited by: J. Saw, DOI 10.1007/978-1-60327-314-5_3,
© Humana Press, a part of Springer Science+Business Media, LLC 2009

it was not until the 1990s that a series of landmark-randomized clinical trials established the efficacy of CEA plus aspirin compared with aspirin alone in preventing stroke in patients with atherosclerotic carotid artery stenosis *(2–7)*. These trials established parameters for revascularization in both symptomatic and asymptomatic diseases. Hence, the current American Heart Association (AHA) guidelines recommend CEA in symptomatic patients with 50–99% stenosis and for asymptomatic patients with 60–99% stenosis if the risks of peri-operative stroke or death are less than 6 and 3%, respectively *(8)*.

The procedural mortality in these surgical trials was low, 0.1% in ACAS *(5)* and 0.6% in NASCET *(2)*. However, many patients were excluded from these studies on the basis of one or more clinical or anatomic criteria that placed them in a high surgical risk category (see Table 1). Analysis of 113,000 'real-world' Medicare patients who underwent CEA in 1992–1993 showed a peri-operative mortality of 1.4% in trial hospitals (institutions participating in NASCET and ACAS) and 1.7–2.5% in non-trial hospitals depending on the annual volume of procedures performed *(9)*. This indicated first that the particular center and experience of the surgeon were important factors in determining outcome; and second, that even at these institutions peri-operative mortality in real-world patients was significantly higher than reported in clinical trials. Several registries and observational series of CEA in high surgical risk patients have corroborated this *(10–13)*, although some authors have criticized some of these high-risk criteria and shown satisfactory results in this patient group *(14, 15)*. Differences in methodology also led to significant variability in the rate of stroke or death. A systematic review of 16,000 patients undergoing CEA between 1980 and 1995 showed that studies in which a neurologist assessed patients after surgery had the highest reported rates of stroke, while those with a single surgeon author had the lowest risk *(16)*. This emphasized the need for uniform independent follow-up to avoid bias in reporting of events. Notably, nearly all major carotid stenting trials and registries in the United States have had independent neurological adjudication of stroke events.

CEA is also associated with adverse events other than death or stroke. These include cranial nerve palsy, hemorrhage, wound infection, and a variety of cardiac, pulmonary, infectious, and other medical complications which, while not life threatening, frequently prolong hospital stay *(17, 18)*. Given these concerns, it was hoped that carotid angioplasty would provide a less-invasive alternative to CEA that might

Table 1
High-Risk Criteria for CEA

Anatomic criteria	Medical comorbidities
Lesion at C2 or higher	Age ≥80 years
Lesion below clavicle	Class III/IV congestive heart failure
Prior radical neck surgery or radiation	Class III/IV angina pectoris
Contralateral carotid occlusion	Left main/≥2-vessel coronary disease
Prior ipsilateral CEA	Urgent (<30 days) heart surgery
Contralateral laryngeal nerve palsy	LV ejection fraction ≤ 30%
Tracheostomy	Recent (<30 days) myocardial infarction
	Severe chronic lung disease
	Severe renal disease

be better tolerated, especially in high surgical risk patients. In 1977, Mathias proposed the idea of percutaneous carotid angioplasty in humans after performing canine experiments *(19)*. In 1980, Kerber reported the first human carotid angioplasty in the proximal carotid artery of a patient undergoing a distal bifurcation endarterectomy *(20)*. During the 1980s further pioneering work was performed by Mathias, Theron, and Kachel (reviewed in *(21)*). This early experience of percutaneous carotid intervention soon established potential pitfalls. In general, carotid plaque is more friable and prone to embolism, and unlike peripheral or even coronary angioplasty, the brain is unforgiving as an end organ. This, coupled with the use of cumbersome, non-dedicated equipment led to high complication rates, and the procedure was initially reserved for palliative treatment in inoperable patients. However, with the arrival of dedicated low-profile tools and the advent of stent technology, early work by Diethrich, Yadav, Wholey, and Roubin suggested that this technique could be an alternative to CEA *(22–26)*. Stents were a key breakthrough – they helped to contain lesion surfaces with potential for thromboembolism, prevent dissections, and reduce restenosis. Nevertheless in these initial trials, peri-procedural stroke rates were still in the range of 5–10% and one randomized clinical trial (RCT) was aborted after enrolling only 17 patients because of an unacceptable stroke rate in the carotid artery stenting (CAS) arm *(27)*.

Early trials were limited by a number of factors: (i) a steep learning curve for the procedure and interventionalists with still limited experience; (ii) balloon-expandable stents, which were at risk of late external compression (these have now been superseded by nitinol self-expanding stents); (iii) inadequate anti-platelet therapy by today's standards; and (iv) lack of neuroprotection. Studies of human CAS have shown that embolic particles consist of atherosclerotic debris, organized thrombus, and calcified material *(28–31)*. Prompted by the observation of a high incidence of distal embolization during CAS, a variety of protection systems were designed to capture and remove debris released during the procedure. Use of these embolic protection devices (EPDs) has become more widespread in subsequent studies.

This chapter aims to review the literature on carotid artery stenting and is organized as follows:

(1) Early large multi-center CAS registries
(2) High surgical risk CAS registries
(3) Trials of CAS vs. CEA
(4) Post-marketing CAS registries
(5) Ongoing trials of CAS vs. CEA

EARLY MULTI-CENTER CAS REGISTRIES

Following initial reports of CAS in the 1990s, a large number of single-center observational studies were published. These had many limitations, including small numbers of patients and relatively short follow-up. There was inconsistent definition of event-rates such as stroke (all stroke vs. ipsilateral stroke), death (all-cause vs. procedure-related), and composite endpoints (e.g., death + stroke + myocardial infarction). Furthermore EPD use was variable and independent neurological assessment was non-uniform in these early studies. To enhance the consistency of data collection, non-randomized, multi-center voluntary registries were created. Although CAS technique and independent oversight were not standardized, three large registries (Pro-CAS, ELOCAS, and the Global Carotid Artery Stent Registry) recorded more than 18,000 procedures in patients from a broad spectrum of surgical risk and provided valuable information on CAS performance and outcomes *(32–34)*.

Pro-CAS

The Prospective Registry of Carotid Artery Angioplasty and Stenting instituted by the German Societies of Angiology and Radiology included 3,267 CAS procedures from 38 centers in Germany, Austria, and Switzerland between 1999 and 2003 *(32)*. The average age of the patients was 70 years and 56% of patients were symptomatic. Overall technical success was 98%. EPD use was only monitored starting October 2000 and was 64% after this. Overall mortality was 0.6%, with permanent stroke in 2.5% and a combined rate of death and permanent stroke in 2.8% although the duration of follow-up was not specified. No clear advantage was demonstrated with EPD use in this non-randomized registry. The rate of neurological complications was moderately higher in symptomatic patients with a 3.1% rate of death and permanent stroke but well within the AHA guidelines of 6% or less, and the rate of 2.4% in asymptomatic patients within the proposed upper limit of 3%.

ELOCAS

The European Long Term Carotid Artery Stenting Registry enrolled 2,172 patients undergoing CAS at four centers in Belgium, Germany, and Italy between 1993 and 2004 *(33)*. The average age was 71 years and 41.6% of patients were symptomatic. Technical success was 99.7 and 85.9% of cases were performed with EPDs. The recruiting centers and interventionalists were highly experienced as reflected by the low combined rate of death plus major stroke of 1.2% at 30 days with no significant difference between symptomatic (1.4%) and asymptomatic patients (1.0%). Long-term follow-up showed death and major stroke rates of 4.1, 10.1, and 15.5% at 1, 3, and 5 years, respectively, with corresponding low binary restenosis rates of 1, 2, and 3.4%. Peri-procedural event rates with and without EPD use were not reported, but in a non-prespecified subgroup analysis, pre-dilatation prior to stent implantation was found to significantly lower the long-term stroke and death rate as compared with direct stenting (2.7% vs. 4.6% at 1 year, $p = 0.0022$). The mechanism proposed was that pre-dilatation remodeled the plaque leading to less extrusion between the stent struts.

The Global Carotid Artery Stent Registry

The Global Carotid Artery Stent Registry was started in 1997 and initially involved 24 major carotid interventional centers in Europe, North America, South America, and Asia. The data were updated annually until September 2002 by which time there was a total of 53 participating centers with 12,392 procedures involving 11,243 patients, 53.2% of whom were symptomatic *(34)*. The technical success rate was 98.9% with the use of neuroprotection in 38.5% (although data on EPD use were only available for 10,974 procedures). The 30-day rates of minor stroke, major stroke, and procedure-related death were 2.14, 1.2, and 0.64%, respectively. Over the 5-year period, the overall rate of all stroke plus procedure-related death at 30 days fell from 5.7 to 3.98%, attributed largely to improvements in equipment, operator experience, and use of neuroprotection. Subset analysis of the 30-day event-rates showed an overall 4.94% stroke/procedure-related death rate in symptomatic patients and

2.95% in asymptomatic patients. In cases performed with neuroprotection, the rate was 2.23% compared with 5.29% among those performed without EPD. This benefit of EPD was seen in both symptomatic (2.70% vs. 6.04%) and asymptomatic (1.75% vs. 3.97%) groups. It was established, however, that there was a steep learning curve for EPD use with centers that had performed 20–50 cases having a 4.04% stroke and death rate compared with 1.56% in centers that had performed more than 500 cases. At 1, 2, and 3 years of follow-up, restenosis rates by carotid duplex were 2.7, 2.6, and 2.4%, and new ipsilateral neurological event rates were observed in 1.2, 1.3, and 1.7%, respectively.

CONTEMPORARY HIGH SURGICAL RISK CAS REGISTRIES

The early voluntary registries described above collected data on CAS in a wide variety of patients with a broad spectrum of surgical risk using non-standardized techniques and equipment. Contemporary, prospective, multi-center registries have focused primarily on safety and efficacy of CAS in high surgical risk patients. These have been largely industry sponsored and conducted as IDE (investigational device exemption) trials to obtain FDA marketing approval in the United States or CE mark approval in Europe for specific carotid stent and EPD platforms. All have had comparable pre-defined inclusion and exclusion criteria, and independent neurological assessment of patients pre- and post-CAS, with oversight by safety and protocol-monitoring committees. Both symptomatic (carotid stenosis >50%) and asymptomatic patients (carotid stenosis >80%) were enrolled. The primary safety end point was typically the combined incidence of death, stroke, and myocardial infarction (MI) at 30 days, with the primary efficacy end point being the above plus the incidence of ipsilateral stroke or death between 31 days and 1 year after CAS. Dual anti-platelet therapy was standard. As these studies were performed in high-risk patients with no control group, a historically weighted estimate of stroke or death of 14–14.5% at 30 days after CEA was used for comparison, although this has attracted strong criticism and been contradicted by other reports *(12, 14, 35, 36)*. Outcome data from the studies described below have been presented at major international meetings, although not all have yet been published in peer-reviewed journals. A summary of these results is shown in Table 2.

ARCHeR

The ARCHeR (AccuLink™ for Revascularization of Carotids in High-Risk patients) trial was a series of three sequential, multi-center, non-randomized prospective registries. ARCHeR 1 and 2 were designed to compare carotid stent therapy using the AccuLink™/AccuNet™ system (Guidant Endovascular, currently Abbott Vascular) with a weighted historical control of CEA in high surgical risk patients. ARCHeR 3 was designed to demonstrate non-inferiority of the 30-day composite end point in comparison to ARCHeR 2. Five hundred and eighty-one patients (24% symptomatic) were consecutively enrolled from 2000 to 2003 at 48 (43 US and 5 non-US) sites in the three phases of the study, which had identical inclusion/exclusion criteria. The AccuLink™ over-the-wire (OTW) self-expanding nitinol stent was used without EPD in ARCHeR 1 and with the AccuNet™ OTW filter EPD in ARCHeR 2. ARCHeR 3 used rapid-exchange versions of both stent and filter systems. The data for each study were presented separately at the American College of Cardiology (ACC) Scientific Sessions in 2004 *(37)* and are shown in

Table 2
High-Risk CAS Registries

	Sponsor	Stent	EPD	Sample size	Symptomatic %	30-day D+S (%)	30-day D+S+MI (%)	1-year outcome (%)[1]	Technical success (%)
ARCHeR pooled	Guidant/Abbott	AccuLink	AccuNet	581	24	6.9	8.3	9.6	>95
ARCHeR 1		AccuLink OTW	None	158	–	6.3	7.6	8.3	–
ARCHeR 2		AccuLink OTW	AccuNet OTW	278	–	6.8	8.6	10.2	–
ARCHeR 3		AccuLink RX	AccuNet RX	145	–	7.6	8.3	–	98.2
BEACH	Boston scientific	Wallstent	FilterWire EX/EZ	747	25.3	2.8	5.8	9.1[2]	96
CABERNET	Boston scientific	EndoTex NexStent	FilterWire EX/EZ	454	24	3.6	3.9	4.5	
CREATE	ev3	Protégé	Spider OTW	419	17.4	5.2	6.2	7.8	97.4
CREATE SpiderRX	ev3	Acculink	SpiderRX	160	–	–	5.6	–	–
MAVErIC 1 + 2	Medtronic	Exponent	GuardWire	498	22[3]	–	5.2		
MAVErIC Int'l	Medtronic	Exponent	InterceptorPlus	51	–	5.7	5.9	11.8	94.2
MO.MA		Any	Mo.Ma	157	19.7	–	5.7	–	96.8
PASCAL		Exponent	Any CE-approved	115	–	–	8	–	–
PRIAMUS		Any	Mo.Ma	416	63.5	4.56	4.56	–	99
SECURITY	Abbott	Xact	Emboshield	305	21	6.89	7.5	8.5	96.7

[1] The 30-day death, stroke, and MI plus ipsilateral stroke 31–365 days unless stated otherwise.
[2] Results from 438 of 480 patients in pivotal group only – 30-day death, stroke, and MI plus ipsilateral stroke/neurological death from 31–365 days.
[3] Proportion of symptomatic patients only available for MAVERiC 2.

Table 2, but have since been published in a pooled format as outcomes were not significantly different *(38)*. The overall 30-day MAE (major adverse event rate) rate of death/stroke/MI was 8.3% (13.1% in symptomatic patients and 6.8% in asymptomatic patients) and that of stroke/death was 6.9% (11.6% in symptomatic patients and 5.4% in asymptomatic patients). The 30-day major stroke rate was 1.5% (4.3% in symptomatic patients and 0.7% in asymptomatic patients). The primary efficacy end point (a composite of 30-day MAE plus ipsilateral stroke between 31 days and 1 year) was seen in 9.6% of patients, which was below the 14.4% historical control comparator. Target lesion revascularization at 1 year was 2.2%. FDA approval was granted in August 2004, making this the first approved carotid stent/embolic protection system in the United States.

BEACH

The Boston Scientific EPI: A Carotid Stenting Trial for High-Risk Surgical Patients (BEACH) was designed to evaluate outcomes of CAS in high-risk patients using the Boston Scientific Carotid Wallstent® and FilterWire EX/EZ systems *(39)*. As with the ARCHeR trial, the hypothesis was that of non-inferiority to CEA using historical control data. The trial design included three groups: a roll-in group of 189 patients, a pivotal group of 480 patients, and a registry group of 78 patients with bilateral carotid stenoses who were treated by staged sequential CAS. Overall, 25.3% of patients were symptomatic. The 30-day composite MAE of all death, stroke, and MI in all 747 patients was 5.8% with no significant difference between the three subgroups. Although symptomatic patients had a higher 30-day stroke rate than asymptomatic patients (7.4% vs. 3.4%, $p = 0.038$), the 30-day composite MAE rates were not significantly different (7.9% vs. 5.0%). The 30-day MAE and mortality rates were higher for patients with medical comorbidities as opposed to anatomic criteria for high surgical risk. There were 34.2% of patients in the pivotal group who underwent procedures for restenosis after prior CEA, and this may have impacted on outcomes as restenotic lesions are generally believed to be more fibrotic and less prone to distal embolization during CAS. The 1-year end point of 30-day MAE plus ipsilateral stroke or neurological death from 31 days to 1 year was 8.9% for the pivotal group with a repeat revascularization rate of 4.7% *(40)*. Longer-term follow-up data have been presented but not published, with a 3-year ipsilateral stroke rate of 7.7%, up from 3.1% at 30 days. The pivotal group data have been submitted to the FDA and approval is currently pending.

CABERNET

The CABERNET (Carotid Artery Revascularization using the Boston Scientific EPI FilterWire EX/EZ and the EndoTex NexStent) trial enrolled 454 high-risk patients from 19 (15 US and 4 non-US) sites. Twenty-four percent of the patients were symptomatic and 20.7% of procedures were performed for restenosis after CEA. The 1- and 3-year data have been presented at TCT 2005 and TCT 2007, respectively. The study analyzed two primary end points. The first primary end point was the 30-day death, stroke, and MI rate, plus ipsilateral stroke from 31 days to 1 year. The composite rate for this end point (in 402 patients) was 4.5%, with a stroke rate of 4.0%. The second primary end point was all death, stroke and MI at 365 days, with a rate of 11.5%. The 30-day composite rate for death, stroke, and MI was 3.9% (death 0.5%, major stroke 1.3%, minor stroke 2.1%, and MI 0.2%). At 3 years, the major stroke rate remained low at 2.8% with an ipsilateral stroke rate of 4.9%. FDA approval for the NexStent/FilterWire platform was obtained in December 2006.

CREATE

The Carotid Revascularization With ev3 Arterial Technology Evolution (CREATE) trial was designed to evaluate the safety and efficacy of the ev3 Protégé carotid stent and the OTW SpiderFX filter protection system for CAS in high-risk patients *(41)*. There were 419 patients enrolled in 32 centers between April and October 2004. There were 7.4% symptomatic patients, and 24% of procedures were performed for restenosis after CEA. The primary composite end point of death, stroke, and MI at 30 days was seen in 6.2% (death 1.9%, all stroke 4.5%, and MI 1%). Multivariate analysis identified duration of filter deployment, symptomatic carotid stenosis, and baseline renal insufficiency as independent predictors of MAE. When the FDA approved the Guidant AccuLink^{TM}/AccuNet^{TM} system in August 2004, the study continued as CREATE 2, or the CREATE SpiderRX arm using the AccuLink^{TM} stent and the rapid-exchange version of the SPIDER filter. There were 160 high-risk patients enrolled and the 30-day composite end point was observed in 5.6% *(42)*. The Protégé stent/SpiderFX EPD system was approved by the FDA in January 2007 and patients are currently being enrolled in the CREATE Post Approval study. The SpiderRX device has received 510(k) clearance from the FDA for use in CAS.

MAVErIC

The MAVErIC (Medtronic Self-Expanding Carotid Stent System with Distal Protection in the Treatment of Carotid Artery Stenosis) trial evaluated the Medtronic Exponent® self-expanding stent and GuardWire® distal balloon occlusion protection device for use in CAS in high-risk patients. Ninety-nine patients from 16 centers were enrolled in MAVErIC 1 (feasibility phase) and 399 patients from 40 centers in MAVErIC 2 (pivotal trial). Twenty-two percent of the pivotal group was symptomatic and 34% were undergoing CAS for restenosis after CEA. The primary end point was the incidence of MAE (death, stroke, and MI) at 1 year. The pooled 30-day results for all 498 patients were presented in 2004, showing an MAE rate of 5.2% (death 1%, stroke 3.6%, and MI 1.8%). The 1-year clinical results from MAVErIC 1 were reported to be unchanged from the 30-day results at 5.1%. These data have not been published and the 1-year results from MAVErIC 2 have never been presented despite completing enrolment in 2003.

The MAVErIC 3 study plans to recruit 413 patients in the United States to evaluate safety and efficacy of the Medtronic Interceptor Plus Carotid Filter system with the Exponent® stent. These data are not available but the smaller MAVErIC International Study which evaluated this platform in 51 patients from 11 centers in Europe, Canada, and the Middle East *(43)* published MAE rates at 30 days of 5.9% (death 2%, stroke 3.9%, and MI 2%) and 11.8% at 1 year (death 3.9%, stroke 5.9%, and MI 5.9%).

MO.MA

The MO.MA registry enrolled 157 patients from 14 European centers from 2002 to 2003 evaluating the performance of the Mo.Ma device (Invatec), which prevents cerebral embolization by proximal endovascular blockage of blood flow with balloon occlusion of the common and external carotid arteries. This study differs slightly from the other registries described in this section in that it was not an IDE trial, was not restricted to a specific stent platform, and did not enroll exclusively high surgical risk patients. However, 75.2% of patients were high-risk and 19.7% symptomatic. Contralateral carotid occlusion was an exclusion criterion, as was severe ECA or proximal CCA disease. Proximal protection success was achieved in 96.8% of patients and in the remaining cases a distal filter was used. The mean duration of flow blockage was 7.6 ± 5.9 minutes and all patients were stented. The published 30-day death and stroke rate was 5.7% (death 0.6%, major stroke 0.6%, minor stroke 4.5%, with no MI) *(44)*.

PASCAL

The PASCAL (Performance and Safety of the Medtronic AVE Self-Expandable Stent in Treatment of Carotid Artery Lesions) study was a non-US multi-center registry of 115 high-risk patients undergoing CAS with the Medtronic Exponent® stent and any CE Mark-approved EPD. The 30-day MAE rate was reported to be 8% *(42)*, although these data remain unpublished.

PRIAMUS

The PRIAMUS study (Proximal Flow Blockage Cerebral Protection during Carotid Stenting) was another non-US trial evaluating the Mo.Ma (Invatec) proximal balloon occlusion EPD system in CAS for high-risk patients *(45)*. There were 416 patients recruited from four Italian centers between 2001 and 2005. There were 63.5% symptomatic patients and >95% had de novo lesions. Unlike the Mo.Ma study *(44)*, contralateral carotid occlusion was not an exclusion factor. The 30-day MAE rate of 4.56% (death 0.48%, major stroke 0.24%, minor stroke 3.84%, with no MI) was similar to other high-risk CAS registries.

SECURITY

The SECURITY trial (Registry Study to Evaluate the Emboshield™ Bare Wire Cerebral Protection System and Xact® Stent in Patients at High Risk for Carotid Endarterectomy) was an Abbott Vascular-sponsored study at 30 sites (29 in the United States and 1 in Australia). There were 305 patients enrolled in the pivotal group, of which 21% were symptomatic. Technical success was observed in 96.7%. The 30-day composite rate of death, stroke, and MI was 7.5% (death 0.98%, major stroke 2.62%, minor stroke 4.26%, and MI 0.66%). The primary end point of 30-day MAE plus ipsilateral stroke from 31 days to 1 year was seen in 8.5% of patients as compared with a weighted historical control of 14% for CEA *(46)*. The results were presented at TCT in 2003 but remain unpublished. Following submission of the data to the FDA, approval was granted in September 2005 making this the second stent/EPD platform approved for use in the United States.

TRIALS OF CAS VS. CEA

The registries of CAS with neuroprotection described above had 30-day MAE rates of between 3.9 and 8.3%, with 1-year rates of 4.5–9.6%. Although at first glance these rates appear relatively high, it should be noted that incidence of myocardial infarction were included along with stroke and death event-rates. These studies also enrolled a heterogenous mixture of symptomatic and asymptomatic patients.

Furthermore all had one or more medical or anatomic criteria for high surgical risk (which would have made them ineligible for NASCET or ACAS) and results were generally superior to the calculated historical comparator values of 14–14.5% for CEA in this population. However, the use of non-randomized data in making comparisons with CEA has been criticized. Evidence from trials directly comparing CAS with CEA are limited, and in some cases, of poor scientific quality. These studies are reviewed below.

The 'Stopped' Trial

The 'Stopped' trial as it has now come to be known was a single-center trial performed in Leicester in the United Kingdom *(27)*. The study was conducted as a prospective, consecutive, randomized trial of CAS vs. CEA for symptomatic severe carotid stenosis >70% and was intended to enroll up to 300 patients starting in 1996. However, the trial was suspended after only 23 patients had been randomized and only 17 patients had received their allocated treatment. This was due to an unacceptable complication rate in the angioplasty arm as five of the seven patients undergoing CAS had a stroke, three of which were disabling at 30 days. By contrast, the 10 CEA procedures performed were uneventful. When this trial commenced, CAS as a technique was still in its infancy and operator experience limited with little or no availability or understanding of the role of EPD. Due to issues of informed consent about peri-procedural risk, the trial could not be restarted even in an amended format. The single-center design and very small size of this early trial precluded any definitive conclusion as to the value of CAS as treatment for carotid stenosis.

CAVATAS

The Carotid and Vertebral Artery Transluminal Angioplasty Study (CAVATAS) was a randomized trial of carotid angioplasty vs. CEA performed at 22 centers in Europe, Canada, and Australia *(47)*. Enrolment took place between 1992 and 1997 but stents were only available after 1994. Ninety percent of patients had symptoms within 6 months of randomization and only 3% of patients were asymptomatic. Two hundred and forty-six patients underwent CEA and 240 underwent angioplasty. High surgical risk patients were excluded and only 26% of angioplasty patients received stents. No cerebral protection was used. The 30-day MAE rate of death plus any stroke was 9.9% in the CEA arm vs. 10% in the angioplasty arm, with comparable rates of death and disabling stroke (6%). At 3-year follow–up, the rate of death or disabling stroke was 14.3% for angioplasty vs. 14.2% for CEA, suggesting equivalence between the two techniques. However, this trial has been criticized due to a number of important limitations. No formal sample size calculations were ever performed and the 30-day MAE rates deemed to be unacceptably high in both arms, especially since high surgical risk patients were excluded. As stent use was infrequent with no cerebral protection, this study's relevance to current practice is limited.

The Wallstent Trial

The Wallstent study was another prematurely discontinued trial of CAS vs. CEA. Two hundred and nineteen patients with low-to-normal surgical risk and symptomatic carotid stenosis >60% were enrolled at multiple sites and randomized to CAS with the Wallstent® endoprosthesis (Boston Scientific) or CEA. EPD was not used. The primary end point of ipsilateral stroke, procedure-related death, or vascular death within 1 year was observed in 12.1% in the stent group vs. 3.6% for CEA ($p = 0.022$). The CAS group also had a higher rate of any stroke plus death at 30 days of 12.1% vs. 4.5% for CEA ($p = 0.049$). CAS was not felt to be equivalent to CEA in symptomatic patients with low-to-normal surgical risk and the trial was terminated prematurely before the planned maximum enrolment of 700 patients following a futility analysis. The study has only been published in abstract form *(48)* and like other early trials such as 'Stopped' and CAVATAS, the results have somewhat limited applicability to current clinical practice given the lack of availability of modern low-profile equipment and lack of EPD use.

Community (Kentucky) Trial

The Community (or Kentucky) trial as it is sometimes known was a single-center randomized comparison of CAS (without EPD) vs. CEA in a community hospital in both symptomatic and asymptomatic patients. In the first study of 104 symptomatic patients with carotid stenosis >70% (Community A), 53 patients were randomized to CAS with the Carotid Wallstent® (Boston Scientific) and 51 to CEA *(49)*. The proportion of high surgical risk patients was not stated but there were few exclusion criteria and the risk spectrum is likely to have been broad. Give the lack of EPD use, event rates were unusually low in both arms with one death in the CEA group and one transient ischemic attach (TIA) in the CAS group, with no strokes recorded. There was a trend toward earlier discharge in CAS patients (1.8 days vs. 2.7 days).

In the second study (Community B), 85 patients with asymptomatic carotid stenosis >80% were randomized to CAS or CEA *(50)*. Again, CAS technical success was 100% and event rates were extremely low with no procedure-related death or stroke in either arm. At 2 years, vessel patency rates were similar with no additional strokes, suggesting equivalence between CAS and CEA. These data have been interpreted with caution, however, given the small size of the trial and the almost complete absence of peri-procedural complications as compared with other studies.

CARESS

The multi-center, prospective, non-randomized CARESS (Carotid Revascularization Using Endarterectomy or Stenting Systems) phase I clinical trial was designed as an equivalence cohort study to determine whether stroke and death rate following CAS with EPD was comparable to CEA and to provide a reliable estimate of the 30-day end point of death plus stroke in the CEA arm for future power calculations for a larger phase II clinical trial *(51, 52)*. The trial was a collaboration between the International Society of Endovascular Specialists, the FDA, the Centers for Medicare and Medicaid Services (CMS), the National Institute of Health (NIH), and industry representatives and performed at 14 centers in the United States. Treatment choice was based on patient and physician preference with a planned enrolment ratio of CEA:CAS of 2:1. Two hundred and fifty-four patients underwent CEA and 143 patients underwent CAS using the monorail Wallstent® (Boston Scientific) and GuardWire Plus EPD (Medtronic). Approximately 85% of patients were high surgical risk and 32% of patients were symptomatic. There was no significant difference in baseline patient characteristics except for a more frequent history of prior carotid revascularization in the CAS group. Kaplan–Meier analysis revealed no significant differences in combined death/stroke rates at 30 days (3.6%

CEA vs. 2.1% CAS) or at 1 year (13.6% CEA vs. 10.0% CAS). Similarly, there was no significant difference in the alternative composite end point of death, stroke, or MI at 30 days (4.4% CEA vs. 2.1% CAS) or 1 year (14.3% CEA vs. 10.9% CAS). The secondary end points of residual stenosis, restenosis, carotid revascularization, or change in quality of life were also not statistically different between the two treatment arms. The composite 1-year event rates were comparable to the rates observed in the ARCHeR, MAVErIC, and CABERNET registries but higher than the stroke rates in NASCET and ACAS, likely reflecting the inclusion of patients with higher surgical risk. The event rates for symptomatic and asymptomatic patients were not reported separately, although a Cox proportional hazards regression did not identify symptomatology as a predictor of MAE. The study concluded that the 30-day and 1-year risk of death, stroke, and MI for CAS with EPD was equivalent to that for CEA in symptomatic and asymptomatic patients with carotid stenosis. Although the trial design has been criticized for the lack of treatment randomization, it has been argued that the study was reflective of broad clinical practice and that the data obtained has paved the way for a larger phase II randomized clinical trial, allowing participation by multiple device manufacturers.

SAPPHIRE

The SAPPHIRE (Stenting and Angioplasty with Protection in Patients at High Risk for Endarterectomy) trial was the first randomized comparison of contemporary CAS with cerebral protection against CEA *(53)*. High-risk patients with symptomatic carotid stenosis >50% or asymptomatic carotid stenosis >80% were recruited from 29 sites in the United States and following review by a local multidisciplinary team consisting of a neurologist, vascular surgeon, and interventionalist were randomized to CAS or CEA. Patients felt to be too high-risk for CEA could be entered into a high-risk CAS registry and patients felt to be unsuitable for CAS could be entered into a high-risk surgical registry. There were 747 patients enrolled, of whom 334 were randomized in the pivotal trial. Three hundred and seven patients underwent their allotted treatment (156 had CAS and 151 had CEA). Four hundred and six patients were entered into the stent registry and seven patients into the surgical registry. In the randomized group, 29.9% of patients undergoing CAS were symptomatic as were 27.7% of CEA patients, and >20% of patients in each arm were undergoing procedures for restenosis.

CAS was performed using the Smart™ or Precise™ nitinol self-expanding stent and AngioGuard™ filter EPD (Cordis Corporation, Johnson & Johnson). The primary end point was a composite of death, stroke, and MI at 30 days plus death or ipsilateral stroke between 30 days and 1 year. Secondary end points included TLR at 1 year, cranial nerve palsy, and access site or wound complications. AngioGuard™ deployment was technically successful in 95.6% of patients in the randomized trial and 91.6% of patients in the CAS registry. In early 2002, enrolment slowed due to the establishment of several of the non-randomized high-risk CAS registries listed previously. The trial was terminated after an interim analysis established that conditions for non-inferiority was met, which was the prespecified design of this trial. On an intention-to-treat basis, the primary end point was seen in 12.2% of CAS patients vs. 20.1% of CEA patients ($p = 0.048$) as shown in Fig. 1.

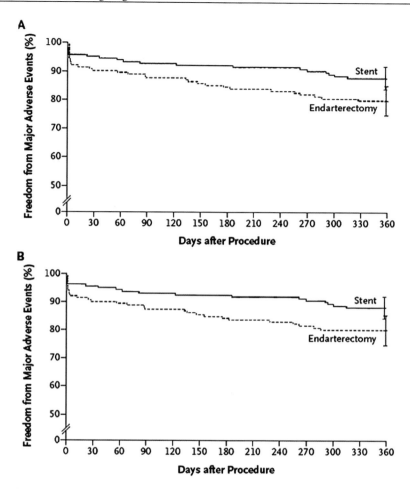

Fig. 1. Freedom from MAE at 1 year in the SAPPHIRE trial. In the intention-to-treat analysis (**Panel A**), the rate of event-free survival at 1 year was 87.8% among patients randomly assigned to carotid stenting, as compared with 79.9% among those randomly assigned to endarterectomy ($p = 0.053$). In the actual-treatment analysis (**Panel B**), the rate of event-free survival at 1 year was 88.0% among patients who received a stent, as compared with 79.9% among those who underwent endarterectomy ($p = 0.048$). I bars represent 1.5 times the SE. (*Reproduced with permission from (53)*).

This was highly significant for non-inferiority of CAS to CEA ($p = 0.004$) but not for superiority ($p = 0.053$). However, if a more conventional end point excluding the cumulative 30-day rate of MI was used, the difference between CAS (5.5%) and CEA (8.4%) was non-significant. The 30-day rates of death, stroke, and MI (on an actual-treatment analysis) were 4.4% for CAS and 9.9% for CEA ($p = 0.06$). For patients with symptomatic carotid stenosis, the primary end point was seen in 16.8% of patients undergoing CAS vs. 16.5% in those undergoing CEA ($p = $ NS), with a 30-day MAE rate of 2.1% for CAS and 9.3% for CEA. For asymptomatic patients, the primary end point and 30-day MAE rates were seen in 9.9 and 5.4% of CAS patients, respectively, vs. 21.5% and 10.2% of CEA patients. The 1-year TLR rates were lower in the CAS group (0.6% vs. 4.3%, $p = 0.04$) as was the incidence of cranial nerve palsy (0% vs. 5.3%, $p = 0.003$). In the high-risk CAS registry of

406 patients, the 30-day MAE rate was 7.8%. In the high-risk CEA registry of seven patients, one patient had a peri-operative MI resulting in a 30-day MAE rate of 14.3%.

Although the SAPPHIRE study is widely accepted as a landmark clinical trial, it has nevertheless attracted a number of criticisms *(54, 55)*. First, over 60% of the 747 patients enrolled were deemed to be too high-risk for CEA based on the reviewing surgeons' opinion and were thus entered into the CAS registry. It has been suggested that this reflected badly on the standard of surgical practice and that lack of a protocol-based exclusion system created a significant bias. The SAPPHIRE authors note, however, that the participating surgeons were more experienced than the US average with a median volume of 30 CEA cases per year and that the incidence of cranial nerve injury was lower than that in NASCET (5.3% vs. 7.6%) where high-risk patients were excluded, attesting to the technical ability of the surgeons in the trial. There has also been widespread discussion of the fact that the difference in the composite end point between the two groups at 1 year was related largely to the greater association of CEA with peri-operative non-Q wave MI. Certainly without inclusion of MI in the end point, no statistical difference would have been observed, although this is defended on the grounds that there is a higher rate of cardiac complications in this patient population with corresponding morbidity and mortality and that exclusion of these events is inappropriate. Additional concerns relate to the high proportion (over a fifth) of patients who had undergone prior ipsilateral carotid revascularization, potentially creating an unfair bias in favor of CAS due to the higher surgical risk in these patients and reduced likelihood of distal embolization during CAS. The early termination of the trial also resulted in a smaller than anticipated sample size, affecting the power of the study to make conclusions about the relative safety and efficacy of CAS vs. CEA. Finally, only 28–29% of patients were symptomatic. Prior studies of CEA vs. medical therapy for asymptomatic carotid stenosis suggest that the natural history of risk of stroke in these patients may not justify either CAS or CEA and that the failure to include a medical therapy arm in a high surgical risk population was a serious flaw. These criticisms also apply to the high-risk CAS registries listed in the previous section, where the majority of patients had asymptomatic carotid stenoses. Nevertheless the results of the study established CAS as a valid alternative to CEA in high-risk patients leading to FDA approval of CAS for this indication.

The long-term 3-year outcomes were recently published, showing no difference in the secondary endpoints (30 day death, stroke, MI or death/stroke from 31 days to 1080 days) between both groups (24.6% CAS vs. 26.9% CEA) *(55b)*. Thus, in summary, SAPPHIRE was a well-conducted randomized comparison between contemporary CAS with EPD versus CEA in high-risk patients, performed by experienced surgeons and interventionalists, coupled with rigorous neurological evaluations throughout the trial. Data from this study supports CAS as an alternative to CEA in high-risk patients, and arguably should be the preferred revascularization strategy in these patients, provided the arch and carotid anatomy is not prohibitive.

EVA-3S

The Endarterectomy Versus Stenting in Patients with Symptomatic Severe Carotid Stenosis (EVA-3S) study was a publicly funded randomized non-inferiority trial comparing stenting with endarterectomy in low-to-normal surgical risk patients with symptomatic carotid stenosis $\geq$60% *(56)*. The trial was performed at 20 academic and 10 non-academic centers in France and it was originally intended to enroll 872 patients. This would have allowed an 80% power to determine whether CAS was inferior to CEA, assuming a 2% non-inferiority margin and 30-day incidence of stroke or death (the primary endpoint) of 5.6% after CEA and 4% after CAS. Eligibility requirements were that vascular surgeons had to have performed at least 25 CEA in the preceding year and that the interventional physician had performed at least 12 lifetime CAS procedures or 35 stenting procedures in the supra-aortic trunks, of which at least 5 were in the carotid artery. Centers without the required interventional experience could still participate provided CAS procedures were proctored by a clinician who did meet the credentialing requirements.

The trial commenced in November 2000 and initially there was no requirement for mandatory EPD use. After January 2003, CAS procedures without EPD use were no longer permitted *(57)*. At this stage 73 patients had undergone completed CAS procedures. Fifty eight patients (79.5%) had an EPD and 15 (20.5%) did not. The adjusted odds ratio (OR) for the 30-day rate of any stroke or death for CAS without EPD (26.7%) vs. CAS with EPD (10.3%) was 2.5 (95% CI, 0.6–10.8). A similar pattern was observed for 30-day death or disabling stroke (13.3% vs. 3.4%, OR 3.8 with 95% CI, 0.5–31.6). Although the limits of the confidence intervals were compatible with no significant difference, due to the threefold difference in event-rates the safety committee recommended that EPD be used routinely in all subsequent CAS procedures. This decision was criticized by some because the trial was not designed to compare CAS safety with and without EPD use, and the numbers involved were small at the time. As stated the difference was not statistically significant and the patients who underwent CAS without EPD use were also older than patients in whom EPD was used (72.7 years vs. 66 years, $p = 0.013$). Furthermore, a number of patients treated without protection developed their stroke not during their procedure but during the first 30 days, and arguably EPD use would not have prevented these events.

In September 2005, after enrolment of 527 patients, the trial was stopped prematurely on the basis of both safety and futility. The 30-day incidence of any stroke or death was 3.9% (95% CI, 2.0–7.2%) after CEA and 9.6% (95% CI, 6.4–14%) after CAS with a relative risk of 2.5 (95% CI, 1.2–5.1). The absolute risk increase was 5.7% and the 95% CI of 2.1–9.3% did not include the 2% limit used to define non-inferiority. The 30-day risk of disabling stroke or death was 1.5% (95% CI, 0.5–4.2%) after CEA and 3.4% after CAS (95% CI, 1.7–6.7%). At 6 months the incidence of any stroke or death was 6.1% after CEA and 11.7% after CAS ($p = 0.02$). There were more systemic complications after endarterectomy and more local access site problems after stenting but these differences were not significant. Cranial nerve injury was more common after CEA (7.7% vs. 1.1%, $p < 0.001$). The trialists concluded that in symptomatic patients with carotid stenosis $\geq$60%, the rates of death and stroke at 1 and 6 months were lower with endarterectomy than with stenting.

Since its publication in 2006 the EVA-3S trial has attracted strong criticism from the interventional community for its perceived limitations. In large part this has focused on the relatively limited experience and credentialing required of the operators (i.e. possibly as little as 5 lifetime CAS procedures) and the fact that two-thirds of sites were initially under tutelage. It is recognized that there is a steep learning curve for CAS *(58, 59)* and this may have biased the results in favor of CEA. The authors point out that the relative risk of stroke or death did not differ significantly among the centers that enrolled fewer than 21 patients vs. those that enrolled more than 40 patients, although this was a narrow spectrum of interventional experience. Similarly, while there was no difference in complication rates between "experienced" interventionalists and those who were tutored during or after training, actual lifetime numbers of the experienced physicians was not specified. The study was also criticized for the fact that the stroke rate in the CAS arm (9.2%) was significantly higher than that in SAPPHIRE (3.6%) although the majority of patients in SAPPHIRE were asymptomatic and thus less likely to have peri-procedural events. In EVA-3S all patients were symptomatic and 45% underwent revascularization within 4 weeks of their qualifying events, resulting in a population at higher risk for stroke. Conversely, patients in SAPPHIRE were all high surgical risk resulting in higher complication rates after CEA but not necessarily to the same extent after CAS. This is supported by the low peri-procedural incidence of MI after CEA of 0.8% in EVA-3S, as compared with SAPPHIRE. The non-uniform use of EPD in the initial stages of the trial has already been discussed, although the interpretation is not straightforward given that technical failure and complications related to EPD use are also related to lack of experience as shown in over 11,000 CAS procedures in the Global Carotid Stent Registry *(34)*.

Another concern raised over the EVA-3S results was that only 85% of CAS patients were on dual anti-platelet therapy post-procedure. The authors comment that the primary end point did not differ significantly between patients who received dual anti-platelet therapy and patients on monotherapy (9% vs. 11.1%), although again the study was not powered to evaluate this. However, a valid point is that this figure may reflect real-world practice and that 100% compliance with dual anti-platelet therapy may not be realistic outside clinical trials. The EVA-3S results were published only 1 week after another study comparing CAS vs. CEA in normal surgical risk patients with symptomatic carotid stenosis – the SPACE trial.

SPACE

The Stent-Supported Percutaneous Angioplasty of the Carotid Artery versus Endarterectomy (SPACE) study was a randomized multi-center trial which aimed to test the hypothesis that CAS was not inferior to CEA for the treatment of severe symptomatic carotid stenosis *(60)*. Patients were eligible if they had a neurological or ocular event within the previous 6 months with an ipsilateral carotid stenosis on ultrasound ($\geq$70%) or angiography ($\geq$50% by NASCET or $\geq$70% by ECST criteria). Patients with restenosis following prior carotid revascularization were excluded. The primary end point was ipsilateral stroke or death between randomization and 30 days after treatment. Secondary 30-day end points included (i) disabling ipsilateral stroke, (ii) any stroke, and (iii) procedural failure. Vascular surgeons were required to have performed 25 consecutive successful carotid endarterectomies, and interventionalists had to show proof of 25 successful percutaneous angioplasties, although these need not be carotid procedures. The null hypothesis was that the difference between the event rates in the CAS group and the CEA group would be 2.5% or more (the non-inferiority margin).

The study was performed in 35 centers in Germany, Austria, and Switzerland between March 2001 and February 2006. By this stage 1,200 patients had been randomized and a pre-specified interim analysis performed. As 17 patients withdrew consent, data from 1,183 patients were available. Fourteen patients allocated to CAS were treated with CEA (crossover rate 2.3%) and 6 patients from the CEA

Table 3
30-Day Outcomes after Treatment in the SPACE Trial

	CAS (n = 599) (%)	CEA (n = 584) (%)	Odds Ratio: CAS/CEA (95% CI)
Primary end point	6.84	6.34	1.09 (0.69–1.72)
Ipsilateral ischemic stroke	6.51	5.14	1.26 (0.77–2.18)[†]
Ipsilateral intracerebral bleeding	0.17	0.86	0.19 (0.004–1.74)[†]
Death	0.67	0.86	0.78 (0.15–3.64)[†]
Secondary end points			
Disabling ipsilateral stroke or death	4.67	3.77	1.25 (0.71–2.22)
Disabling ipsilateral stroke	4.01	2.91	1.39 (0.74–2.62)
Any stroke	7.51	6.16	1.24 (0.79–1.95)
Any stroke or death	7.68	6.51	1.19 (0.75–1.92)
Procedural failure	3.17	2.05	1.56 (0.71–3.56)[†]

[*]CI on differences of two binomial proportions based on the standardized statistic and inverting two 1-sided tests.
[†]Exact CI. Adapted from *(60)*.
Disabling stroke was defined as a score of 3 or more on the modified Rankin scale. CAS, carotid artery stenting; CEA, carotid endarterectomy.

group were treated with CAS (crossover rate 1%). Eighteen patients in the CAS group and 12 patients in the CEA group were not treated but all were included in an intention-to-treat analysis. EPD were used in only 27% of patients. The 30-day rate of death or ipsilateral stroke was 6.84% with CAS and 6.34% with CEA. On the basis of a non-inferiority analysis and problems with funding, the trial was stopped prematurely. The primary and secondary end point data are shown in Table 3.

The absolute difference between CAS and CEA was 0.51% (90% CI −1.89 to 2.91%). The authors' rationale for the use of 90% confidence intervals was the one-sided 5% significance level chosen for the sample size calculations. Although the one-sided *p*-value for non-inferiority was 0.09, as the upper 90% confidence interval of 2.91% was greater than the pre-specified equivalence threshold of 2.5% the authors concluded that the null hypothesis could not be rejected and that the trial failed to prove non-inferiority of CAS to CEA. Not surprisingly, the SPACE trial has been strongly criticized for its confusing statistical design and interpretation of the data, as well as for limitations related to technical issues and clinical end points. These are set out below.

Study Design and Power: The non-inferiority design of the SPACE trial meant that a sample size of 1,900 was required based upon an expected 30-day event-rate (death or stroke) of 5%, using 80% power, a one-sided alpha of 5%, and a non-inferiority margin of 2.5%. However, after inclusion of only 1,200 patients the trial was stopped prematurely, as the very small difference between the groups meant a much larger number of patients needed to be enrolled (~2,500) and also due to lack of funding. Re-calculation using the actual event-rate confirmed that it was tremendously underpowered to test its null hypothesis (conditional power of only 52%). The 90% confidence interval of −1.89 to 2.91 for the absolute difference of 0.51% between CAS and CEA also crosses zero suggesting the difference is non-significant or uncertain. Furthermore, the authors did not specify their rationale for the assumption of a 5% event-rate, and as the actual event-rate was 6.6% the predetermined absolute non-inferiority margin of 2.5% used may have been too restrictive.

Technical Issues: As with EVA-3S, the low use of EPD was also criticized. Although no dedicated randomized controlled trial of CAS with or without EPD has been performed, non-randomized registry data strongly suggest lower stroke event-rates with cerebral protection *(34, 61)*. Although this contention is not universal, many interventionalists believe that the use of an EPD is indispensable with contemporary CAS and that most experienced interventionalists can deploy an EPD safely with minimal extra time. The rate of EPD use of only 27% in SPACE could alone explain the higher 30-day death or stroke event-rate with CAS over CEA. The SPACE authors did not specify if there were criteria that mandated the use of EPD during CAS, and although a comparison of event-rates between those who received EPD vs. no EPD during CAS was provided (event-rate 7% in both groups), this was not a pre-specified analysis, and was not adjusted (e.g., EPD use may have been reserved for higher risk characteristics). In an echo of the criticisms of EVA-3S, the technical experience of the interventionalists in SPACE has been called into question, as the average carotid stent experience of these operators was not stated. Although proof of at least 25 successful consecutive percutaneous angioplasties was required, these did not have to be carotid stent procedures, and thus the credentialing requirements appear inappropriate. Likewise, many carotid interventionalists who do not use EPD routinely are often less experienced, particularly with the use of such devices, raising the possibility that the infrequent use of EPD in this study was also partially due to inexperienced operators. By comparison, the CREST trial required that interventionalists have at least 30 prior carotid stent procedures, and go through at least 3 lead-in CAS cases prior to enrolling patients into the randomized phase.

Clinical Endpoints: Although the primary end point (death or stroke) used in this study was relevant and comparable to prior CEA studies, data on peri-procedural MI, cranial nerve palsy, and wound complications were not collected. While the issue is controversial, it could nonetheless be argued that these are appropriate secondary safety end points, which should be evaluated in a non-inferiority study, and that failure to do so may have undermined the potential benefits of CAS in comparison to the "gold-standard" of CEA.

Criticisms and justifications notwithstanding, the results of the EVA-3S and SPACE trials have to some extent reduced the swing of the pendulum from CEA toward CAS created by the SAPPHIRE study. Certainly CAS has not yet been shown to be superior or even equivalent to CEA for low-surgical risk patients. The limitations of these trials, however, have prevented their conclusions from being accepted by the majority of the interventional community and the consensus is that further clarification is required from currently ongoing trials such as CREST, ACT-1, ICSS (CAVATAS-2) ACST-2, and TACIT. Although these results are awaited, a number of meta-analyses on the available trial data have been performed.

Meta-analyses of CAS vs. CEA Trial Data

A Cochrane systematic review of randomized trials comparing CAS with CEA included five studies – the 'Stopped', Wallstent, CAVATAS, Community (A and B), and SAPPHIRE trials – from 1998 to 2004, with a total of 1,269 patients, 75% of which were symptomatic *(62)*. Analysis of 30-day safety data found no significant difference in the odds ratio of treatment-related death or any stroke (OR 1.33, 95% CI 0.86–2.04), death or disabling stroke, death, any stroke, or MI for CAS as compared with CEA, although there was a trend toward higher event rates with CAS. At 1 year, there was no difference between the two treatments in the rate of death or any stroke (OR 1.01, 95% CI 0.71–1.44). Endovascular treatment also significantly reduced the risk of cranial nerve injury. However, there was marked heterogeneity in trial methodology with limited use of stents in CAVATAS and non-routine use of EPD in four out of five of the studies. In addition, patient inclusion was different between the trials with varying proportions of symptomatic and high surgical risk patients. Consequently the authors concluded that while the data suggested that event rates between CAS and CEA were comparable, the wide confidence intervals meant that it was not possible to confidently exclude a difference in favor of one treatment.

A more recent meta-analysis by Gurm et al evaluated safety of CAS for patients with symptomatic carotid stenosis *(63)*. Five studies with 2,122 patients were analyzed, including the Wallstent, Community A, SAPPHIRE (symptomatic patient data extracted), and the recently published EVA-3S and SPACE trials, and summary risk ratios (RRs) calculated. There was no significant difference in risk of 30-day mortality (RR 0.57, 95% CI 0.22–1.47), stroke (RR 1.64, 95% CI 0.67–4.00), disabling stroke (RR 1.67, 95% CI 0.50–5.62), death and stroke (RR 1.54, 95% CI 0.81–2.92), or death and disabling stroke (RR 1.19, 95% CI 0.57–2.51) among patients randomized to CAS as compared to CEA. A restriction of the analysis to only the SAPPHIRE, EVA-3S, and SPACE trials resulted in the same conclusion. There was a trend toward lower mortality with CAS, but a lower stroke rate with CEA, although again confidence intervals were wide due to differences in patient selection and trial methodology.

Another review assessing short-term outcomes for protected carotid angioplasty with stents included 26 studies published between 2002 and 2004, with 2,992 patients treated *(64)*. Fifty-six percent of patients were symptomatic. The pooled peri-procedural rate of any stroke at 30 days was 2.4% ± 0.3% (95% CI). The 30-day major stroke rate was 0.6% ± 0.2% (95% CI) with a 30-day minor stroke rate of 1.1% ± 0.2% (95% CI). Although the majority of these studies were not randomized comparisons of CAS with CEA, but case series with heterogeneity of patient selection, devices, and adjuvant medical therapy, the 30-day stroke rates were low and within the limits specified by the AHA guidelines.

POST-MARKET SURVEILLANCE (PMS) REGISTRIES

While there can be no doubt that randomized controlled trials produce the highest quality scientific and clinical data, there have been relatively few such studies evaluating protected CAS and these have had a number of limitations as discussed above. While several studies are ongoing, these results may not be available for some years. However, as a condition of device approvals, the FDA mandated that the device experience be monitored outside of the clinical trial setting post-approval. These registries can be rich sources of important 'real-world' data on CAS given that the number of patients in various PMS registries is over 10,000 patients. A number of these studies are ongoing and three (CAPTURE, CASES-PMS, and EXACT) have been presented or published. These are reviewed below.

CAPTURE

Following FDA approval of the RX AccuLink™ stent/RX AccuNet™ EPD system (Guidant Corporation, now Abbott Vascular) in 2004 on the basis of data from the ARCHeR studies, the CAPTURE (Carotid RX AccuLink™/AccuNet™ Post-Approval Trial to Uncover Unanticipated or Rare Events) PMS study was setup. This was designed to assess (i) the safety of CAS by physicians with varying levels of experience as a measure of the adequacy of physician training and (ii) the identification of rare or unexpected device-related complications. Three hundred and fifty-three physicians at 144 sites participated. Interventional physicians were placed in three groups according to their level of experience, although as a minimum requirement had to have performed at least 25 selective carotid angiograms, 10 peripheral procedures with self-expanding stents, and 10 procedures with 0.014″ systems. All interventionalists underwent mandatory manufacturer-conducted hands-on training and less experienced physicians underwent a structured 2-day carotid training program including didactic and simulator-based training. Data from the first 3,500 patients enrolled between October 2004 and March 2006 have now been published *(65)*. Although no explicit inclusion/exclusion criteria were specified, selection based on device indications was encouraged, i.e., high surgical risk patients with symptomatic (>50%) or asymptomatic (>80%) carotid stenosis. Approximately 14% of patients were symptomatic and 23.7% were ≥80 years of age.

The primary end point (a composite of death, stroke and MI at 30 days) was seen in 6.3% (95% CI 5.5–7.1%) and did not differ significantly among the three operator experience levels (5.3, 6.0, and 7.4% from most to least experienced) when adjusted for case mix. The primary end point event rate was 12% in symptomatic patients and 5.4% in asymptomatic patients, higher than recommended by AHA guidelines but the majority of patients were high surgical risk. Preliminary data for the CAPTURE-2 PMS study which began enrolling at 195 sites in March 2006 was presented at ACC 2007. In 597 patients (of which 11.1% were symptomatic), the 30-day rate of death or any stroke was 5.2% overall with a rate of 9.1% in symptomatic patients and 4.7% in asymptomatic patients *(66)*. Up to 10,000 patients may be enrolled in this registry.

CASES-PMS

Although the SAPPHIRE trial provided evidence for the effectiveness of CAS with distal embolic protection using the Precise™ stent and AngioGuard™ filter (Cordis, Johnson & Johnson) in high-risk patients, it was not known if similar outcomes could be achieved by physicians expert in endovascular procedures but possessing a wide range of experience in CAS or in use of the AngioGuard™ EPD. To address these questions the CAS with Embolic Protection Surveillance – Post Marketing Study (CASES-PMS) was initiated *(67)*. There were 1,493 high-risk patients (21.8% symptomatic) enrolled at 73 sites from August 2003 to October 2005. As in the CAPTURE study, all physicians underwent additional education in up to five training modules depending on their level of experience.

The primary end point of death, stroke, or MI at 30 days was 5.0%, which compared favorably to the 6.3% rate obtained from the stent cohort in the SAPPHIRE trial. Symptomatic patients had a composite event-rate of 6.2% and the asymptomatic patients an event rate of 4.7%. Technical success with the AngioGuard™ device was

98%. As with CAPTURE, the CASES-PMS study also concluded that with a comprehensive training program, CAS could be performed in the community setting with safety and efficacy similar to that achieved in the original device-approval studies.

EXACT

The Emboshield™ and Xact® Post Approval Carotid Stent Trial (EXACT) studied post-marketing data on 1,500 high-risk patients (9.9% were symptomatic) enrolled from 128 sites who underwent CAS with the Xact® stent and Emboshield™ EPD (Abbott Vascular) following completion of the pivotal SECURITY trial. The 30-day results were presented at ACC 2007. The composite end point of death, stroke, and MI occurred in 4.6% – an improvement on the 7.5% reported in the SECURITY trial, although the patients in SECURITY were older and a larger proportion (21%) were symptomatic. Results for both symptomatic and asymptomatic patients are shown in Table 4. Unlike CAPTURE and CASES-PMS, however, a significant difference in the 30-day death and stroke rate was seen between the most experienced (Level 1) operators (3.2%) and the least experienced (Level 3) operators (8.8%).

As demographic and methodological differences exist between the original IDE studies (ARCHeR, SAPPHIRE, and SECURITY) and their corresponding PMS registries (CAPTURE, CASES, and EXACT), statistical comparisons between the study outcomes cannot be made directly. Nevertheless the data do indicate that with appropriate training, CAS can be performed in the community setting with complication rates that appear to be declining over time and are at least comparable if not better than the original pivotal studies (Tables 2 and 4). Ongoing PMS studies include CAPTURE-2, CHOICE, and PROTECT (Abbott Vascular), SAPPHIRE WW (Cordis, Johnson & Johnson), CREATE PAS (ev3), and SONOMA (Boston Scientific). If enrollment targets are achieved, these studies will recruit up to 28,000 patients undergoing CAS *(42)*.

Table 4
30-Day Outcomes from PMS Registries

	CAPTURE (%)	CAPTURE-2 (%)	CASES (%)	EXACT (%)
Death, stroke, and MI	6.3	–	5	4.6
Death and any stroke				
All patients	5.7	5.2	–	4.5
Symptomatic patients	10.6	9.1	–	8.6
Asymptomatic patients	4.9	4.7	–	4.0
Death and disabling stroke				
All patients	2.9	1.3	–	1.8
Symptomatic patients	–	1.5	–	2.9
Asymptomatic patients	–	1.3	–	1.7

ONGOING TRIALS OF CAS VS. CEA

CREST

The Carotid Revascularization Endarterectomy versus Stent Trial (CREST) is currently the largest randomized clinical trial (RCT) comparing CAS to CEA.

Sponsored by the US National Institute of Neurological Disorders (NINDS)/ National Institute of Health (NIH) with assistance from Abbott Vascular, the trial spent several years in the planning and development stage before enrollment of the first patient in December 2000 *(68, 69)*. After a mandatory lead-in phase for operators and centers to meet start-up and credentialing requirements, a total of 2,500 patients will be recruited in the United States and Canada. Patients at high risk for either CEA or CAS will be ineligible, unlike the SAPPHIRE trial and most of the device-approval registries. It was originally intended to enroll only symptomatic patients with carotid stenosis ($\geq$50% on angiography or $\geq$70% by ultrasound or CT/ MRA), but in 2004 the trial was expanded to include asymptomatic patients (carotid stenosis $\geq$60% by angiography or $\geq$70% by ultrasound or $\geq$80% by CT/MRA) *(70)*. This was done in order to (i) improve the rate of enrollment which was initially slow and (ii) widen generalizability of the results following the favorable results of the Asymptomatic Carotid Surgery Trial (ACST) published earlier that year *(7)*. Inclusion and exclusion criteria are otherwise similar to those in the cardinal CEA trials – NASCET and ACAS – as well as the recent EVA-3S and SPACE trials. The investigational devices used in the CAS arm of the study are the RX AccuLink™ stent and RX AccuNet™ EPD (Abbott Vascular) and the primary end point is the composite of death, stroke, and MI at 30 days, plus ipsilateral stroke in the follow-up period.

All participating interventionalists are required to undergo a rigorous credentialing process with a minimum of 30 lifetime procedures (with up to 20 cases using the AccuLink™/AccuNet™ system) and are approved only after careful case review by a multidisciplinary interventionalist panel. As of August 1, 2007, 1,549 patients had been enrolled in the lead-in phase of the trial, a measure of the scrutiny applied. Results from the first 749 patients treated with CAS in the lead-in phase of CREST have been published *(71)*. The 30-day stroke and death rate overall was 4.41% but for octogenarians this rose to 12.1%, while the corresponding rate for patients <80 years of age was 3.23%. The higher complication rate in this elderly population was not mitigated by adjustment for symptomatic status, use of EPD, gender, stenosis severity, or the presence of distal arterial tortuosity. Although the number of octogenarians involved was small (99 patients) and this was a lead-in phase of the study, similar findings have been reported by other studies *(72, 73)*. The German ALKK registry found no excess complication rate in octogenarians although increasing age (as a continuous variable) was a predictor of in-hospital death or stroke *(74)*. Other studies have reported no significant increase in complications with elderly patients *(75, 76)*, although until further data are available, caution should be exercised before recommending CAS in patients over 80 years of age, especially if asymptomatic.

Within the CREST study proper, a total of 113 centers (106 in the United States and 7 in Canada) were approved with 1,925 patients (1,056 symptomatic, 869 asymptomatic) enrolled as of 1 August 2007 *(77)*. And as of July 10, 2008, the study had completed enrolment of 2,516 patients into the main study, and results are anticipated in the near future.

ICSS/CAVATAS-2

The International Carotid Stenting Study (ICSS or CAVATAS-2) is an academic international multi-center RCT coordinated by the Institute of Neurology in London, UK. It plans to randomize 1,500 patients with symptomatic carotid stenosis >50% (by NASCET criteria) who are suitable for both CAS and CEA in a 1:1 fashion *(78)*. The primary outcome will be long-term survival free of disabling stroke. Secondary outcome measures will be any stroke, death, or MI at 30 days, treatment-related cranial nerve palsy or hematoma, or restenosis $\geq 70\%$ on ultrasound, stroke, or TIA during follow-up. The coordinators of the EVA-3S, SPACE, and ICSS trials have announced their intention to analyze the pooled data from these trials when ICSS is complete. As of July 31, 2007, 1,298 patients had been enrolled and recruitment is expected to reach target in the first half of 2008.

ACT-1

The Asymptomatic Carotid Stenosis Stenting versus Endarterectomy Trial (ACT-1) is an Abbott Vascular-sponsored Phase III multi-center trial of CAS vs. CEA in asymptomatic patients *(79)*. The devices used in the CAS arm will be the Xact stent and Emboshield Pro EPD (Abbott Vascular). The study started in April 2005 and plans to randomize 1,658 patients in North America to CAS or CEA on a 3:1 basis. Patients over 80 years old or at high risk for CAS or CEA are excluded. The primary outcome measures are the composite occurrence of death, stroke, or MI at 30 days, and ipsilateral stroke between 31 days and 1 year.

ACST-2

The 5-year results of the Asymptomatic Carotid Surgery Trial (ACST-1) published in 2004 showed a reduced stroke and peri-operative death rate of 6.42% in asymptomatic patients with severe carotid stenosis treated with early CEA, as compared to 11.78% in patients who had CEA deferred ($p = 0.00001$) *(7)*. Following on from this, the ACST-2 trial plans to randomize 5,000 asymptomatic low-risk patients with carotid stenosis 1:1 to CAS or CEA *(80)*. The trial is jointly funded by the UK Health Technology Assessment program with assistance from the BUPA foundation. The primary end points will be (i) the 30-day composite rate of death, stroke and MI; and (ii) long-term freedom from stroke up to 5 or more years. Enrollment started in July 2007.

TACIT

The Transatlantic Asymptomatic Carotid Intervention Trial is a Phase III multi-center RCT designed to determine the optimal therapy for patients with asymptomatic carotid stenosis $\geq 60\%$ *(81)*. Due to advances in medical therapy since ACAS and ACST, concerns have been voiced that carotid revascularization in asymptomatic patients may no longer be appropriate. TACIT will therefore randomize patients to not only CAS and CEA but also best medical therapy (BMT) in an approximate 1:1:1 fashion. The study is organized by the Society of Interventional Radiology Foundation, C-operative Alliance for Interventional Radiology Research (CAIRR), and the Cardiovascular and Interventional Radiology Society of Europe, with industry sponsorship anticipated. They plan to enroll 3,700 patients from a minimum of 100 sites in the United States and Europe and evaluate peri-procedural death and stroke outcomes out to 5 years.

CONCLUSION

In summary, considerable advances have been made in the development of CAS as a treatment for atherosclerotic carotid stenosis. Increased operator experience and training have been coupled with improvements in technique and design of dedicated low-profile equipment, and the use of cerebral protection is becoming widespread. As a rival to CEA, the evidence in favor of CAS is most robust and established in high surgical risk patients. While results from large registries have reported acceptable outcomes for CAS, initial randomized trial data (although fraught with limitations) were disappointing for low-risk patients. Results from ongoing better-designed and rigorous large randomized trials are anticipated to address the utility of CAS in standard and low-risk patients.

REFERENCES

1. Eastcott H, Pickering G, Rob C. Reconstruction of internal carotid artery in a patient with intermittent attacks of hemiplegia. Lancet 1954;267:994–996.
2. NASCET Investigators. Beneficial effect of carotid endarterectomy in symptomatic patients with high-grade carotid stenosis. North American Symptomatic Carotid Endarterectomy Trial Collaborators. N Engl J Med 1991;325:445–453.
3. ECST Investigators. Randomized trial of endarterectomy for recently symptomatic carotid stenosis: final results of the MRC European Carotid Surgery Trial (ECST). Lancet 1998;351:1379–1387.
4. Mayberg MR, Wilson SE, Yatsu F, Weiss DG, Messina L, Hershey LA, Colling C, Eskridge J, Deykin D, Winn HR. Carotid endarterectomy and prevention of cerebral ischemia in symptomatic carotid stenosis. Veterans Affairs Cooperative Studies Program 309 Trialist Group. JAMA 1991;266:3289–3294.
5. ACAS Investigators. Endarterectomy for asymptomatic carotid artery stenosis. Executive Committee for the Asymptomatic Carotid Atherosclerosis Study. JAMA 1995;273:1421–8.
6. Hobson RW, 2nd, Weiss DG, Fields WS, Goldstone J, Moore WS, Towne JB, Wright CB. Efficacy of carotid endarterectomy for asymptomatic carotid stenosis. The Veterans Affairs Cooperative Study Group. N Engl J Med 1993;328:221–227.
7. Halliday A, Mansfield A, Marro J, Peto C, Peto R, Potter J, Thomas D. Prevention of disabling and fatal strokes by successful carotid endarterectomy in patients without recent neurological symptoms: randomised controlled trial. Lancet 2004;363:1491–1502.
8. Sacco RL., Adams R, Albers G, Alberts MJ, Benavente O, Furie K, Goldstein LB, Gorelick P, Halperin J, Harbaugh R, Johnston SC, Katzan I, Kelly-Hayes M, Kenton EJ, Marks M, Schwamm LH, Tomsick T. Guidelines for prevention of stroke in patients with ischemic stroke or transient ischemic attack: a statement for healthcare professionals from the American Heart Association/American Stroke Association Council on Stroke: co-sponsored by the Council on Cardiovascular Radiology and Intervention: the American Academy of Neurology affirms the value of this guideline. Stroke 2006;37, 577–617.
9. Wennberg DE, Lucas FL, Birkmeyer JD, Bredenberg CE, Fisher ES. Variation in carotid endarterectomy mortality in the Medicare population: trial hospitals, volume, and patient characteristics. JAMA 1998;279:1278–1281.
10. Goldstein LB, Samsa GP, Matchar DB., Oddone EZ. Multicenter review of preoperative risk factors for endarterectomy for asymptomatic carotid artery stenosis. Stroke 1998;29:750–753.
11. McCrory DC, Goldstein LB, Samsa GP, Oddone EZ, Landsman PB, Moore WS, Matchar DB. Predicting complications of carotid endarterectomy. Stroke 1993;24:1285–1291.
12. Ouriel K, Hertzer NR, Beven EG, O'Hara PJ, Krajewski LP, Clair DG, Greenberg RK., Sarac TP, Olin JW, Yadav JS. Preprocedural risk stratification: identifying an appropriate population for carotid stenting. J Vasc Surg 2001;33:728–732.
13. Wong JH, Findlay JM, Suarez-Almazor ME. Regional performance of carotid endarterectomy. Appropriateness, outcomes, and risk factors for complications. Stroke 1997;28:891–898.
14. Gasparis AP, Ricotta L, Cuadra SA, Char DJ, Purtill WA, Van Bemmelen PS, Hines GL, Giron F, Ricotta JJ. High-risk carotid endarterectomy: fact or fiction. J Vasc Surg 2003;37:40–46.
15. Lepore MR, Jr, Sternbergh WC, 3rd, Salartash K, Tonnessen B, Money SR. Influence of NASCET/ ACAS trial eligibility on outcome after carotid endarterectomy. J Vasc Surg 2001;34:581–586.
16. Rothwell PM, Slattery J, Warlow CP. A systematic review of the risks of stroke and death due to endarterectomy for symptomatic carotid stenosis. Stroke 1996;27:260–265.
17. Ferguson GG, Eliasziw M, Barr HW, Clagett GP, Barnes RW, Wallace MC, Taylor DW, Haynes RB, Finan JW, Hachinski VC, Barnett HJ. The North American Symptomatic Carotid Endarterectomy Trial : surgical results in 1415 patients. Stroke 1999;30:1751–1758.

18. Paciaroni M, Eliasziw M, Kappelle LJ, Finan JW, Ferguson GG, Barnett HJ. Medical complications associated with carotid endarterectomy. North American Symptomatic Carotid Endarterectomy Trial (NASCET). Stroke 1999;30:1759–1763.
19. Mathias K. A new catheter system for percutaneous transluminal angioplasty (PTA) of carotid artery stenoses. Fortschr Med 1977;95:1007–1011.
20. Kerber CW, Cromwell LD, Loehden OL. Catheter dilatation of proximal carotid stenosis during distal bifurcation endarterectomy. AJNR Am J Neuroradiol 1980;1:348–349.
21. Kachel R. Results of balloon angioplasty in the carotid arteries. J Endovasc Surg 1996;3:22–30.
22. Diethrich EB, Ndiaye M, Reid DB. Stenting in the carotid artery: initial experience in 110 patients. J Endovasc Surg 1996;3:42–62.
23. Jordan WD, Jr, Schroeder PT, Fisher WS, McDowell HA. A comparison of angioplasty with stenting versus endarterectomy for the treatment of carotid artery stenosis. Ann Vasc Surg 1997;11:2–8.
24. Jordan WD, Jr, Voellinger DC, Fisher WS, Redden D, McDowell HA. A comparison of carotid angioplasty with stenting versus endarterectomy with regional anesthesia. J Vasc Surg 1998;28, 397–402; discussion 3.
25. Yadav JS, Roubin GS., Iyer S, Vitek J, King P, Jordan WD, Fisher WS. Elective stenting of the extracranial carotid arteries. Circulation 1997;95:376–381.
26. Roubin GS, New G, Iyer SS, Vitek JJ, Al-Mubarak N, Liu MW, Yadav J, Gomez C, Kuntz RE. Immediate and late clinical outcomes of carotid artery stenting in patients with symptomatic and asymptomatic carotid artery stenosis: a 5-year prospective analysis. Circulation 2001;103:532–537.
27. Naylor AR, Bolia A, Abbott RJ, Pye IF, Smith J, Lennard N, Lloyd AJ, London NJ, Bell PR. Randomized study of carotid angioplasty and stenting versus carotid endarterectomy: a stopped trial. J Vasc Surg 1998;28, 326–334.
28. Angelini A, Reimers B, Della Barbera M, Sacca S, Pasquetto G, Cernetti C, Valente M, Pascotto P, Thiene G. Cerebral protection during carotid artery stenting: collection and histopathologic analysis of embolized debris. Stroke 2002;33, 456–461.
29. Mathur A, Roubin GS, Iyer SS, Piamsonboon C, Liu MW, Gomez CR, Yadav JS, Chastain HD, Fox LM, Dean LS, Vitek JJ. Predictors of stroke complicating carotid artery stenting. Circulation 1998;97:1239–1245.
30. Ohki T, Marin ML, Lyon RT, Berdejo GL, Soundararajan K, Ohki M, Yuan JG, Faries PL, Wain RA, Sanchez LA, Suggs WD, Veith FJ Ex vivo human carotid artery bifurcation stenting: correlation of lesion characteristics with embolic potential. J Vasc Surg 1998;27:463–471.
31. Reimers B, Corvaja N, Moshiri S, Sacca S, Albiero R, Di Mario C, Pascotto P, Colombo A. Cerebral protection with filter devices during carotid artery stenting. Circulation 2001;104:12–15.
32. Theiss W, Hermanek P, Mathias K, Ahmadi R, Heuser L, Hoffmann FJ, Kerner R, Leisch F, Sievert H, von Sommoggy S. Pro-CAS: a prospective registry of carotid angioplasty and stenting. Stroke 2004;35:2134–9.
33. Bosiers M, Peeters P, Deloose K, Verbist J, Sievert H, Sugita J, Castriota F, Cremonesi A. Does carotid artery stenting work on the long run: 5-year results in high-volume centers (ELOCAS Registry). J Cardiovasc Surg (Torino) 2005;46:241–247.
34. Wholey MH, Al-Mubarek N. Updated review of the global carotid artery stent registry. Catheter Cardiovasc Interv 2003;60:259–266.
35. Mackey WC. Invited commentary. J Vasc Surg 2006;44, 268–269.
36. Reed AB, Gaccione P, Belkin M, Donaldson MC, Mannick JA, Whittemore AD, Conte MS. Preoperative risk factors for carotid endarterectomy: defining the patient at high risk. J Vasc Surg 2003;37:1191–1199.
37. Gray W, for the ARCHeR Investigators. ARCHeR Trial. In: American College of Cardiology Annual Scientific Sessions; New Orleans, LA; 2004.
38. Gray WA, Hopkins LN, Yadav S, Davis T, Wholey M, Atkinson R, Cremonesi A, Fairman R, Walker G, Verta P, Popma J, Virmani R, Cohen DJ. Protected carotid stenting in high-surgical-risk patients: the ARCHeR results. J Vasc Surg 2006;44, 258–268.
39. White CJ, Iyer SS, Hopkins LN, Katzen BT, Russell ME. Carotid stenting with distal protection in high surgical risk patients: the BEACH trial 30 day results. Catheter Cardiovasc Interv 2006;67:503–512.
40. Iyer SS, White CJ, Hopkins LN, Katzen BT, Safian R, Wholey MH, Gray WA, Ciocca R, Bachinsky WB, Ansel G, Joye JD, Russell ME. Carotid artery revascularization in high-surgical-risk patients using the Carotid WALLSTENT and FilterWire EX/EZ: 1-year outcomes in the BEACH Pivotal Group. J Am Coll Cardiol 2008;51:427–434.

41. Safian RD, Bresnahan JF, Jaff MR, Foster M, Bacharach JM, Maini B, Turco M, Myla S, Eles G, Ansel GM. Protected carotid stenting in high-risk patients with severe carotid artery stenosis. J Am Coll Cardiol 2006;47:2384–2389.

• • 42. Endovascular Today. CAS clinical trial and registry update. Endovascular Today 2007;6:76–79.

43. Hill MD, Morrish W, Soulez G, Nevelsteen A, Maleux G, Rogers C, Hauptmann KE, Bonafe A, Beyar R, Gruberg L, Schofer J. Multicenter evaluation of a self-expanding carotid stent system with distal protection in the treatment of carotid stenosis. AJNR Am J Neuroradiol 2006;27:759–765.

44. Reimers B, Sievert H, Schuler GC, Tubler T, Diederich K, Schmidt A, Rubino P, Mudra H, Dudek D, Coppi G, Schofer J, Cremonesi A, Haufe M, Resta M, Klauss V, Benassi A, Di Mario C, Favero L, Scheinert D, Salemme L, Biamino G. Proximal endovascular flow blockage for cerebral protection during carotid artery stenting: results from a prospective multicenter registry. J Endovasc Ther 2005;12:156–165.

45. Coppi G, Moratto R, Silingardi R, Rubino P, Sarropago G, Salemme L, Cremonesi A, Castriota F, Manetti R, Sacca S, Reimers B. PRIAMUS – proximal flow blockage cerebral protection during carotid stenting: results from a multicenter Italian registry. J Cardiovasc Surg (Torino) 2005;46:219–227.

• 46. Xact® Carotid Stent System – P040038. Summary of Safety and Effectiveness data. 2005. Accessed at http://www.fda.gov/cdrh/pdf4/p040038.html

47. CAVATAS Investigators. Endovascular versus surgical treatment in patients with carotid stenosis in the Carotid and Vertebral Artery Transluminal Angioplasty Study (CAVATAS): a randomised trial. Lancet 2001;357:1729–1737.

48. Alberts MJ. Results of a Multicenter Prospective Randomized Trial of Carotid Artery Stenting vs. Carotid Endarterectomy. Abstracts of the International Stroke Conference 2001;32:325-d.

49. Brooks WH, McClure RR, Jones MR, Coleman TC, Breathitt L. Carotid angioplasty and stenting versus carotid endarterectomy: randomized trial in a community hospital. J Am Coll Cardiol 2001;38:1589–1595.

50. Brooks WH, McClure RR, Jones MR, Coleman TL, Breathitt L. Carotid angioplasty and stenting versus carotid endarterectomy for treatment of asymptomatic carotid stenosis: a randomized trial in a community hospital. Neurosurgery 2004;54:318–324; discussion 24–25.

51. CARESS Steering Committee. Carotid revascularization using endarterectomy or stenting systems (CARESS): phase I clinical trial. J Endovasc Ther 2003;10:1021–1030.

52. CaRESS Steering Committee. Carotid Revascularization Using Endarterectomy or Stenting Systems (CaRESS) phase I clinical trial: 1-year results. J Vasc Surg 2005;42:213–219.

53. Yadav JS, Wholey MH, Kuntz RE, Fayad P, Katzen BT, Mishkel GJ, Bajwa TK, Whitlow P, Strickman NE, Jaff MR, Popma JJ, Snead DB, Cutlip DE, Firth BG, Ouriel K. Protected carotid-artery stenting versus endarterectomy in high-risk patients. N Engl J Med 2004;351:1493–1501.

54. Cambria RP. Stenting for carotid-artery stenosis. N Engl J Med 2004;351:1565–1567.

55. LoGerfo FW. Carotid stents: unleashed, unproven. Circulation 2007;116:1596–1601; discussion 601.

56. Mas JL, Chatellier G, Beyssen B, Branchereau A, Moulin T, Becquemin JP, Larrue V, Lievre M, Leys D, Bonneville JF, Watelet J, Pruvo JP, Albucher JF, Viguier A, Piquet P, Garnier P, Viader F, Touze E, Giroud M, Hosseini H, Pillet JC, Favrole P, Neau JP, Ducrocq X. Endarterectomy versus stenting in patients with symptomatic severe carotid stenosis. N Engl J Med 2006;355:1660–1671.

57. Mas JL, Chatellier G, Beyssen B. Carotid angioplasty and stenting with and without cerebral protection: clinical alert from the Endarterectomy Versus Angioplasty in Patients with Symptomatic Severe Carotid Stenosis (EVA-3S) trial. Stroke 2004;35:e18–20.

58. Ahmadi R, Willfort A, Lang W, Schillinger M, Alt E, Gschwandtner ME, Haumer M, Maca T, Ehringer H, Minar E. Carotid artery stenting: effect of learning curve and intermediate-term morphological outcome. J Endovasc Ther 2001;8:539–546.

59. Verzini F, Cao P, De Rango P, Parlani G, Maselli A, Romano L, Norgiolini L, Giordano G. Appropriateness of learning curve for carotid artery stenting: an analysis of periprocedural complications. J Vasc Surg 2006;44, 1205–1211; discussion 11–12.

60. Ringleb PA, Allenberg J, Bruckmann H, Eckstein HH, Fraedrich G, Hartmann M, Hennerici M, Jansen O, Klein G, Kunze A, Marx P, Niederkorn K, Schmiedt W, Solymosi L, Stingele R, Zeumer H, Hacke W. 30 day results from the SPACE trial of stent-protected angioplasty versus carotid endarterectomy in symptomatic patients: a randomised non-inferiority trial. Lancet 2006;368:1239–1247.

61. Kastrup A, Groschel K, Kraph H, Brehm B, Dichgans J, Schulz J. Early outcome of carotid angioplasty and stenting with and without cerebral protection devices. A systematic review of the literature. Stroke 2003;34:813–819.

62. Coward LJ, Featherstone RL., Brown MM. Safety and efficacy of endovascular treatment of carotid artery stenosis compared with carotid endarterectomy: a Cochrane systematic review of the randomized evidence. Stroke 2005;36:905–911.

63. Gurm HS, Nallamothu BK, Yadav J. Safety of carotid artery stenting for symptomatic carotid artery disease: a meta-analysis. Eur Heart J 2008 Jan; 29(1):113–119.

64. Burton KR, Lindsay TF. Assessment of short-term outcomes for protected carotid angioplasty with stents using recent evidence. J Vasc Surg 2005;42:1094–1100.

65. Gray WA, Yadav JS, Verta P, Scicli A, Fairman R, Wholey M, Hopkins LN, Atkinson R, Raabe R, Barnwell S, Green R. The CAPTURE registry: results of carotid stenting with embolic protection in the post approval setting. Catheter Cardiovasc Interv 2007;69:341–348.

66. Adams GL, Mills JS, Melloni C, Allen LA, Jolicoeur EM, Wang T, Chan M, Majidi M, Lopes RD. Highlights from the 56th annual scientific sessions of the American College of Cardiology: March 25 to 27, 2007, Atlanta, Georgia. Am Heart J 2007;154:247–259.

67. Katzen BT, Criado FJ, Ramee SR, Massop DW, Hopkins LN, Donohoe D, Cohen SA, Mauri L. Carotid artery stenting with emboli protection surveillance study: thirty-day results of the CASES-PMS study. Catheter Cardiovasc Interv 2007;70:316–323.

68. Hobson RW, 2nd. CREST (Carotid Revascularization Endarterectomy versus Stent Trial): background, design, and current status. Semin Vasc Surg 2000;13:139–143.

69. Hobson RW, 2nd, Howard VJ, Brott TG, Howard G, Roubin GS, Ferguson RD. Organizing the Carotid Revascularization Endarterectomy versus Stenting Trial (CREST): National Institutes of Health, Health Care Financing Administration, and industry funding. Curr Control Trials Cardiovasc Med 2001;2:160–164.

70. Hughes S, Roberts J, Brott T, Hobson RW, 2nd, Sheffet A. The CREST trial update. Endovascular Today 2004; September, 76–7.

71. Hobson RW, 2nd, Howard VJ, Roubin GS, Brott TG, Ferguson RD, Popma JJ, Graham DL, Howard G. Carotid artery stenting is associated with increased complications in octogenarians: 30-day stroke and death rates in the CREST lead-in phase. J Vasc Surg 2004;40:1106–1111.

72. Chastain HD, 2nd, Gomez CR, Iyer S, Roubin GS, Vitek JJ, Terry JB, Levine RL. Influence of age upon complications of carotid artery stenting. UAB Neurovascular Angioplasty Team. J Endovasc Surg 1999;6:217–222.

73. Kastrup A, Schulz JB, Raygrotzki S, Groschel K, Ernemann U. Comparison of angioplasty and stenting with cerebral protection versus endarterectomy for treatment of internal carotid artery stenosis in elderly patients. J Vasc Surg 2004;40:945–951.

74. Zahn R, Ischinger T, Hochadel M, Zeymer U, Schmalz W, Treese N, Hauptmann KE, Seggewiss H, Janicke I, Haase H, Mudra H, Senges J. Carotid artery stenting in octogenarians: results from the ALKK Carotid Artery Stent (CAS) Registry. Eur Heart J 2007;28:370–375.

75. Longo GM, Kibbe MR, Eskandari MK. Carotid artery stenting in octogenarians: is it too risky? Ann Vasc Surg 2005;19:812–816.

76. Shawl F, Kadro W, Domanski MJ, Lapetina FL, Iqbal AA, Dougherty KG, Weisher DD, Marquez JF., Shahab ST. Safety and efficacy of elective carotid artery stenting in high-risk patients. J Am Coll Cardiol 2000;35:1721–1728.

77. Hughes SE, Meelee T, Longbottom M, Aheffet AJ, Brott TG, Hobson R, 2nd W. CREST Update. Endovascular Today 2007;6(9):71–74.

78. ICSS – International Carotid Stenting Study. Accessed at www.cavatas.com

79. ACT I: Asymptomatic Carotid Stenosis, Stenting Versus Endarterectomy Trial. Accessed at http://www.clinicaltrials.gov/ct2/show/NCT00106938?term = asymptomatic + carotid + stenosis&rank = 3#locn

80. Asymptomatic Carotid Surgery Trial (ACST-2). A large, simple randomised trial to compare carotid endarterectomy versus carotid artery stenting to prevent stroke. Accessed at www.acst.org.uk

81. Transatlantic Asymptomatic Carotid Intervention Trial (TACIT) website. Accessed at http://www.sirfoundation.org/tacit.shtml

II LABORATORY SETUP AND BACKGROUND NONINVASIVE IMAGING

4 Catheterization Laboratory: X-Ray Equipment, Imaging Modalities and Programs, and Radiation Safety

David A. Wood, MD
and Anthony Y. Fung, MBBS

CONTENTS

ABSTRACT

Choosing the correct equipment and utilizing the most appropriate imaging modalities will not only improve the planning and performance of interventional cerebrovascular procedures, but also limit the radiation exposure for both the patient and laboratory personnel. Digital subtraction angiography remains the gold standard technique for assessing both lesion severity and plaque characteristics during cerebrovascular interventions. No single acquisition mode, however, will provide the best image quality and anatomical information in all situations. It is the operator's responsibility to understand these differences and employ strategies to both maximize image quality and limit radiation exposure to ensure patient and staff safety.

Keywords: Image intensifier; Digital flat-panel detector system; Acquisition modes; Digital subtraction angiography; Roadmap; Radiation safety

Acknowledgement: Carsten Stevenson

From: *Contemporary Cardiology: Carotid Artery Stenting: The Basics*
Edited by: J. Saw, DOI 10.1007/978-1-60327-314-5_4,
© Humana Press, a part of Springer Science+Business Media, LLC 2009

INTRODUCTION

Choosing the correct equipment and utilizing the most appropriate imaging modalities will not only improve the planning and performance of interventional cerebrovascular procedures, but also limit the radiation exposure for both the patient and laboratory personnel. This chapter will provide an overview of imaging equipment (image intensifier, digital flat-panel detector (DFP) systems, and biplane), intravascular contrast agents, and imaging programs [digital subtraction angiography (DSA), bolus chase, roadmap, fluoroscopy loop store, panel detector contouring, last image hold and virtual collimation]. It presents a framework for understanding when to utilize different imaging modalities. Radiation injury is an important early and late procedural complication, and methods to limit stochastic and deterministic effects are important for both patient and operator safety. This chapter will also review basic radiation principles and discuss techniques to limit exposure.

A complete discussion of x-ray physics, imaging technology, and radiopathology is beyond the scope of the current chapter. For more details, readers are referred to a recent intersociety clinical competency statement *(1)* and standard textbooks in the field *(2–4)*. A procedural description of aortic arch and four-vessel cerebrovascular angiography is reviewed separately in Chapter 10.

IMAGING EQUIPMENT

Image quality has a significant impact on planning and performing cerebrovascular interventions. Before discussing the advantages and disadvantages of different imaging equipment and modalities, it is important to understand the factors that influence image quality: spatial resolution, noise, and contrast resolution. Spatial resolution is the ability to see very small objects. Typically the measurement is done by using a device that tests lines per millimeter. The more lines per millimeter you can see, the higher the resolution. Noise is any image data that are transferred to the detector that is not part of the patient anatomy. Noise can be caused by scattered radiation from the patient, from the x-ray photons being sent "off course" from hitting high-density objects within the patient's body, or can be induced by the detector's own electronic array. In the digital world, noise is inversely related to detector efficiency. The higher the efficiency of the detector for a given dose, the lower the noise level. Contrast resolution is the ability to distinguish objects of very similar contrast makeup. Higher contrast resolution makes it easier to distinguish soft tissue objects of similar density.

Detective quantum efficiency (DQE) is used to measure the "imaging performance" of a detector. DQE is a way of quantifying spatial resolution, noise, and contrast resolution. The measurement is taken for both fluoroscopy and record acquisition (discussed below) and displayed as a percentage. Improved DQE results in either improved image quality or a reduction in radiation dose for the same image quality.

Before selecting the imaging equipment, it is important to decide if the laboratory will be utilized for a variety of applications (coronary, peripheral, and cerebrovascular) or used solely for carotid stenting. Most cardiovascular interventional laboratories are designed to perform a variety of procedures and utilize an x-ray cinefluoroscopic system to generate images. A collimated x-ray beam of appropriate intensity and quality is projected through the patient at a desired angle to generate a usable visible light image. Major differences in types of equipment are most evident in x-ray detection and recording. Image intensifiers have been utilized since the 1950s *(5)*. The modulated x-ray beam emerging from the patient enters the image intensifier and is detected by a cesium iodide fluorescent layer *(6)*. The electron image is converted back into a visible light image when the electrons interact with the output screen. A variety of magnification modes can be generated with a wide range of fields of view. A larger field of view is often essential for both peripheral and intracranial angiography. In contrast, digital flat-panel (DFP) detector systems often have a broader dynamic range and better dosimetric performance. Although the dose efficiency of a DFP system is thought to be similar to a modern image intensifier, the newest generation of DFP systems may be able to attain a high DQE with a 28% lower effective dose. Another important difference occurs when an image is zoomed. With image intensifier systems every step up in magnification (decrease in field of view) doubles the effective radiation dose. This occurs because of the relationship between the input phosphor and the output phosphor – magnifying the image decreases the size of the input phosphor and thus makes the image appear larger. The reduction in size of the input phosphor requires an increase in dose to display the same brightness. DFP systems do not have input and output phosphors; consequently, there is not a drastic increase in dose (only about 15% each step) as the image is zoomed. Although the intrinsic spatial resolution does not increase with zoom, the digitally magnified image on the monitor may provide better detailed coupling to the observer's eye. Although an image intensifier may be more versatile in a multiuse laboratory, DFP systems offer a variety of features that maximize image quality and reduce effective radiation dose.

The standard cinefluoroscopic system is mounted on a C-arm semicircular support with an x-ray tube at one end and an image detection system (image intensifier or DFP) at the opposite end (Figs. 1 and 2). A biplane system incorporates two orthogonal C-arms and allows visualization of the structure from two different angles simultaneously. This may reduce both x-ray exposure and contrast load for neurovascular procedures.

INTRAVASCULAR CONTRAST AGENTS

Contrast agents are used to define vascular anatomy. The original high-osmolar ionic contrast media were Na+/meglumine salts of substituted tri-iodobenzoic acid *(6)*. Low osmolality contrast media (both ionic and non-ionic) emerged in the late 1980s. The newest class of iso-osmolar contrast medium (Iodixanol [Visipaque, GE Healthcare, Buckinghamshire, UK]) is a non-ionic dimer with six iodine atoms per molecule and an osmolarity similar to blood.

High-osmolar contrast agents may cause sensations of warmth, discomfort, and headache, and thus, an iso-osmolar agent is often utilized for peripheral and cerebral angiography due to its lower incidence of side effects. In the elderly patients, diabetics, and patients with underlying renal dysfunction, the use of iso-osmolar contrast may also decrease the risk of contrast-induced nephropathy (CIN) *(7)*. An arbitrary range of a relative 25–50% increase in serum creatinine levels 48–72 h from baseline or an absolute increase of 0.5–1.0 mg/dL have been proposed as definitions for CIN.

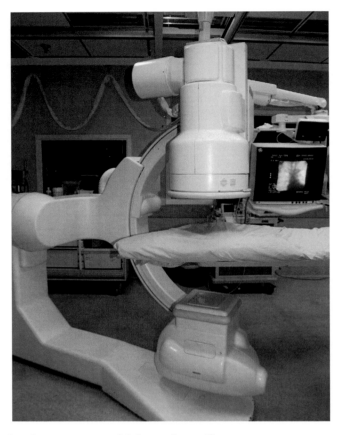

Fig. 1. A conventional x-ray system with image intensifier.

Many patients undergoing carotid artery stenting have multiple comorbidities and thus the risk of CIN should be considered in every patient. The best way to prevent CIN is to identify patients at risk and to provide adequate peri-procedural hydration. The role of various drugs in the prevention of CIN is still controversial and warrants future studies *(7)*.

IMAGING MODALITIES AND PROGRAMS

Although obtaining the correct imaging equipment is important, understanding the different acquisition modes in angiography will have the greatest impact on image quality and radiation exposure. The ideal angiographic system would produce high-quality cine and fluoroscopic images at the lowest reasonably achievable dose. However, no single acquisition mode will provide the best image quality and anatomical information in all situations.

Fluoroscopy is used in all modes of angiography. This acquisition type has the lowest dose and the lowest image quality of all acquisition modes *(1)*. Fluoroscopy is the most significant contributor to radiation dose during an interventional procedure; therefore, reducing the dose during fluoroscopy has the greatest impact on total procedural dose. Pulse rates of 15 and 30 pulses per second are commonly used. Most fluoroscopy can be performed in low-dose mode at 15 frames per second (fps).

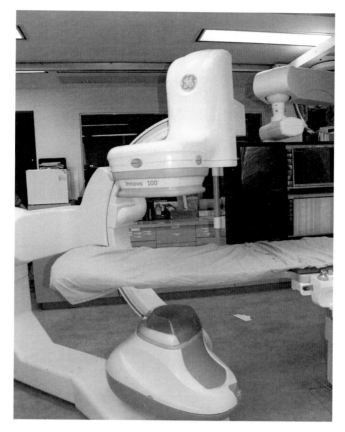

Fig. 2. An x-ray system with digital flat-panel technology.

A transition to 30 fps will usually improve image quality, which is sometimes necessary in large-sized patients. It is important to remember that reducing the frame rate from 30 to 15 fps does not cut the radiation dose in half. The pulse width (maximum exposure time for each pulse of fluoro) is usually higher at lower frame rates. Consequently, although the dose is reduced when switching from 30 to 15 fps, the "dose per frame" is actually higher and gives better image quality at lower dose as long as the visual smoothness of the transition between frames is maintained.

Fluoro loop store, panel detector contouring, last image hold, and virtual collimation can all improve image quality and limit radiation exposure during fluoroscopy. Fluoro loop store is a method of retrospectively storing the last fluoroscopic event. This allows the operator to record events at lower dose. A modern fluoro loop system should be able to store 30 s of fluoroscopy. With improved fluoroscopic DQE, large portions of an interventional procedure can be stored at one-fifth the x-ray exposure. Patient detector contouring can also lower the radiation dose to both the patient and the operator. Modern systems have a sensor that will keep the detector at an optimal distance during acquisition. This not only decreases radiation dose but also improves image quality by reducing geometric distortion. Last image hold presents the last acquired fluoroscopic frame on the video monitor, thus providing an opportunity to study the image without continuing the exposure. Collimating an image reduces the amount of scattered radiation and decreases the area being irradiated. Virtual collimation allows the operator to collimate from the last image on the monitor and can further decrease radiation exposure during fluoroscopy *(1)*.

Record mode or "cine" involves unsubtracted acquisition at a high frame rate (usually 15 or 30 fps) (Fig. 3). Higher x-ray input dose rates are used to reduce image noise and optimize clinical visualization. Although this acquisition type has the second lowest "radiation dose per frame", it remains approximately 15 times greater than for fluoroscopy.

Digital subtracted angiography (DSA) acquisition mode remains the gold standard technique for assessing both lesion severity and plaque characteristics during cerebrovascular interventions (Fig. 4). Images are first acquired without injection of contrast media. The DSA sequence requires the acquisition to start prior to injection of the contrast media. This is necessary to allow a mask image to be used as a negative image to remove the background from the positive vascular images. Only the injected vasculature is visible in the final subtracted images. This type of acquisition has the highest "radiation dose per frame". The images can be presented subtracted or masked. It is critical that the patient remains immobilized with an adequate breath hold and a head collar during DSA. This acquisition mode is dedicated to non-moving structures and thus the acquisition rate is lower than that used in cardiac acquisition. Choosing the correct frame rate is not only important to capture all of the relevant vascular structures but also to ensure that the patient is not subjected to unnecessarily high frame rates. Typical arterial

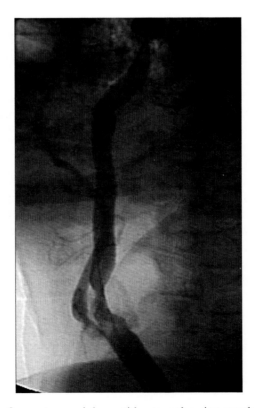

Fig. 3. Cine angiogram of an extracranial carotid artery showing overlapping bony structures.

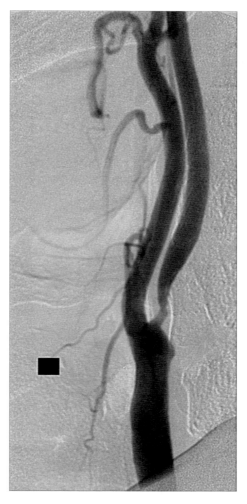

Fig. 4. Digital subtraction angiography of an extracranial carotid artery showing subtraction of the bony structures.

frame rates are 2–4 fps for cerebrovasculature and 2–5 fps for the aortic arch. Virtually all vascular structures (except for coronary arteries) can be imaged with DSA.

The unsubtracted "low-dose" mode is another acquisition alternative. Many systems have an unsubtracted mode that is a cross between a cine and unsubtracted DSA mode. The frame rate is usually much lower than cine but at a lower radiation level than DSA. The images are not subtracted and this allows the operator to pan the table to follow an injection in the vasculature.

Bolus chase acquisition mode is used primarily for femoral "run-off" studies. The system typically acquires a series of masks, starting at the abdomen or pelvis and ending at the feet, before acquiring the same series of images with injected contrast. The acquisitions can be done bilaterally or a single leg at a time. The systems either utilize "table motion" or "gantry motion" to move up and down the legs.

Roadmap fluoroscopic imaging involves generating a static fluoro image with contrast and then superimposing live fluoroscopic images over the stored image. This gives a "roadmap" of the vessel and lesion and allows catheters to be delivered to the correct location with minimal irradiation and contrast use.

RADIATION SAFETY

For both interventionalists and patients, the occupational radiation dose received should be minimized without compromising appropriate patient care. This concept is referred to as ALARA (as low as reasonably achievable) *(8)*. ALARA includes the following principles: there is no known absolutely safe dose of ionizing radiation; the smaller the dose, the less the risk of an adverse effect; and incremental radiation exposures have cumulative effects *(9)*. Radiation injuries are induced by two mechanisms. The stochastic mechanism is caused by unrepaired radiation damage to the DNA of even a single cell. The deterministic mechanism is caused by radiation acutely killing a large number of cells. Although all laboratory personnel are exposed to a degree of stochastic risk, deterministic effects (cataracts, skin burns) should never occur in an interventional setting.

Three groups of factors affect the dose delivered to the patient during an invasive cardiovascular procedure: equipment-related factors, patient-related factors, and procedural-related factors. Readers are referred to the 2004 ACCF/AHA/HRS/ SCAI clinical competency statement for a complete discussion of both the above parameters and currently used metrics to measure the effects of radiation *(1)*. In general, minimizing patient exposure will limit the stochastic effects for both the operator and the catheterization laboratory personnel. Two parameters of dose – the dose at the interventional reference point (IRP) and the dose-area product (DAP) – are useful for characterizing patient exposure. Currently available interventional fluoroscopic equipment determines real-time estimates of the instantaneous and cumulated values for these dose factors. The unit's indication of these cumulated values provides valid indicators of a patient's dose and consequent risk for radiation-induced effects.

Effective dose may be expressed in terms of rems (or the System Internationale unit sievert) *(1)*. The average background radiation exposure is approximately 0.1 rem per year. Interventional cardiologists receive another 0.004–0.016 rem per case. The maximum recommended exposure by the National Council on Radiation Protection and Measurement (NCRPM) is 5 rems per year for the total body *(10)*. Over an individual's lifetime, the accumulated maximum dose should be no greater than the accumulated rem exposure × age (or a maximum of 50 rems).

Basic principles for minimizing radiation exposure include the following:

1. Minimize beam-on time, both for fluoroscopy and acquisition.
2. Use optimal beam collimation.
3. Position the x-ray source and image receptor optimally.
4. Use the least degree of image magnification required for accurate interpretation.
5. Understand and utilize the x-ray dose-reduction features provided by the x-ray unit.
6. Vary the site of the radiation entrance port.
7. Record the estimated dose delivered to the patient.
8. Maintain x-ray equipment in good repair and calibration.
9. Select x-ray units with sophisticated dose-reduction and monitoring features *(11)*.

Despite these recommendations, interventional cardiologists working in high-volume catheterization laboratories often have collar badge exposures that exceed currently recommended levels *(12)*. It is ultimately the operator's responsibility to ensure the safety of both the patient and the laboratory personnel.

CONCLUSIONS

Choosing the correct equipment and utilizing the most appropriate imaging modalities will not only improve the planning and performance of interventional cerebrovascular procedures but also limit the radiation exposure for both the patient and the laboratory personnel. Digital subtraction angiography remains the gold standard technique for assessing both lesion severity and plaque characteristics during cerebrovascular interventions. It is the operator's responsibility to understand the different acquisition modes and employ strategies to both maximize image quality and limit radiation exposure to ensure patient and staff safety.

REFERENCES

1. Hirshfeld JW, et al. ACCF/AHA/HRS/SCAI clinical competence statement on physician knowledge to optimize patient safety and image quality in fluoroscopically guided invasive cardiovascular procedures. J Am Coll Cardiol 2004;44:2259–2282.
2. Balter S. Interventional Fluoroscopy, Physics, Technology, Safety. John Wiley, New York; 2001.
3. Hall EJ. Radiobiology for the Radiologist. 4th Ed. JB Lippincott, Philadelphia, PA;1994.
4. Bushberg J, Seibert JA, Ledidholdt EM, Boone JM. The Essential Physics of Medical Imaging. 2nd Ed. Williams & Wilkins, Baltimore, MD; 2002.
5. Sones FM Jr. Cine-cardio-angiography. Pediatr Clin North Am 1958;5:945–979.
6. Baim DS. Chapter 2: Cineangiographic imaging, radiation safety, and contrast agents. In: Grossman's Cardiac Catheterization, Angiography, and Intervention. 7th Ed. Lippincott Williams and Wilkins, Philadelphia, PA; 2006.
7. Pucelikova T, Dangas G, Mehran R, Contrast-Induced nephropathy. Catheter Cardiovasc Interv 2008;71:62–72.
8. National Council on Radiation Protection and Measurements. Report 105. Radiation Protection for Medical and Allied Health Personnel. National Council on Radiation Protection and Measurements, Bethesda, MD;1989.
9. Koenig TR, Mettler FA, Wagner LK. Skin injuries from fluoroscopically guided procedures: part 2, review of 73 cases and recommendations for minimizing dose delivered to patient. AJR Am J Roentgenol 2001;177:13–20.
10. Bashore et al. ACC/SCA&I Clinical expert consensus document on catheterization laboratory standards. J Am Coll Cardiol 2001;37(8):2170–2214.
11. Medical electrical equipment, part 2-43. Particular requirements for the safety of x-ray equipment for interventional procedures. Geneva: International Electrotechnical Commission, 2000; IEC report 60601.
12. McKetty MH. Study of radiation doses to personnel in a cardiac catheterization laboratory. Health Phys 1996 Apr;70(4):563–567.

5

Noninvasive Imaging of the Extracranial Carotid Circulation

Jonathon Leipsic, MD

CONTENTS

ABSTRACT

Technological advances have revolutionized vascular noninvasive imaging over the past two decades. There are now several options aside from conventional angiography to image carotid artery stenosis. These modalities are constantly evolving, and this chapter will review CT angiography, MR angiography, and carotid Doppler for noninvasive carotid artery imaging.

Keywords: Carotid ultrasound; CT angiography; MR angiography

INTRODUCTION

Over the last two decades, technological advances have revolutionized vascular noninvasive imaging. When previously the only option of choice was conventional angiography, there are now several options to assess stenosis that go even further in characterizing and imaging atherosclerosis. These modalities are constantly evolving and this chapter will review the modalities commonly used at the present time in the evaluation of carotid disease.

CT ANGIOGRAPHY

In recent years, there have been rapid advances in computed tomographic (CT) technology and image post-processing. CT angiography has steadily improved by decreasing section thickness and increasing scan speed and has emerged as a

From: *Contemporary Cardiology: Carotid Artery Stenting: The Basics*
Edited by: J. Saw, DOI 10.1007/978-1-60327-314-5_5,
© Humana Press, a part of Springer Science+Business Media, LLC 2009

powerful tool in neurovascular imaging. With availability of modern 64-multidetector scanners in clinical practice, true isotropic imaging is achievable, allowing for imaging in all planes and for robust post-processing techniques to create images comparable to those acquired with catheter angiography. Achieving optimal image quality relies on two factors: CT angiographic technique (scan protocol, contrast protocol, image reconstruction) and data visualization technique (image post-processing) *(1)*.

CT Technique

A prerequisite for adequate vascular imaging is using the appropriate technique for the clinical question at hand. The three major technical factors that are at the core of all vascular CT protocols are scan speed, spatial resolution, and contrast administration.

INFLUENCE OF SCAN SPEED

Examination of the whole length of the carotid arteries from the aortic arch to the circle of Willis requires a scan range of approximately 250 mm. The total time of acquisition depends on the type of scanner used. With modern 64-detector scanner technology, this could be imaged in 4 s, allowing phase-resolved imaging. The higher number of detectors in use also improves through-plane resolution by reducing detector width. Typical in-plane and through-plane resolution of 0.5–0.7 mm is achievable using modern systems, thus providing isotropic data and multiplanar imaging.

CONTRAST INJECTION PROTOCOLS

Short scan times require short contrast agent injections. Rapid injection rates and highly concentrated contrast agents (iodine, 350–370 mmol/mL) are preferable. Timing of the contrast bolus is required to ensure optimal imaging *(1)*. Various proprietary techniques (CARE bolus, Smart Prep, and Sure Start) are all commonly used and fast techniques to aid in contrast timing. Using these techniques, imaging commences when adequate opacification of the carotid circulation is noted. Alternatively, a test bolus method can be used in which an enhancement histogram is generated to assess peak enhancement following the injection of a 10 cc test bolus.

Image Reconstruction

In an attempt to reduce noise, images can be reconstructed slightly thicker than the detector. Overlapping image reconstruction should be performed to improve 3D post-processing. Overlap of anywhere from 50–75% of the detector width is generally recommended. Image post-processing techniques include multiplanar reformats (MPR), maximum intensity projections (MIP), and shaded surface display and volume rendering.

Multiplanar reformats create views in various planes without sacrificing resolution (Fig. 1). The interrogation of axial imaging alone yields high sensitivity but poor specificity for the detection of stenotic lesions *(2)*. Furthermore, it is well established in the literature that stenosis measurement on a single plane leads to misclassification of stenoses *(3)*. One particular advantage of MPR is that it provides the opportunity to directly compare the stenotic region with the normal

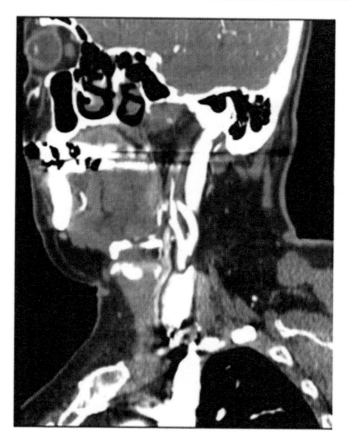

Fig. 1. Sagittal multiplanar reformat of the left carotid artery displayed on a narrow window display.

internal carotid artery more distally. Sagittal oblique views are especially helpful at evaluating the patency of the lumen, particularly in the setting of dense calcification (Figs. 2 and 3).

Maximum intensity projections are created by displaying only the highest attenuation. This technique sacrifices depth information for increased conspicuity of the vessel in question. The loss of depth perception does come with limitations, in particular, overlapping vessels that can obscure luminal assessment and hide stenoses (4). MIP is still the most common technique used in carotid evaluation, as it is part of the standard post-processing software on most modern CT scanners (Fig. 4).

Shaded surface display (SSD) shows the first layer of voxels within defined thresholds (in Hounsfield units), leading to the visualization of the surface of all structures that fulfill threshold conditions (5). Unlike MIP, the "depth" information is preserved but the "attenuation" information is lost with SSD. Arteries will vary in caliber depending on the thresholds that are selected, and a moderate stenosis could be misinterpreted as an occlusion (6). The strength and purpose of SSD is to provide a quick visual roadmap of the course of the vessel being interrogated.

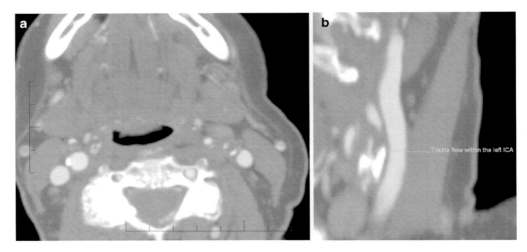

Fig. 2. (A) Axial CT angiographic image displaying a tight stenosis of the left ICA with residual trickle flow on the basis of calcified and non-calcified plaque. (B) Sagittal oblique reformat displaying the same findings.

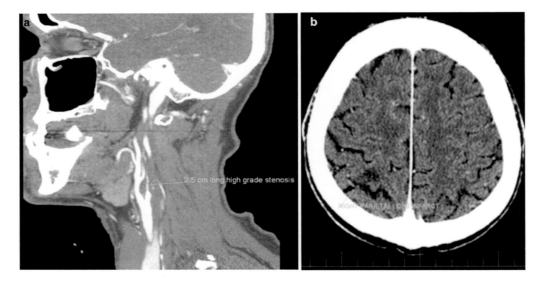

Fig. 3. (A) High-grade non-calcified right ICA stenosis. (B) Complicating right parietal lobe infarct.

Volume rendering (VR) principally allows the integration of all available information from a volumetric data set (Fig. 5) *(7)*. Groups of voxels within defined attenuation thresholds are selected, and color as well as "opacity" is assigned. Allowing opacity leads to transparent images and vice versa. Unlike MIP and SSD images, VR images are created not from a single layer of voxels, but from all voxels that meet the selection criteria. With this technique, it is possible to demonstrate a calcified internal carotid artery (ICA) or the circle of Willis together with the skull base in different colors. VR is the best choice for 3D imaging of the extracranial and intracranial vessels.

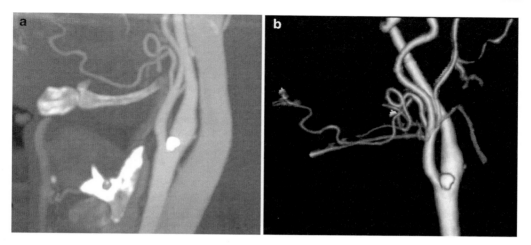

Fig. 4. (A) Sagittal oblique MIP image of the left ICA with nodular calcified plaque. The plaque is more conspicuous because of the technique, but MIP imaging should not be the primary technique in stenosis assessment. (B) A volume-rendered image of the same carotid artery.

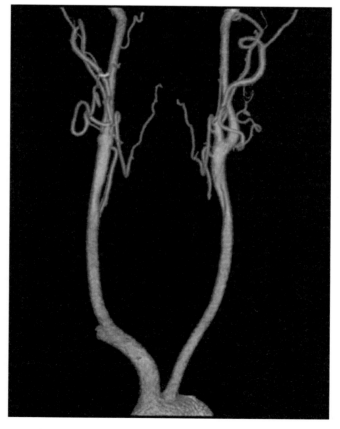

Fig. 5. Superb anatomical delineation is the strength of volume rendering as shown by this coronal volume-rendered image of both carotids.

Image Interpretation

Data analysis must start with the inspection of source images, preferably on a workstation that allows for multiplanar reformatting. The axial assessment allows for direct comparison to the contralateral carotid artery. Occlusion and calcified stenosis and thrombosis of one carotid artery can be easily compared to the other side. Occlusion is usually easily identified by a lack of contrast enhancement. In the absence of calcifications, coronal and oblique MIP projections will typically allow for adequate initial analysis. When calcifications obscure a stenosis, axial source images or curved multiplanar reformatted images are most helpful in the evaluation of stenosis *(8)*.

CT Artifacts

Like in other body areas, CT angiographic imaging of the carotid circulation is associated with a number of known artifacts. The most commonly encountered in the carotid circulation is beam hardening related to heavily calcified plaque within the carotid arteries themselves, or secondary to dental amalgam. This rarely renders the imaging non-diagnostic. However, it does limit the value of certain post-processing techniques like volume rendering and shaded surface display *(9)*. These dense materials result in dark streaks distally as they significantly attenuate the radiation beam. A second source of artifact is motion-related to patient swallowing or movement, voluntary or otherwise. Patients must be coached appropriately to suspend breathing and swallowing to ensure optimal image acquisition.

Validation Studies of CT Angiography

Recently, a new body of literature has arisen assessing the accuracy of CTA of the carotid circulation *(10, 11)*. Unfortunately most of these studies predated the development of multidetector CT scanners. Several authors have reported multidetector CT use exclusively for the preoperative evaluation of patients *(12)*. These studies were criticized for the lack of correlative catheter angiography, but no unexpected surgical findings or adverse outcomes were encountered. With modern techniques and advanced CT scanner technology, diagnostic images are achievable rapidly and without the risks associated with catheter studies *(13)*. CT in many ways not only correlates well with catheter angiography, but offers a more complete assessment particularly in the evaluation of eccentric stenoses and plaque evaluation. Initial attempts at plaque evaluation have been somewhat limited by the spatial resolution of the scanner technology available. CT may visualize the lipid core on the basis of its lower density, but there remains considerable variability of this finding *(14)*.

MR ANGIOGRAPHY

The carotid arteries are well suited for MR assessment (Fig. 6). Unlike the heart, which poses greater challenges due to motion and longer acquisition times, the neck is stationary and provides few limitations for image acquisition. High-sensitivity neck coils depict carotid anatomy with excellent detail. The two most commonly used sequences for carotid imaging are time-of-flight (TOF) and contrast-enhanced magnetic resonance angiography (CE-MRA) (Figs. 7 and 8). TOF relies upon imaging of non-saturated blood into the imaging volume. CE-MRA consists of

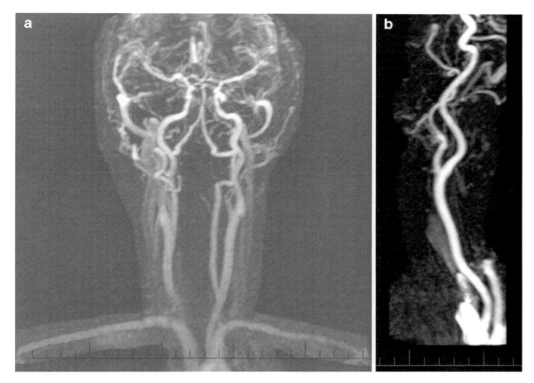

Fig. 6. (A) Coronal MIP MRI reformat of both carotid arteries. **(B)** Sagittal MIP reconstruction of the left carotid artery.

imaging the distribution of contrast material, not of blood motion *(15)*. TOF can be further characterized as 2D TOF and 3D TOF *(16)*. The distinction depends on whether the angiogram is constructed from multiple thin sections or from a slab. A hybrid of 2D and 3D TOF techniques uses multiple overlapping thin section acquisitions (MOTSA) (Fig. 9) *(17)*. All of these sequences have been shown to be successful in estimating carotid stenosis with individual strengths and weaknesses.

Time-of-Flight MRA

Since its introduction in the late 1980s, carotid MRA has developed into a robust clinical tool for assessment of carotid stenosis. The first technique used routinely was conventional 2D TOF. In 2D TOF one obtains a sequential series of transaxial slices through the neck extending from the thoracic inlet to the base of the skull. Tissues that are stationary are exposed to pulsed radio waves, are "saturated", and become dark. Flowing blood that enters a slice between radiofrequency pulses have not been saturated and will therefore be bright. Each slice is acquired completely before moving on. For adequate resolution, slice thickness should be less than 2 mm. A moving saturation band is put in place to suppress signal from the jugular veins.

The 3D TOF provides finer resolution than 2D TOF imaging with slice acquisition typically 1 mm in thickness (Fig. 10). This is achieved by acquiring a thick slab

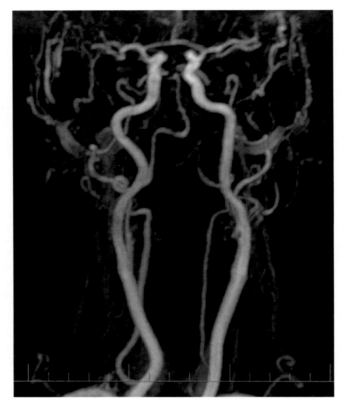

Fig. 7. Coronal contrast-enhanced MRA of both carotid arteries.

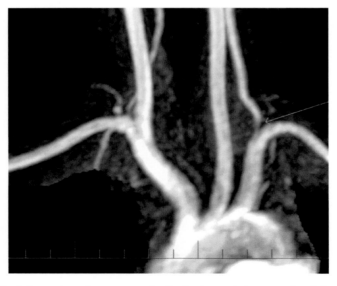

Fig. 8. MRI MIP of the arch and great vessels displaying a tight stenosis of the origin of the left vertebral artery (*arrow*).

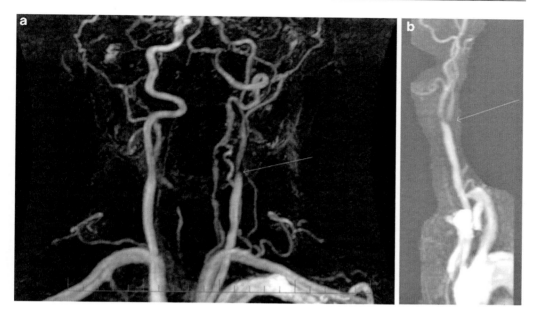

Fig. 9. (A) Coronal reformat of a MOTSA MRA displaying a tight stenosis of the left ICA. **(B)** Sagittal reformat, which shows the stenosis better.

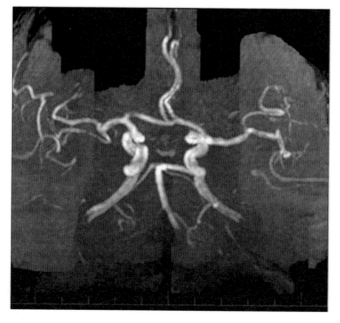

Fig. 10. 3D TOF MRA of the circle of Willis in a patient with renal failure in whom gadolinium is contraindicated.

transaxially through the bifurcation and partitioning the data set with a second phase-encoding gradient *(18)*. As in 2D TOF, a saturation band is placed to eliminate jugular venous signal. This technique is limited due to its motion sensitivity and large volume coverage required for imaging.

In MOTSA, the angiogram is built like a puzzle with multiple thin slabs. Each slab is divided into thin partitions and the thin slabs allow blood to traverse the volume and refresh the signal between radiofrequency pulses. Each slab partially overlaps the volume acquired by prior slab. This does result in a relatively inefficient acquisition with long acquisition times in the order of 10 min.

Contrast-Enhanced MRA

CE-MRA has proven to be a very effective and fast way of noninvasively imaging the carotid arteries. The study is less sensitive to artifact and is the test of choice for patients who cannot lie still. The technique involves injection of a small gadolinium contrast bolus in a peripheral arm vein. Upon arrival in the carotid arteries a fast 3D gradient-echo sequence is obtained. CE-MRA is based on the combination of rapid 3D imaging and the T1-shortening effect of intravenously infused paramagnetic contrast. These agents greatly shorten the T1 of blood resulting in very bright signal intensity on T1-weighted sequences. The acquisition slab may be then oriented in a coronal plane to cover the entire length of the carotid circulation from the neck through the circle of Willis. The time of acquisition is approximately 20 s and requires rather significant patient cooperation, i.e., no swallowing or moving throughout the examination.

CE-MRA is best done on modern machines with strong gradients of 20 mT/m or greater. The stronger gradients allow for more rapid imaging and often cuts imaging time below 20 s. The shorter acquisition times allow for lower contrast volumes. Typically 20–30 cc of gadolinium is required. Like in all noninvasive angiography, signal to noise improves with higher injection rates.

The last technical development in recent years has been the development of parallel imaging techniques *(19)*. These are based on an optimal utilization of redundant information from multiple phased array coils and allow a reduction in the time-consuming phase-encoding steps required to spatially encode MR signal. High spatial resolution images can be acquired in a shortened time often by a factor of 2–4. Parallel imaging is now a mainstay of modern MRA and is used in conjunction with a variety of techniques including CE-MRA. The main limitation is that of somewhat reduced signal-to-noise ratio.

Gadolinium

Gadolinium-based contrast agents have been used for decades in other MRI applications. Gadolinium has seven unpaired electrons in its outer shell and hastens T1 relaxation, thereby increasing signal in the area of interest. Gadolinium alone is cytotoxic but not when combined with a chelating agent. Gadolinium has minimal nephrotoxicity and anaphylaxis risk. Several Food and Drug Administration (FDA)-approved gadolinium preparations have been used for over a decade and the safety profile is far more favorable than iodinated contrast. A prior study of high-dose gadolinium in a population with a high prevalence of baseline renal insufficiency showed no renal failure associated with its administration *(20)*. The rate of allergic reactions is extremely low and is largely limited to mild nausea, vomiting, and urticaria. The rate of serious allergic reactions was less than 0.01% *(21)*.

Any updated review about MRA, in particular CE-MRA, must include a brief discussion about nephrogenic systemic fibrosis (NSF) *(22)*. On May 23, 2007, the

FDA updated a previously issued public health advisory after receiving 90 reports of patients with at least moderate renal dysfunction, gadolinium exposure, and subsequent development of NSF, a dermatologic condition that is characterized by severe and progressive skin induration *(23)*. The proposed association between gadolinium and NSF has been further solidified by recent reports of gadolinium isolated up to 11 months following administration in biopsy specimens of patients with NSF *(24)*. The updated advisory suggests that the risk of gadolinium-based MRI contrast agents increases the risk for NSF in patients with acute or chronic severe renal insufficiency (GFR < 30 mL/min) or acute renal insufficiency of any severity due to hepatorenal syndrome. The risk of developing NSF among patients with mild or moderate renal insufficiency or normal renal function is not known.

MRA Validation

Subsequent to the publication of the NASCET trial, a series of validation studies were launched to determine the least costly and most accurate means of evaluating carotid stenosis. Early studies compared 3D TOF and MOTSA with catheter angiography *(23, 24)*. The median sensitivity was 0.93 and the median specificity 0.88. Studies comparing CE-MRA and catheter angiography have shown very similar results *(25, 26)*. Unfortunately, validation studies performed in the past used catheter angiography as the gold standard. The issue with this assumption is that any errors made in measurement during catheter angiography were assumed to be errors in MRA. Since catheter angiography only has a reproducibility of 94% *(27)*, one can deduce that sensitivities and specificities are actually better than reported. In the last 10 years there have been several reports that suggest MRA correlates better with surgical specimens than catheter angiography *(28, 29)*. The discrepancies noted between MRA and catheter angiography are now usually attributed to the inability of catheter angiography to appreciate the smallest diameter when the stenosis is elliptical or complex in shape. Recent literature has shown that catheter angiography often underestimates the severity of the lesion by not viewing it from the most stenotic direction particularly without rotational angiography *(29)*. MR historically has been said to overestimate the severity of stenosis but the evidence is now suggesting that MR is more accurate in stenosis assessment than catheter studies. Information about the shape of the plaque, which can be seen on MRA but not catheter angiography, is also ignored in the validation studies. However, only catheter angiography has been shown to reduce the incidence of strokes through large-scale clinical trials. Clinical trials of the scale of NASCET have never been undertaken using MRA *(30)*. Nevertheless, revascularization decision utilizing MRA alone (with assumed correspondent stenosis severity with catheter angiography) is usually presumed to be adequate.

CAROTID ULTRASONOGRAPHY

Sonography with Doppler has been used for many years to evaluate the carotid arteries. In fact, ultrasound interrogation of the carotid arteries predates the randomized trials in the 1980s comparing endarterectomy to medical management for carotid stenosis. Unlike the other noninvasive carotid imaging tests, ultrasound is very operator and technique dependent. A number of technical factors can affect the accuracy of carotid and Doppler sonography: Doppler angle, sample volume box, color Doppler sampling box, and color gain *(31)*. The extensive technical factors that are intrinsic to reliable image acquisition go beyond the scope of this chapter but should be considered when reviewing provided images.

The normal carotid wall appears hypoechoic on gray-scale imaging. An inner white line noted lining the inner margin of the wall is formed by the interface of the wall and the blood within the lumen. This sonographic morphology of the carotid wall is seen to greatest advantage in the common carotid artery (CCA) and to a lesser extent in the internal and external carotid arteries. Normally the thickness of the hyperechoic line is less than 0.9 mm. Increasing wall thickness is said to be the first sign of the development of atherosclerosis. Examples of carotid plaques are illustrated in Figs. 11, 12, 13, 14 and 15.

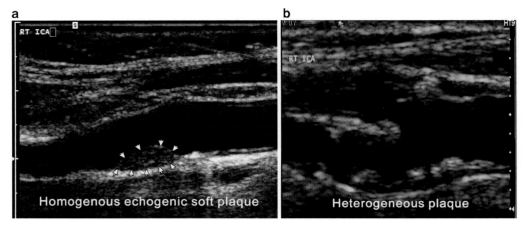

Fig. 11. (A) Soft plaque – homogeneous echogenicity of non-shadowing non-calcified plaque. **(B)** Heterogeneous plaque. *Gray-scale* ultrasound image shows a heterogeneous plaque in the proximal right ICA. Note the irregular surface of the plaque, which contains echogenic and echolucent areas. This type of plaque is considered unstable with the potential for inducing a transient ischemic attack or cerebrovascular accident.

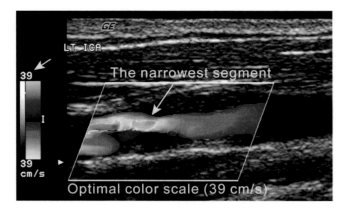

Fig. 12. Color Doppler image obtained with the optimal color scale setting showing the region of highest velocity, which corresponds to the narrowest segment of the ICA. Velocity sampling should be performed at this site.

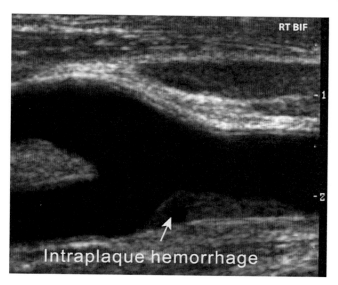

Fig. 13. Intraplaque hemorrhage – *gray-scale* ultrasound image shows a plaque containing an echo-poor area (*arrow*), which may be due to hemorrhage or lipids. In contrast to fat deposits, intraplaque hemorrhage is associated with a rapid increase in the size of the plaque.

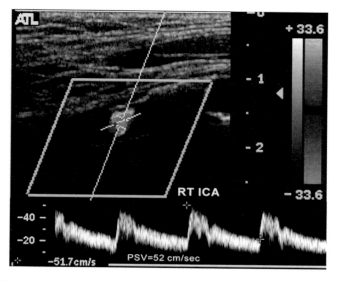

Fig. 14. Calcified shadowing plaque – pulsed-wave Doppler image of the right ICA obtained immediately distal to a circumferential shadowing. Plaque shows no sign of turbulence, and the PSV is within normal limits. Therefore, there is unlikely to be a significant stenosis behind the calcified plaque.

When performing carotid sonographic examinations, the technician needs to first distinguish the ICA from the external carotid artery (ECA). Like other parenchymal organs, the brain has a strikingly low arterial resistance with broad systolic peaks and well-maintained diastolic flow throughout the cardiac cycle *(32)*. The

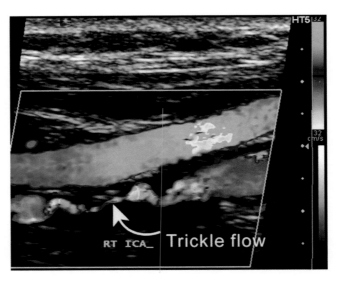

Fig. 15. Trickle flow in the ICA. Color Doppler image shows a narrow patent channel (the string sign) in the right ICA. This finding is suggestive of near occlusion of the ICA.

ECA supplies the scalp, muscles, and face, which have a higher resistance arterial flow. The ECA can also be distinguished as it is more anteromedially located and is smaller in size with multiple side branches.

Determination of carotid stenosis is estimated generally by both gray-scale and color Doppler. Peak systolic velocity (PSV) of the ICA and gray-scale assessment are felt to be the most accurate. If the degree of narrowing is indeterminate, then secondary parameters such as ICA/CCA ratios and ICA end-diastolic velocities (EDV) are considered. Sonographic features of severe ICA or CCA stenosis may include any of the following: PSV of greater than 230 cm/s, a significant amount of visible plaque (>50% lumen diameter reduction on a gray-scale image), color aliasing despite high color velocity setting (>100 cm/s), spectral broadening, post-stenotic turbulence, end-diastolic velocity greater than 100 cm/s, and ICA/CCA PSV ratio of greater than 4.0.

Given the limitations of duplex ultrasound (DUS) and the lack of standardization between laboratories, the Society of Radiologists in Ultrasound convened and produced a consensus document addressing the performance and interpretation of DUS *(32)*. They recommended that all carotid artery imaging should include gray-scale ultrasound, color Doppler, and spectral Doppler. There should be particular attention to obtain the Doppler waveform with an angle of insonation ≤60°. The sample volume should be placed at the area of greatest stenosis (at site of highest velocity). Furthermore, they recommend that the interpretation of stenosis severity should be based primarily on the ICA PSV and the presence of plaque on gray-scale or color Doppler. If the PSV is thought to be unreliable due to technical reasons, then the ICA/CCA ratio and ICA EDV may be used. The consensus document recommendation on classification of stenosis severity is shown in Table 1.

Table 1
The Society of Radiologists in Ultrasound Consensus for Carotid Artery
Stenosis Classification

Stenosis severity	PSV	Plaque visualization	ICA/CCA ratio	EDV
Normal	<125 cm/s	No plaque	<2.0	<40 cm/s
<50%	<125 cm/s	Intimal thickening or visible plaque ≤50%	<2.0	<40 cm/s
50–69%	125–230 cm/s	Visible plaque ≥50%	2.0–4.0	40–100 cm/s
≥70% to near occlusion	>230 cm/s	Narrowed lumen with plaque ≥50%	>4.0	>100 cm/s
Near occlusion	Undetectable, low, or high flow	Severely narrowed lumen	Variable	Variable
Total occlusion	No flow	No lumen	–	–

Adapted from (32).
CCA, common carotid artery; EDV, end-diastolic velocity; ICA, internal carotid artery; PSV, peak systolic velocity.

Other Applications for Carotid Sonography

The intimal media thickness (IMT) of the extracranial carotid arteries is a measurable index of the presence of atherosclerosis (33, 34). The IMT of the CCA is thought to be associated with risk factors for stroke. The bifurcation IMT and the presence of plaque are more directly associated with risk factors for ischemic heart disease (35). IMT measurements must be obtained fastidiously from gray-scale images, not color Doppler imaging. A high-frequency linear transducer with harmonics to reduce near-field artifacts should be used. Measurements can be taken at the near or far wall of the CCA or ICA with only the echogenic intima and echolucent media included in the measurement.

Plaque morphology can also be characterized by carotid ultrasound (imaging plaque location, internal characteristics, and surface features). Plaques can be characterized as homogeneous and heterogeneous. Homogeneous plaques may be fibrous or calcified and tend to have uniform internal architecture and a smooth surface contour. Heterogeneous plaques and ulcerated plaques are felt to be unstable or friable with the potential for embolic cerebrovascular events (36). These symptomatic plaques have lower calcium content but larger amounts of intraplaque hemorrhage and lipid, which makes them hypoechoic (36). Hypoechoic plaques are also more likely to be symptomatic (37).

Plaque ulceration may be detected by demonstrating eddy flow within the plaque depressions at color Doppler imaging (38). Color flow within plaque burden implies ulceration assuming other confounding artifacts like inappropriate color scale setting and motion are not present. It should be noted that color and power Doppler can be quite difficult or impossible in the setting of circumferential calcified plaque.

Carotid Near and Total Occlusion

As the distinction of near versus total carotid occlusion is clinically very important, the number of false-positive diagnoses of complete occlusion needs to be extremely low. A number of technical adaptations can be used to help discern these two entities; however, ultimately a confirmatory CT or MR angiogram is needed to confirm the diagnosis *(39, 40)*. The sonographic hallmark of near-total carotid occlusion is the "string sign" or "trickle flow" at color Doppler imaging. In a total ICA occlusion, on the other hand, there is a characteristic "to-and-fro" flow pattern with a "thud flow" appearance at color Doppler imaging. Other findings of carotid occlusion include direct visualization of thrombus at gray-scale imaging, absent flow at color Doppler imaging, and a damped resistive flow in the CCA at power Doppler imaging.

RECOMMENDATIONS REGARDING IMAGING

The work-up of suspected carotid artery stenosis should begin with ultrasound in an experienced and accredited laboratory. This is recommended due to the ready availability, the lack of ionizing radiation, the noninvasive nature, and the low cost of the test. If the ultrasound indicates a >70% lesion, and there is no suggestion of a tandem lesion on the basis of waveform, some actually advocate proceeding directly to surgery. However, given the multiple limitations of DUS, such practice may lead to unnecessary revascularization procedure. Moreover, there are often technical limitations like calcified shadowing plaque, deep course of the ICA, discordant gray-scale and contralateral disease that may make further imaging necessary. Although Doppler ultrasound in isolation is the most cost-effective presurgical algorithm, confirmation of a surgical lesion with MRA or CTA is usually prudent and often necessary.

The choice between CTA and MRA is not an absolute one. The decision often depends on the preference and strengths of the imaging department of the local hospital. CTA is the test of choice for patients post-carotid stenting and for those patients who cannot lie still. MRA is the test of choice if the patient has received iodinated contrast in the last 24 hours, has a known allergy to CT dye, and for those where thorough brain imaging is required. Assuming DUS and CTA/MRA are in agreement, there is felt to be little need for catheter angiography, unless of course the patient is undergoing carotid stenting (where catheter angiography will be performed as part of the procedure), as opposed to carotid endarterectomy.

REFERENCES

1. Higgins CB, Roos A. MRI and CT of the Cardiovascular System 2nd ed. Lippincott Williams & Wilkins. Philadelphia, PA; 2006.
2. Josephson SA, BryantSO, Mak HK, et al. Evaluation of carotid stenosis using CT angiography in the initial evaluation of stroke and TIA. Neurology 2004;63(3):457–460.
3. Nonent M, Serfaty JM, Nighossian N, et al. Concordance rate differences of three non-invasive imaging techniques to measure carotid stenosis in routine clinical practice. Stroke 2004;35:682.
4. Zuiderveld K. Visualisation of multimodality medical volume data using object oriented methods. Utrecht University, Utrecht, the Netherlands; 1995.

5. Tomandl B, Klotz E, et al. Comprehensive Imaging of Ischemic Stroke with Multidetector CT. Radiographics 2003;23:565–592.

6. Takahashi M, Ashtari M, Papp Z, et al. CCT angiography of carotid bifurcation: artefacts and pitfalls in shaded-surface display. AJR 1997;168:813–817.

7. Rubin GD, Beaulieu CF, Argiro V, et al. Perspective volume rendering of CT and MR images: applications for endoscopic imaging. Radiology 1996;199:321–330.

8. Anderson GB, Ashforth R, Steinke DE, et al. CT angiography for the detection and characterization of carotid artery bifurcation disease. Stroke 2000;31:2168–2174.

9. Zhang Z, Berg MH, Ikonen AE. Carotid artery stenosis: reproducibility of automated 3D CT angiography analysis method. Eur Radiol 2004;14(4):665–672.

10. Marcu CD, Ladam-Marcus VJ, et al. Carotid arterial stenosis: evaluation at CT Angiography with volume rendered technique. Radiology 1999;211: 775–780.

11. Anderson GB, Ashforth R, et al. CT Angiography for the detection and characterization of carotid artery bifurcation disease. Stroke 2000;31:2168–2174.

12. Katano H, Kato K, Umemura A, et al. Perioperative evaluation of carotid endarterectomy by 3-D CT angiography with refined reconstruction. Br J Neurosurg 2004;18(2):138–148.

13. Josephson SA, Bryant SO, et al Evaluation of carotid stenosis using CT angiography in the initial evaluation of stroke and TIA. Neurology 2004;63:457–460.

14. Walker LJ, Ismail A, McMeekin W, et al. Tomography angiography for the evaluation of carotid atherosclerotic plaque correlation with the histopathology of endarterectomy specimens. Stroke 2002;33:977.

15. Parker DL, Yuan C, Blatter DD. MR Angiography Multiple Thin Slab 3D Acquisition. Mag Reson Med 1991;17:434–451.

16. Rubinstein D. MR Imaging and the evaluation of extracranial carotid stenosis. AJR 1994;163: 1213–1214.

17. Leyendecker J, et al. Parallel MR Imaging: a user's guide. Radiographics 2005;25:1279–1297.

18. Prince MR, Arnoldus C, Frisoli JK. Nephrotoxicity of high-dose gadolinium compared with iodinated contrast. J Magn Reson Imaging 1996;6:162–166.

19. Murphy KP, Szopinski KT, Cohan RH, et al. Occurrence of adverse reactions to gadolinium-based contrast material and management of patient sat increased risk: a survey of the American Society of Neuroradiology Fellowship Directors. Acad Radiol 1999;6:656–664.

20. U.S. Food and Drug Administration Information for Health Professionals: Gadolinium-based contrast agents for magnetic resonance imaging (marketed as Magnevist, Multihance, Omniscan, Optimark, Prohance). Available at: http://www.fda.gov/cder/drug/Infosheets/HCP/gcca_200705HCP.pdf. Last update May 23,2007. Accessed July 24,2007.

21. Mendoza FA, Artlett CM, Sandorfi N, Latinis K, et al. Description of 12 cases of nephrogenic fibrosing dermopathy and review of the literature. Semin Arthritis Rheum 2006 Feb;35(4)208–210.

22. Kuo PH, Kanal E, et al. Gadolinium based MR contrast agents and nephrogenic systemic fibrosis. Radiology 2007;242:647–649.

23. Korogi Y, Takahashi M, Mabuchi N, et al. Intracranial vascular stenosis and occlusion: diagnostic accuracy of 3D, Fourier transform, TOF MR angiography. Radiology 1994;193: 187—193.

24. Nicholas GG, Osborne MA, Jaffe JW, et al. Carotid artery stenosis: preoperative evaluation in a community hospital. J Vascular Surg 1995;22:9–16.

25. Slosman F, Stolpen AH, et al. Gadolinium enhanced MR angiography of the carotid arteries. J Neuroimaging 1998;8:195–200.

26. Gagne PJ, Matchett J, Macfarland D, et al. Can the NASCET technique for measuring carotid stenosis be reliably applied outside the trial? J Vascular Surgery 1996;24:449–455.

27. Young GR, Sandercock PA, Slattery J, et al. Observer variation in the interpretation of intra-arterial angiograms and the risk of inappropriate decisions about carotid endarterectomy. J Neurol Neurosurg Psychiatry 1996;60:152–157.

28. Benes V, Netuka D, Mandys V, et al. Comparison between degree of carotid stenosis observed at angiography and histological examination. Acta Neurochir 2004;146(7):671–677.

29. Elgersma OE, Wust AFJ, et al. Multidirectional depiction of internal carotid artery stenosis: three-dimensional time-of-flight MR angiography versus rotational and conventional digital subtraction angiography. Radiology 2000;216:511–516.

30. Cloft HJ, Murphy KJ, et al. 3D Gadolinium enhanced MR angiography of the Carotid Arteries. Magn Reson Imaging 1996;14:593–600.

31. Tahmasepbour M, Cooperberg P, et al. Sonographic examination of the carotid arteries. Radiographics 2005;25:1561–1575.
32. Grant EG, Benson CB, et al. Carotid artery stenosis: gray scale and Doppler Ultrasound diagnosis-Society of Radiologists in Ultrasound Consensus Conference. Ultrasound Q; 2003:19(4):190–198.
33. O'Leary DH, Polak JF. Intima-media thickness: a tool for atherosclerosis imaging and event prediction. Am J Cardiol 2002;90:18L–21L.
34. Baldassarre D, Amato M, Bondioli A, et al. Carotid artery intima-media thickness measured by ultrasonography in normal clinical practice correlates well with atherosclerosis risk factors. Stroke 2000;31:2426–2430.
35. Ebrahim S, Papcosta O, Whincup P. Carotid plaque, intima-media thickness, cardiovascular risk factors, and prevalent cardiovascular disease in men and women. Stroke 1999;30:841–850.
36. Polak JF, Shemanski L, O'Leary DH, et al. Hypoechoic plaque at US of the carotid artery: an independent risk factor for incident stroke in adults aged 65 years or older. Radiology 1998; 208(3):649–654.
37. Sabetai MM, Tegos TJ, et al. Hemispheric symptoms and carotid plaque echomorphology. J Vascular Surgery 2000;31 (1):39–49.
38. Furst H, Hart WH, Jansen I, et al. Colour flow Doppler sonography in the identification of ulcerative plaques in patients with high-grade carotid artery stenosis. AJNR 1992;13:1581–1587.
39. Chen CJ, Lee TH, Tseng YC, et al. Multi-slice CT angiography in diagnosing total versus near occlusions of the internal carotid artery: comparison with catheter angiography. Stroke 2004; 35(1):83–85.
40. Masaryk TJ, Modic MT, Ruggiere PM, et al. Three-dimensional gradient-echo imaging of the carotid bifurcation: preliminary clinical experience. Radiology 1989;171:801–806.

III PATIENT AND OPERATOR PREPARATION FOR CAROTID STENTING

6 Pre-procedural Patient Preparation

Adil Al-Riyami, MD
and Jacqueline Saw, MD, FRCPC

CONTENTS

ABSTRACT

Carotid artery stenting is accepted as a less invasive alternative to carotid endarterectomy in high-risk patients. Careful patient preparation, examination, and documentation of their neurological status and outcomes are important for procedural safety. Optimizing medical therapy peri-procedurally, especially antiplatelet agents and anticoagulants, is paramount to CAS success.

Keywords: Neurological examination; NIH stroke scale; Antiplatelet therapy; Anticoagulation

INTRODUCTION

The pre-procedural management of patients prior to carotid artery stenting (CAS) is important to facilitate safe execution of the procedure. Prior to embarking on the procedure, the operator must review the patient's clinical history, physical examination, baseline carotid ultrasound, and noninvasive angiography (CT or MR angiography) in detail. Patients should fulfill the indications for carotid revascularization and lack contraindications for CAS (see Chapter 7). The procedure and its potential complications should be thoroughly explained to the patient. The

From: *Contemporary Cardiology: Carotid Artery Stenting: The Basics*
Edited by: J. Saw, DOI 10.1007/978-1-60327-314-5_6,
© Humana Press, a part of Springer Science+Business Media, LLC 2009

estimated 30-day death or stroke (major or minor) event rate is approximately 2–5%, and the estimated myocardial infarction (MI) event rate is 0–2% (see Chapter 14). The frequencies of other complications are listed in Chapter 14, Table 1. Although the reported major complications of death, stroke, and MI with CAS vary with different studies, it is generally lower in patients who were asymptomatic, considered low risk for surgery, and in whom emboli protection devices were used.

We will begin with a brief discussion of the pertinent neurological examination at baseline, followed by the management of medications peri-procedurally. The contemporary use of antiplatelet agents and anticoagulants with CAS will also be reviewed.

BASELINE NEUROLOGICAL EXAMINATION

The key objective of performing CAS is to decrease the incidence of future stroke events. Unfortunately, the procedure itself carries a small but significant risk of neurological complications mainly consequent to cerebral embolization. Fortunately, only a minute proportion of procedural embolization actually results in neurological deficits. In the study by Lacroix, among 60 patients who underwent carotid endarterectomy (CEA) and 61 patients who underwent CAS, although subclinical MRI-proven lesions occurred in 42.6% of patients, only 3.3% suffered clinical strokes *(1)*. Nevertheless, cerebral embolization is a frequent event and it is imperative that a quick but thorough neurological examination be performed before and after any carotid interventional procedure (including diagnostic carotid angiography). In fact, a neurological consult prior to and following the procedure is recommended.

The neurological examination should include assessment of

- Higher cerebral functions
- Cranial nerves
- Gross motor and sensory functions
- Reflexes and coordination

A detailed description of a comprehensive neurological examination is beyond the scope of this chapter; however, a concise neurological examination is described in Chapter 15. To facilitate comparisons between patients and between neurological status pre- and post-procedures, operators are encouraged to utilize scoring systems to record neurological status. Several scoring systems have been developed to aid communication between neurologists and neurosurgeons. These scoring systems help quantify functional disabilities after an adverse neurological event. These scores have been used in many studies and were found to correlate with stroke outcomes following a neurological event. When compared with several other scoring systems, the National Institute of Health Stroke Scale (NIHSS) score was found to best predict 3 month outcomes *(2)*.

NIH Stroke Scale

The clinical expert committee on CAS recommended using the NIH Stroke Scale score in patients undergoing carotid interventional procedures *(3)*. The NIHSS score should be ascertained before the procedure, immediately after the procedure, and 24 h later. It should also be re-evaluated whenever a change in neurological status is suspected.

The NIHSS includes a series of 15-item detailed questions and tasks that the patient has to follow (Table 1). These tasks evaluate all the higher mental, motor, and sensory functions listed above, specifically the level of consciousness, language, extraocular movement, visual field loss, motor strength, ataxia, dysarthria, sensory loss, and neglect. Each task is scored from 3 to 5 grades, with 0 being normal, and the maximum worse score is 42.

Table 1
NIH Stroke Scale Scoring System

NIH Stroke Scale	Record score in the order listed, do not go back and change scores. Test should take 5–8 min
(1a) Level of consciousness	0 = Alert; keenly responsive 1 = Not alert; but arousable by minor stimulation to obey, answer, or respond 2 = Not alert; requires repeated stimulation to attend, or is obtunded and requiresstrong or painful stimulation to make movements (not stereotyped) 3 = Responds only with reflex motor or autonomic effects or totally unresponsive, flaccid, and areflexic
(1b) Level of consciousness questions: Patient is asked age and the month. Patients unable to speak (unless due to aphasia) are given score of 1	0 = Answers both questions correctly 1 = Answers one question correctly 2 = Answers neither question correctly
(1c) Level of consciousness commands: Patient is asked to open and close the eyes and then to grip and release the non-paretic hand. Other one-step commands okay	0 = Performs both tasks correctly 1 = Performs one task correctly 2 = Performs neither task correctly
(2) Best gaze: Test horizontal eye movements only	0 = Normal 1 = Partial gaze palsy; gaze is abnormal in one or both eyes, but forced deviation or total gaze paresis is not present 2 = Forced deviation or total gaze paresis not overcome by the oculocephalic maneuver
(3) Visual: Testing visual fields by confrontation, using finger counting or visual threats	0 = No visual loss 1 = Partial hemianopia 2 = Complete hemianopia 3 = Bilateral hemianopia (blind including cortical blindness)

(Continued)

Table 1
(Continued)

NIH Stroke Scale	Record score in the order listed, do not go back and change scores. Test should take 5–8 min
(4) Facial palsy: Ask patient to show teeth or raise eyebrows and close eyes	0 = Normal symmetrical movements 1 = Minor paralysis (flattened nasolabial fold, asymmetry on smiling) 2 = Partial paralysis (total or near-total paralysis of lower face) 3 = Complete paralysis of one or both sides (absence of facial movement in the upper and lower face)
(5) Motor arm: Test for arm drifting (at 90° if sitting, or 45° if supine). Drift is scored if arm falls within 10 s	0 = No drift; limb holds 90° (or 45°) for full 10 s 1 = Drift; limb holds 90° (or 45°), but drifts down before full 10 s; does not hit bed or other support 2 = Some effort against gravity; limb cannot get to or maintain (if cued) 90° (or 45°), drifts down to bed, but has some effort against gravity 3 = No effort against gravity; limb falls 4 = No movement UN = Amputation or joint fusion, explain: _____ 5a. Left arm 5b. Right arm
(6) Motor leg: Test drift in legs by holding the leg at 30° (always tested supine). Drift is scored if the leg falls before 5 s	1 = Drift; leg falls by the end of the 5-s period but does not hit bed 2 = Some effort against gravity; leg falls to bed by 5 s, but has some effort against gravity 3 = No effort against gravity; leg falls to bed immediately 4 = No movement UN = Amputation or joint fusion, explain: _____ 6a. Left leg 6b. Right leg
(7) Limb ataxia: Perform the finger–nose–finger and heel–shin tests on both sides, and ataxia is scored only if present out of proportion to weakness	0 = Absent 1 = Present in one limb 2 = Present in two limbs UN = Amputation or joint fusion, explain: _____
(8) Sensory: Test sensation or grimace to pinprick, or withdrawal from noxious stimulus in the obtunded or aphasic patient	0 = Normal; no sensory loss 1 = Mild-to-moderate sensory loss; patient feels pinprick is less sharp or is dull on the affected side; or there is a loss of superficial pain with pinprick, but patient is aware of being touched 2 = Severe to total sensory loss; patient is not aware of being touched in the face, arm, and leg

(Continued)

**Table 1
(Continued)**

NIH Stroke Scale	*Record score in the order listed, do not go back and change scores. Test should take 5–8 min*
(9) Best language: Patient is asked to describe what is happening in the attached picture, to name the items on the attached naming sheet, and to read from the attached list of sentences. See items on www.ninds.nih.gov web site	0 = No aphasia; normal 1 = Mild-to-moderate aphasia; some obvious loss of fluency or facility of comprehension, without significant limitation on ideas expressed or form of expression. Reduction of speech and/or comprehension, however, makes conversation about provided materials difficult or impossible. For example, in conversation about provided materials, examiner can identify picture or naming card content from patient's response 2 = Severe aphasia; all communication is through fragmentary expression; great need for inference, questioning, and guessing by the listener. Range of information that can be exchanged is limited; listener carries burden of communication. Examiner cannot identify materials provided from patient response 3 = Mute, global aphasia; no usable speech or auditory comprehension
(10) Dysarthria: Patient asked to read or repeat words from the attached list. See items on www.ninds.nih.gov web site	0 = Normal 1 = Mild-to-moderate dysarthria; patient slurs at least some words and, at worst, can be understood with some difficulty 2 = Severe dysarthria; patient's speech is so slurred as to be unintelligible in the absence of or out of proportion to any dysphasia, or is mute/anarthric UN = Intubated or other physical barrier, explain:_____
(11) Extinction and inattention (formerly neglect): Simultaneously touch patients bilaterally, and test both visual fields concurrently	0 = No abnormality 1 = Visual, tactile, auditory, spatial, or personal inattention or extinction to bilateral simultaneous stimulation in one of the sensory modalities 2 = Profound hemi-inattention or extinction to more than one modality; does not recognize own hand or orients to only one side of space

Adapted from www.ninds.nih.gov.

ADJUSTING MEDICATIONS PRIOR TO THE PROCEDURE

Patients presenting for carotid revascularization are typically on several classes of medications for concomitant diseases. Several of these medications should be adjusted prior to CAS and can be classified into two categories. The first category pertains to generic medications that should be withheld or adjusted prior to any invasive procedure utilizing parenteral contrast agents (e.g., coronary angiography, contrast CT scans, carotid angiography). The second category is specific for carotid artery interventions.

Medication Adjustment Prior to Contrast Agents Use

Medications that can worsen renal function and the risk of contrast-induced nephropathy (CIN) include aminoglycoside antibiotics, anti-cancer rejection medications, and non-steroidal anti-inflammatory drugs (NSAIDs). These medications should be withheld whenever possible. Angiotensin-converting enzyme inhibitors (ACEI) can be continued but should not be started or the dose increased peri-procedurally until renal function has stabilized. Adequate hydration is important in preventing CIN, but the decision to withhold diuretics should be made on an individual patient basis.

The role of oral *N*-acetyl cysteine (NAC) in preventing CIN remains controversial; however, many interventionalists routinely administer it peri-procedurally as it is considered harmless. Typically, NAC 600 mg twice daily is given the day before and the day of the procedure for a total of four doses. There are conflicting data regarding the efficacy of this regimen, with some studies showing marked improvement *(4)* while others show no benefit *(5, 6)*. Higher doses of NAC (1,200 mg) may provide added protection to hydration with normal saline. In addition, the use of low-osmolarity or iso-osmolar non-ionic contrast media in patients with moderate to severe renal dysfunction (creatinine >2.5 mg/dl or >220 μmol/l) receiving large doses of contrast media (>140 ml) *(7)* may reduce the incidence of CIN.

Although metformin does not increase the risk of CIN, it has the potential of causing lactic acidosis should renal dysfunction occurs. If renal function is normal prior to the procedure, metformin should be withheld the day of the procedure and resumed 48 h post-procedure if renal function remains normal. If renal function is abnormal prior to the procedure, then metformin should be withheld 48 h prior to the procedure and resumed 48 h post-procedure if renal function remains unchanged *(8)*.

Major bleeding events can be life threatening in percutaneous invasive procedures. Access site bleeding has been extensively documented with percutaneous coronary interventions (PCI), and such data can be extrapolated to CAS procedures with the same precautions observed. Overall, access site bleeding has been reported in 3% of CAS procedures *(9)*. For patients on warfarin pre-procedure, it should be withheld for 3–5 days to achieve an INR < 2.0 prior to CAS. If withholding anticoagulation is not feasible (e.g., high-risk mechanical valves), bridging with heparin is recommended to minimize the duration of anticoagulation.

Medication Adjustment Prior to Carotid Intervention

The neurological status of a patient can be affected by central nervous system medications that can cause drowsiness or excitation. These centrally acting medications should not be started or their doses increased prior to the interventional procedure. Mild sedatives such as benzodiazepines can be administered to alleviate the anxiety associated with CAS; however, its use is usually avoided as prompt recognition of the neurological status throughout the procedure is imperative. Stronger sedatives should not be used for the same reason.

Hemodynamic depression in the form of reflex bradycardia and hypotension commonly occurs when balloon dilatation of the carotid bulb is performed. This is usually transient and resolves spontaneously. Medications that act by increasing atrioventricular (AV) nodal blockade such as beta-blockers and non-dihydropyridine calcium channel blockers can theoretically increase the incidence and duration of this reaction. On the other hand, withholding such medications could result in reflex tachycardia and hypertension, which has been associated with increased risk of adverse outcomes in CAS *(10)*. In fact, in a multivariate analysis by Gupta et al. which aimed at identifying the predictors of hemodynamic compromise during CAS, the use of beta-blockers did not have an effect on the development of hemodynamic depression. Therefore, there are no specific recommendations regarding withholding AV-blocking agents at this point *(11)*.

USE OF ANTIPLATELET AGENTS PRIOR TO AND FOLLOWING CAS

Aspirin

Acetylsalicylic acid (ASA) is the most commonly used antiplatelet medication. It acts by irreversibly inhibiting cyclooxygenase enzyme required for the production of thromboxane A2 from arachidonic acid. Thromboxane A2 stimulates platelets, eventually leading to the formation of a platelet-rich thrombus. The use of aspirin has been demonstrated to prevent strokes in patients with previous strokes and in those who are at high risk for stroke. In addition, the benefit of using aspirin in carotid intervention was realized early in the surgical literature *(12)*.

Endothelial injury resulting from expanding a stent in a diseased vessel stimulates platelet-rich thrombus formation with potential downstream showering and embolic strokes. This was known early in the development of angioplasty techniques *(13)*. It is recommended that aspirin 75–325 mg be started at least 4 days prior to the stent procedure and continued indefinitely in the absence of contraindications. Higher doses of aspirin are not recommended since it does not confer any added protection, but may instead cause more side effects *(14)*.

Thienopyridines

The thienopyridines inhibit platelets via a different pathway from aspirin. They inhibit platelet aggregation by irreversibly blocking ADP receptors on the platelet surface. The first thienopyridine to be developed was ticlopidine. However, clopidogrel is now the agent that is almost exclusively used given its safety profile. Ticlopidine unfortunately causes severe but reversible neutropenia in <1% of patients *(15)* and thrombotic thrombocytopenia purpura in <0.1% *(16)*. Clopidogrel was shown to be superior to aspirin alone in preventing ischemic events in the CAPRIE (Clopidogrel versus Aspirin in Patients at Risk for Ischemic Events) and CURE (Clopidogrel in Unstable angina to prevent Recurrent Events) trials and to be comparable in efficacy to ticlopidine plus aspirin *(17)*. In the CURE trial, the addition of clopidogrel to aspirin resulted in a non-significant 14% reduction in stroke risk for acute coronary syndrome patients.

Prasugrel is a novel thienopyridine that is more potent than the above-mentioned agents. It is also more efficacious against recurrent ischemic events in patients with acute coronary syndrome undergoing percutaneous coronary interventions *(18)*. However, it was associated with more bleeding events, and its role in CAS has not been evaluated.

The use of dual antiplatelet therapy has been adopted early in CAS practices. The use of a thienopyridine (ticlopidine or clopidogrel) in addition to aspirin has been studied in a registry of 162 consecutive patients undergoing CAS. Clopidogrel was found to be superior to ticlopidine in preventing the composite 30-day rate of death, stroke, transient ischemic attack, and MI in this study (4.3 versus 13%) *(19)*. Furthermore, dual antiplatelet therapy did not increase the incidence of intracranial hemorrhage in these patients. Therefore, it is routinely recommended that patients be started on dual antiplatelet therapy prior to CAS using aspirin and clopidogrel *(20)*. However, there are clinicians who question whether this regimen is superior to aspirin plus extended-release dipyridamole *(21)*. Nevertheless, the 2007 clinical expert consensus document on carotid stenting recommends 300–600 mg loading dose of clopidogrel followed by 75 mg daily for at least 4 days prior to the procedure, in conjunction with aspirin *(3)*.

The combination of heparin and aspirin (intravenous heparin for 24 h, and aspirin indefinitely) was found to increase the risk of bleeding (4 versus 2%) and stent thrombosis (2 versus 0%) compared to the combination of ticlopidine and aspirin (both agents for 30 days, then aspirin indefinitely) following CAS *(22)*. Therefore, dual antiplatelet therapy remains the preferred therapy compared to prolonged heparin infusion for CAS.

The duration of continuing dual antiplatelet therapy post-CAS has not been specifically studied. Nonetheless, extrapolating from coronary stenting literature, it seems reasonable to continue dual antiplatelet therapy for at least 30 days. Certainly, premature discontinuation of one or both antiplatelet drugs can result in subacute thrombosis of the newly placed stent *(23)*. In the study by Bhatt et al. *(18)*, clopidogrel was continued for 4 weeks in addition to aspirin. In the PCI-CURE and CREDO (Clopidogrel for the Reduction of Events During Observation) studies, continuation of dual antiplatelet therapy beyond 30 days resulted in further reduction in the occurrence of cardiovascular events in patients with coronary artery disease. The CHARISMA (Clopidogrel for High Atherothrombotic Risk and Ischemic Stabilization, Management, and Avoidance) trial, which included high atherothrombotic risk patients, showed no benefit of long-term dual antiplatelet therapy (median 28 months), but with increased risk of bleeding *(24)*. However, in a prespecified subgroup analysis of CHARISMA, there was a reduction in stroke with the dual antiplatelet regimen. Furthermore, patients with established prior MI, ischemic stroke, or symptomatic peripheral arterial disease (CAPRIE-like population) may also benefit from long-term dual antiplatelet therapy *(25)*. Whether long-term dual antiplatelet therapy in patients undergoing CAS will continue protection against adverse neurological outcomes remains to be studied.

USE OF ANTICOAGULANTS WITH CAS

Use of Unfractionated Heparin (UFH)

As with coronary stenting procedures, the use of anticoagulation during CAS is mandatory. Heparin binds with circulating anti-thrombin causing a conformational change, rendering it a 1000 times more active in inhibiting thrombin, which is a key element in thrombus formation. UFH should be administered at an initial dose of 50 units/kg intravenous bolus, and then supplemented with extra boluses to achieve a peak activated clotting time (ACT) between 250 and 300 s. Inadequate anticoagulation with too low an ACT may cause acute thrombosis of the deployed stent and of the embolic protection device. Over anticoagulation may result in bleeding complications at the access site, intracranial hemorrhage, and need for blood transfusions. In a retrospective analysis of 605 patients who underwent CAS procedures at the Cleveland Clinic Foundation who had peak ACT documented during the procedure, there was a U-shaped relationship between ACT and adverse outcomes (Fig. 1). A peak ACT between 250 and 299 s was associated with a 72.1% lower combined event rate of death, stroke, or MI at 30 days compared with an ACT of 300–350 s *(26)*. This protective effect of achieving an ACT of 250–299 s was especially noted when glycoprotein (GP) IIb/IIIa inhibitors were not used (HR 0.14 versus 0.64 with GP IIb/IIIa inhibitors).

Use of Low Molecular Weight Heparins (LMWH)

UFH remains the preferred choice in most interventional procedures given its low cost, the ability to monitor the degree of anticoagulation with a bedside ACT, and the complete reversibility with protamine sulfate. However, a significant proportion of interventional laboratories have started using low molecular weight heparins (LMWH) or direct thrombin inhibitors as anticoagulants, particularly for coronary procedures. Several trials evaluating the use of LMWH in coronary interventions have been conducted, and these showed that LMWH with or without concomitant GP IIb/IIIa inhibitors administered during PCI were comparable to that of UFH *(27)*. The largest study of UFH versus LMWH was the SYNERGY (Superior Yield of the New strategy of Enoxaparin, Revascularization and Glycoprotein IIb/IIIa Inhibitors) trial in which 10,027 patients with acute coronary

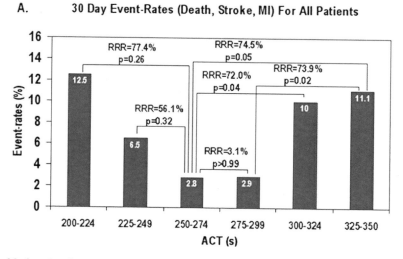

Fig. 1. The 30-day death, stroke, or myocardial infarction event rate of patients who underwent carotid artery stenting with unfractionated heparin, showing a U-shaped relationship between adverse outcomes and ACT. Printed with permission from *(26)*.

syndrome were randomly assigned to open-labeled UFH or enoxaparin. There was no difference in the primary outcome of all-cause death or nonfatal MI during the first 30 days after randomization and secondary outcomes of ischemic events with PCI *(28)*.

One of the key concerns regarding the use of LMWH with interventional procedures is the occurrence of catheter and equipment thrombosis, and acute vessel thrombosis and closure. There have been several reports of these complications in the literature even despite therapeutic anti-Xa levels in some of these cases *(29, 30)*. In the study by Dana et al., macroscopic thrombus was observed on PCI equipment in 6 of 122 patients (5%) who underwent PCI within 8 h of subcutaneous heparin. This occurred despite all patients having documented therapeutic anti-factor-Xa levels at the time of PCI and despite pretreatment with aspirin and clopidogrel *(29)*. This relatively infrequent but potentially catastrophic complication with LMWH use during PCI has diminished the acceptance of LMWH as the sole anticoagulant for PCI. Given this limitation, and the paucity of literature on LMWH use in CAS, it is not recommended to routinely administer LMWH as the sole anticoagulant with CAS.

Direct Thrombin Inhibitors

Direct thrombin inhibitors, mainly bivalirudin, have also been used as alternatives to heparin plus GP IIb/IIIa inhibitors for coronary stenting. In the ACUITY (Acute Catheterization and Urgent Intervention Triage strategY) trial, bivalirudin was compared to heparin plus GP IIb/IIIa inhibitors in patients with acute coronary syndrome undergoing coronary interventions. Bivalirudin was equivalent to the combination therapy in preventing adverse ischemic events with a significant reduction in bleeding *(31)*.

There are limited data on the use of bivalirudin with CAS procedures, although interventionalists have become increasingly familiar with this agent through their use with PCI procedures, and hence extrapolated its efficacy and safety to carotid procedures. Lin et al. described a retrospective analysis of their single-center experience with 200 CAS procedures in 186 consecutive patients *(32)*. They compared the results and complications of the first 50 cases with the second, third, and fourth groups of 50 cases of CAS. Bivalirudin was used instead of intravenous heparin after the first 54 patients. They attributed the significantly lower hemorrhagic complications (0 versus 6%) in the latter 100 patients to bivalirudin use. There are, however, several factors to be taken into account. First, the heparin bolus used (100 units/kg) was higher than what is typically used (50 units/kg). Second, they did not report the peak ACT in their analysis, a major factor in bleeding complications as previously mentioned. Third, the bleeding complications could also have been a result of the increased experience gained by the operators in performing more CAS procedures. And lastly, the peri-procedural control of hypertension and other hemodynamic controls has changed during that period.

In another study, Folmar et al. performed 42 CAS procedures via the radial approach with the use of procedural bivalirudin *(33)*. Procedural success was 83% with only one stroke event 24 h after the procedure. Given these limited data, larger prospective and randomized trials will be necessary to evaluate the efficacy and safety of bivalirudin in comparison to UFH for CAS.

Use of Glycoprotein IIb/IIIa Inhibitors

The use of GP IIb/IIIa inhibitors in coronary interventions had been extensively studied in randomized trials and was shown to reduce adverse ischemic outcomes. In contrast, their use in CAS procedures had only been evaluated in a few small studies. Kapadia et al. reported on the use of abciximab in 128 patients undergoing CAS at the Cleveland Clinic. These patients were compared to 23 patients who did not receive adjuvant abciximab. The rate of procedural events was less frequent in the abciximab group compared to the control group (1.6 versus 8%) *(34)*. This experience, though, was not replicated in other studies and large registries where the reduction in ischemic events was counterbalanced by an increase in intracerebral bleeding *(35, 36)*. In a small prospective randomized study involving 74 consecutive patients undergoing CAS, abciximab was administered to half the patients. The incidence of ischemic complications was not different between the two groups (19% abciximab group versus 8% control group, $P>0.05$).

At this juncture, routine use of GP IIb/IIIa inhibitors is not recommended with CAS. Larger prospective randomized studies are needed to identify subsets of patients who may benefit from GP IIb/IIIa inhibitors during CAS and the optimal dosing to reduce the bleeding complications inherent to the addition of these agents.

CONCLUSION

Carotid artery stenting is an accepted less invasive alternative to carotid endarterectomy in high-risk patients. Careful patient preparation, examination, and documentation of their neurological status and outcomes are important to enable comparison with carotid endarterectomy. Optimizing antiplatelet and anticoagulant therapy with CAS is paramount to inhibit platelets to reduce peri-procedural ischemic events, without compromising safety with respect to bleeding complications.

REFERENCES

1. Lacroix V, Hammer F, Astarci P, Duprez T, Grandin C, Cosnard G, Peeters A, Verhelst R. Ischemic cerebral lesions after carotid surgery and carotid stenting. Eur J Vasc Endovasc Surg 2007;33(4):430–435.
2. Muir KW, Weir CJ, Murray GD, Povey C, Lees KR. Comparison of neurological scales and scoring systems for acute stroke prognosis. Stroke 1996;27:1817–1820.
3. Bates ER, Babb JD, Casey DE, Jr, et al. ACCF/SCAI/SVMB/SIR/ASITN 2007 clinical expert consensus document on carotid stenting: a report of the American College of Cardiology Foundation Task Force on Clinical Expert Consensus Documents (ACCF/SCAI/SVMB/SIR/ASITN Clinical Expert Consensus Document Committee on Carotid Stenting). J Am Coll Cardiol 2007;49:126–170.
4. Tepel M, van der Giet M, Schwarzfeld C, Laufer U, Liermann D, Zidek W. Prevention of radiographic-contrast-agent-induced reductions in renal function by acetylcysteine. N Engl J Med 2000;343:180–184.
5. Webb JG, Pate GE, Humphries KH, Buller CE, Shalansky S, Al Shamari A, Sutander A, Williams T, Fox RS, Levin A. A randomized controlled trial of intravenous N-acetylcysteine for the prevention of contrast-induced nephropathy after cardiac catheterization: lack of effect. Am Heart J 2004;148(3), 422–429.
6. Hoffmann U, Fischereder M, Kruger B, Drobnik W, Kramer BK. The value of N-acetylcysteine in the prevention of radiocontrast agent-induced nephropathy seems questionable. J Am Soc Nephrol 2004;15:407–410.
7. Briguori C, Colombo A, Violante A, et al. Standard vs double dose of N-acetylcysteine to prevent contrast agent associated nephrotoxicity. Eur Heart J 2004;25:206–211.

8. Thomsen HS, Morcos SK. Contrast media and metformin: guidelines to diminish the risk of lactic acidosis in non-insulin-dependent diabetics after administration of contrast media. ESUR Contrast Media Safety Committee. Eur Radiol 1999;9:738–740.

9. Taha MM, Sakaida H, Asakura F, et al. Access site complications with carotid angioplasty and stenting. Surg Neurol 2007;68:431–437.

10. Abou-Chebl A, Yadav JS, Reginelli JP, Bajzer C, Bhatt D, Krieger DW. Intracranial hemorrhage and hyperperfusion syndrome following carotid artery stenting: risk factors, prevention, and treatment. J Am Coll Cardiol 2004;43(9):1596–1601.

11. Gupta R, Abou-Chebl A, Bajzer CT, Schumacher HC, Yadav JS. Rate, predictors, and consequences of hemodynamic depression after carotid artery stenting. J Am Coll Cardiol 2006;47:1538–1543.

12. Edwards WH, Edwards WH, Jr, Mulherin JL, Jr, Jenkins JM. The role of antiplatelet drugs in carotid reconstructive surgery. Ann Surg 1985;201:765–770.

13. Murray PD, Garnic JD, Bettmann MA. Pharmacology of angioplasty and intravascular thrombolysis. AJR Am J Roentgenol 1982;139:795–803.

14. Collaborative meta-analysis of randomized trials of antiplatelet therapy for prevention of death, myocardial infarction, and stroke in high risk patients. BMJ 2002; 324:71–86.

15. Hass WK, Easton JD, Adams HP, Jr, et al. A randomized trial comparing ticlopidine hydrochloride with aspirin for the prevention of stroke in high-risk patients. Ticlopidine Aspirin Stroke Study Group. N Engl J Med 1989;321:501–507.

16. Bennett CL, Davidson CJ, Raisch DW, Weinberg PD, Bennett RH, Feldman MD. Thrombotic thrombocytopenic purpura associated with ticlopidine in the setting of coronary artery stents and stroke prevention. Arch Intern Med 1999;159:2524–2528.

17. Bertrand ME, Rupprecht HJ, Urban P, Gershlick AH. Double-blind study of the safety of clopidogrel with and without a loading dose in combination with aspirin compared with ticlopidine in combination with aspirin after coronary stenting: the clopidogrel aspirin stent international cooperative study (CLASSICS). Circulation 2000;102:624–629.

18. Wiviott SD, Braunwald E, McCabe CH, et al. Prasugrel versus clopidogrel in patients with acute coronary syndromes. N Engl J Med 2007;357:2001–2015.

19. Bhatt DL, Kapadia SR, Bajzer CT, et al. Dual antiplatelet therapy with clopidogrel and aspirin after carotid artery stenting. J Invasive Cardiol 2001;13:767–771.

20. Chaturvedi S, Yadav JS. The role of antiplatelet therapy in carotid stenting for ischemic stroke prevention. Stroke 2006;37:1572–1577.

21. Kramer J, Abraham J, Teven CM, Jones PA. Role of antiplatelets in carotid artery stenting. Stroke 2007;38:14.

22. Dalainas I, Nano G, Bianchi P, Stegher S, Malacrida G, Tealdi DG. Dual antiplatelet regime versus acetyl-acetic acid for carotid artery stenting. Cardiovasc Intervent Radiol 2006;29:519–521.

23. Buhk JH, Wellmer A, Knauth M. Late in-stent thrombosis following carotid angioplasty and stenting. Neurology 2006;66:1594–1596.

24. Bhatt DL, Fox KA, Hacke W, et al. Clopidogrel and aspirin versus aspirin alone for the prevention of atherothrombotic events. N Engl J Med 2006;354:1706–1717.

25. Bhatt DL, Flather MD, Hacke W, et al. Patients with prior myocardial infarction, stroke, or symptomatic peripheral arterial disease in the CHARISMA trial. J Am Coll Cardiol 2007;49:1982–1988.

26. Saw J, Bajzer C, Casserly IP, et al. Evaluating the optimal activated clotting time during carotid artery stenting. Am J Cardiol 2006;97:1657–1660.

27. Wong GC, Giugliano RP, Antman EM. Use of low-molecular-weight heparins in the management of acute coronary artery syndromes and percutaneous coronary intervention. JAMA 2003;289:331–342.

28. Ferguson JJ, Califf RM, Antman EM, et al. Enoxaparin vs unfractionated heparin in high-risk patients with non-ST-segment elevation acute coronary syndromes managed with an intended early invasive strategy: primary results of the SYNERGY randomized trial. JAMA 2004;292: 45–54.

29. Buller CE, Pate GE, Armstrong PW, O'Neill BJ, Webb JG, Gallo R, Welsh RC. Catheter thrombosis during primary percutaneous coronary intervention for acute ST elevation myocardial infarction despite subcutaneous low-molecular-weight heparin, acetylsalicylic acid, clopidogrel and abciximab pretreatment. Can J Cardiol. 2006 May 1;22(6):511–515.

30. Dana A, Nguyen CM, Cloutier S, Barbeau GR. Dana Macroscopic thrombus formation on angioplasty equipment following antithrombin therapy with enoxaparin. Catheter Cardiovasc Interv. 2007 Nov 15;70(6):847–853.

31. Stone GW, McLaurin BT, Cox DA, et al. Bivalirudin for patients with acute coronary syndromes. N Engl J Med 2006;355:2203–2216.
32. Lin PH, Bush RL, Peden EK, et al. Carotid artery stenting with neuroprotection: assessing the learning curve and treatment outcome. Am J Surg 2005;190(6):850–857.
33. Folmar J, Sachar R, Mann T. Transradial approach for carotid artery stenting: a feasibility study. Cath Cardiovasc Interv 2007;69:355–361.
34. Kapadia SR, Bajzer CT, Ziada KM, et al. Initial experience of platelet glycoprotein IIb/IIIa inhibition with abciximab during carotid stenting: a safe and effective adjunctive therapy. Stroke 2001;32:2328–2332.
35. Qureshi AI, Suri MF, Ali Z, et al. Carotid angioplasty and stent placement: a prospective analysis of perioperative complications and impact of intravenously administered abciximab. Neurosurgery 2002;50:466–473; discussion 73–75.
36. Zahn R, Ischinger T, Hochadel M, et al. Glycoprotein IIb/IIIa antagonists during carotid artery stenting: results from the carotid artery stenting (CAS) registry of the Arbeitsgemeinschaft Leitende Kardiologische Krankenhausarzte (ALKK). Clin Res Cardiol 2007;96:730–737.

7 Patient Selection for Carotid Stenting

Juhana Karha, MD
and Deepak L. Bhatt, MD, MPH, FACC

CONTENTS

ABSTRACT

The goal in treating carotid artery atherosclerotic disease is to reduce the risk of stroke. Three therapeutic options for management of carotid disease exist: medical therapy, carotid artery stenting, and carotid endarterectomy. Clinical and anatomic characteristics of the individual patient dictate which of these options should be chosen. This chapter will review the indications and contraindications to carotid artery stenting.

Keywords: Indications; Contraindications; Reimbursement; Training requirement; Credentialing

INTRODUCTION

The goal in treating carotid artery atherosclerotic disease is to reduce the risk of stroke. Three therapeutic options for management of carotid disease exist: medical therapy, carotid artery stenting (CAS), and carotid endarterectomy (CEA). Clinical

From: *Contemporary Cardiology: Carotid Artery Stenting: The Basics*
Edited by: J. Saw, DOI 10.1007/978-1-60327-314-5_7,
© Humana Press, a part of Springer Science+Business Media, LLC 2009

and anatomic characteristics of the individual patient dictate which of these options should be chosen. Certainly, even if a revascularization procedure is performed, medical therapy with antiplatelet and cholesterol-lowering medications remains critically important.

In contemplating carotid revascularization, it is important to recognize that the annual stroke risk with a severe carotid artery stenosis is 2–4% in the absence of symptoms, and in excess of 10% if the patient has sustained a recent stroke or transient ischemic attack (TIA). These risk levels serve as benchmarks that cannot be exceeded as one considers an invasive revascularization procedure.

The question about choosing between medical therapy, CAS, and CEA can be framed by considering the following variables: (1) the patient's symptomatic status and the severity of the carotid lesion, (2) the presence of clinical features that increase the risk of the procedure (the so-called high-risk features), and (3) the stroke rate associated with the procedure. Patients with symptoms of anterior circulation ischemia of the corresponding hemisphere, either a stroke or a TIA, stand to gain more from revascularization compared to asymptomatic patients with a similar diameter carotid stenosis. A multitude of clinical variables may place a patient at high risk for one procedure, thus making the other procedure the preferred approach.

ATHEROTHROMBOTIC RISK PROFILE IN PATIENTS WITH CEREBROVASCULAR DISEASE

It is important to note that patients with cerebrovascular disease have many of the conventional atherothrombotic risk factors. The international Reduction of Atherothrombosis for Continued Health (REACH) registry included 18,843 patients with cerebrovascular disease *(1)*. These patients from 44 different countries had a high prevalence of diabetes mellitus (37.4%), hypertension (83.3%), dyslipidemia (58.2%), obesity or overweight status (63.1%), and either former or current tobacco use (52.9%) *(1)*. Reflecting the importance of a global approach to a patient with cerebrovascular disease, 40% of the REACH registry patients with cerebrovascular disease also had either coronary artery disease or peripheral arterial disease *(1)*. Unfortunately, many of these 18,843 patients were not being treated for their risk factors: 18.2% were not treated with an antiplatelet agent, 38.7% were not treated with a lipid-lowering agent, 5.9% of those with elevated blood pressure did not receive anti-hypertensive therapy, and 17.8% of the diabetics did not receive medical therapy for diabetes mellitus *(1)*. It appears that having undergone a CEA increases the likelihood for a patient to be receiving antiplatelet agents and statin drugs *(2)*. It is encouraging that the revascularization procedure may in the real world practice provide an opportunity for the health care professionals and the patient to institute these important therapies.

The 1-year data from the REACH registry highlight the very high incidence of adverse cardiovascular outcomes among patients with cerebrovascular disease. The 1-year event rate of a combined end point of cardiovascular death, myocardial infarction, or stroke was 6.47%, and if this end point also included hospitalization for an atherothrombotic event, the rate was even higher at 14.53% *(3)*.

CAROTID ENDARTERECTOMY

Initial studies evaluating the efficacy of carotid artery revascularization were the North American Symptomatic Carotid Endarterectomy Trial (NASCET) *(4, 5)*, European Carotid Surgery Trial (ECST) *(6, 7)*, Asymptomatic Carotid Atherosclerotic Study (ACAS) *(8)*, and Asymptomatic Carotid Surgery Trial (ACST) *(9)* (Table 1). The NASCET and ECST studies showed that CEA was superior to medical therapy among symptomatic patients with a carotid stenosis of 51–99% *(5, 7)*. A pooled analysis of 6,092 of these patients revealed a 28% relative risk reduction in the incidence of ipsilateral stroke at 5 years among patients with a diameter stenosis of 50–69% (95% confidence interval (CI) for the relative risk reduction: 14–42%, $p = 0.002$) *(10)*. Patients with a diameter stenosis of 70–99%

Table 1
Trials of Carotid Endarterectomy (CEA) vs. Medical Management

Trial	n	Inclusion criteria	Primary end point	Finding
NASCET *(4)*	659	70–99% stenosis in symptomatic (stroke) carotid artery	Ipsilateral stroke at 2 years	Absolute risk reduction of 17% favoring CEA, $p < 0.001$
NASCET *(5)*	2,226	50–69% stenosis in symptomatic (stroke or transient ischemic attack) carotid artery	Ipsilateral stroke at 5 years	Absolute risk reduction of 6.5% favoring CEA, $p = 0.045$
ECST *(6)*	778	70–99% stenosis in symptomatic (stroke or transient ischemic attack) carotid artery	Perioperative death or any stroke at 3 years	Absolute risk reduction of 9.6% favoring CEA, $p < 0.01$
ECST *(7)*	3,024	80–99% stenosis in symptomatic (stroke or transient ischemic attack) carotid artery	Major stroke or death at 3 years	Absolute risk reduction of 11.6% favoring CEA, $p = 0.001$
ACAS *(8)*	1,662	60–99% stenosis in an asymptomatic carotid artery	Ipsilateral stroke at a median of 2.7 years + any perioperative stroke	Absolute risk reduction of 5.9% favoring CEA, $p < 0.05$
ACST *(9)*	3,120	60–99% stenosis in an asymptomatic carotid artery	Any stroke or perioperative death at 5 years	Absolute risk reduction of 5.4% favoring CEA, $p < 0.0001$

Table 2
High-Risk Features with Carotid Endarterectomy

Anatomic high-risk features	Clinical high-risk features
High lesion location (at or above C2)	Age ≥ 80 years
Low lesion location (below the clavicle)	Severe congestive heart failure (class III–IV)
Prior radical neck surgery or radiation	Severe angina pectoris (class III–IV)
Contralateral carotid artery occlusion	Two to three vessel coronary artery disease
Prior ipsilateral carotid endarterectomy	Left main trunk coronary artery disease
Contralateral laryngeal nerve palsy	Need for urgent heart surgery in the next 30 days
Tracheostomy	Left ventricular ejection fraction ≤ 30%
	Myocardial infarction within the last 30 days
	Severe renal insufficiency
	Severe chronic lung disease

derived an even greater benefit with a 48% relative reduction in the risk of ipsilateral stroke at 5 years (95% CI: 36–60%, $p = 0.00001$) *(10)*. In reviewing the symptomatic CEA data, the patients who derived the most benefit (with CEA) were elderly men with hemispheric, not ocular, symptoms.

Similar to the symptomatic patients, CEA was beneficial among asymptomatic patients with stenosis >60% in the ACAS and ACST trials *(8, 9)*. The relative risk reduction in favor of CEA was 31%, but interestingly, and in contrast with the symptomatic population, there was no association between stenosis severity and postoperative outcome. The clinical features which are associated with an adverse perioperative outcome with CEA have been termed the high-risk criteria (Table 2). These include both anatomic features and clinical comorbidities. Anatomical high-risk criteria include high lesion location (at or above C2), low lesion location (below the clavicle), prior radical neck surgery or radiation, contralateral carotid artery occlusion, prior ipsilateral CEA, contralateral laryngeal nerve palsy, and tracheostomy. Medical comorbidities include age of 80 years or greater, severe (class III or IV) congestive heart failure, severe (class III or IV) angina pectoris, coronary artery disease involving two or three vessels or the left main trunk, need for urgent heart surgery in the upcoming 30 days, depressed left ventricular systolic function (ejection fraction of 30% or less), recent myocardial infarction (within 30 days), severe chronic lung disease, or severe renal disease.

CAROTID ARTERY STENTING VS. CAROTID ENDARTERECTOMY

The early comparisons of CAS with CEA were colored by poor interventional technology, lack of embolic protection, and operator inexperience and did not come out favorably for CAS. The trials comparing CAS vs. CEA are shown in Table 3. The landmark trial establishing carotid stenting as an alternative to CEA was the Stenting and Angioplasty with Protection in Patients at High Risk for Endarterectomy (SAPPHIRE) study, which compared CAS and CEA among high-risk patients *(11)*. This randomized trial utilized contemporary carotid stenting techniques including embolic protection. The primary end point of 30-day death, myocardial infarction, or stroke plus 12-month neurological death or ipsilateral stroke was similar for the two treatment strategies: 12.2 vs. 20.1% for CAS and CEA,

Table 3
Trials of Carotid Artery Stenting (CAS) vs. Carotid Endarterectomy (CEA)

Trial	n	Inclusion criteria	Primary end point	Finding
SAPPHIRE *(11)*	334	50–99% stenosis in a symptomatic carotid artery or 80–99% stenosis in an asymptomatic carotid artery	30-day death, myocardial infarction, or stroke plus death or ipsilateral stroke between 31 days and 1 year	Primary end point was similar: 12.2% (CAS) vs. 20.1% (CEA), $p = 0.053$
EVA-3S *(12)*	527	60–99% stenosis in a symptomatic carotid artery	30-day rate of death or stroke	Primary end point was higher with CAS: 9.6% (CAS) vs. 3.9% (CEA), $p = 0.01$
SPACE *(14)*	1,200	70–99% stenosis in a symptomatic carotid artery	30-day rate of death or ipsilateral ischemic stroke	Primary end point was similar: 6.8% (CAS) vs. 6.3% (CEA), $p = 0.09$

respectively, $p = 0.053$ for superiority, $p = 0.004$ for noninferiority *(11)*. It is important to note, however, that numerically there were fewer myocardial infarctions and deaths in the CAS arm of the trial. These differences, like the primary end point, failed to reach statistical significance. The secondary end points which did favor CAS demonstrated less target vessel revascularization and cranial nerve palsy.

The recent publication of two trials involving low-risk symptomatic patients with severe carotid stenosis has complicated the evaluation of CAS vs. CEA in carotid revascularization. Endarterectomy versus Angioplasty in Patients with Symptomatic Severe Carotid Stenosis (EVA-3S) trial was a French trial which employed endovascular operators of more variable experience, thus making its interpretation difficult *(12)*. However, the 30-day rate of death or stroke was considerably higher in the CAS arm compared to CEA: 9.6 vs. 3.9%, $p = 0.01$. A similar issue of less operator experience with carotid stenting, as well as non-mandatory embolic protection, has also been raised in the evaluation of the Stent-Supported Percutaneous Angioplasty of the Carotid Artery versus Endarterectomy (SPACE) trial, a study which resulted in the 30-day rate of death or stroke of 6.8% for CAS and 6.3% for CEA, one-sided p-value for noninferiority = 0.09 *(13, 14)*.

Ongoing studies comparing CAS and CEA in low-risk patients include Carotid Revascularization Endarterectomy vs. Stent Trial (CREST) *(15, 16)*, the International Carotid Stenting Study (ICSS or CAVATAS II) *(17)*, the Asymptomatic Carotid Stenosis Stenting vs. Endarterectomy Trial (ACT I) *(18)*, and the Second Asymptomatic Carotid Surgery Trial (ACST-2) *(19)*. A study design of CAS vs. medical therapy among asymptomatic patients will be used in the upcoming Transatlantic Asymptomatic Carotid Intervention Trial (TACIT) *(20)*.

In addition to the randomized trials, a number of registries on carotid artery stenting in high-risk patients have been completed *(21)*. These registries have employed different stents, embolic protection devices, and operator backgrounds. Of the ones that have used 30-day death, stroke, or myocardial infarction as the primary end point, the outcome has ranged between 3.8 and 8.5%. The BEACH and CREATE studies are representative examples of these registries. The Boston Scientific EPI: A Carotid Stenting Trial for High-Risk Surgical Patients (BEACH) study included 747 high-risk patients and demonstrated a technical success rate of 98.2% and 30-day combined end point of death, stroke, or myocardial infarction of 5.8% *(22)*. The incidence of neurological death or ipsilateral stroke between day 31 and 1 year was 3.1% *(23)*. The BEACH investigators compared the composite of these two end points (8.9%) with a calculated estimate for CEA outcome in similar patients (12.6%), and by this methodology demonstrated noninferiority *(23)*. The Carotid Revascularization with ev3 Arterial Technology Evolution (CREATE) study of 419 high-risk patients noted a technical success rate of 97.4% and a 30-day incidence of death, stroke, or myocardial infarction of 6.2% *(24)*. A number of registries are currently in progress, including Carotid Acculink/Accunet Post Approval Trial to Uncover Rare Events (CAPTURE) 2 *(25)*, Emboshield and Xact Post Approval Carotid Stent Trial (EXACT) *(26)*, Use of the FiberNet® Emboli Protection Device in Carotid Artery Stenting (EPIC) *(27)*, Evaluation of the Medtronic AVE Self-expanding Carotid Stent System with Distal Protection in the Treatment of Carotid Stenosis (MAVErIC)-III *(28)*, Performance and Safety of the Medtronic AVE Self-Expandable Stent in the Treatment of Carotid Artery Lesions (PASCAL), Stenting of High-risk Patients Extracranial Lesions Trial with Embolic Removal (SHELTER) *(29)*, and Vivexx Carotid Revascularization Trial (VIVA) *(30)*.

SPECIAL POPULATIONS

The data are conflicting regarding the optimal revascularization strategy for elderly patients with carotid artery disease. Whereas the SAPPHIRE study demonstrated a favorable outcome for elderly patients undergoing CAS compared with CEA *(11)*, the CREST study showed that octogenarians had a higher incidence of death and stroke with CAS compared to CEA (leading to discontinuation of the study in this population) *(16)*. It appears that the risk of complications is higher among women undergoing CEA compared to men *(31)*. This results in smaller overall benefit with the CEA operation among women, a gender difference that has not been noted for CAS. Patients who undergo coronary artery bypass graft (CABG) operation are at high risk of perioperative stroke if they have had a prior cerebrovascular event (either TIA or stroke). Their risk is increased 4-fold *(32)*. To further highlight the issue of carotid disease and CABG, asymptomatic patients with carotid artery stenosis >75% have a 10-fold increase in perioperative stroke *(32)*. As a general rule, carotid and coronary revascularization should be done in staged fashion, and not during the same procedure. Complication rates are lower when carotid revascularization precedes CABG. If clinically feasible, CABG should be delayed by 1 month following CAS while the patient receives aspirin plus clopidogrel therapy.

A special situation for which CAS is well suited is carotid artery dissection with residual ischemia. Many dissections, however, heal completely without angioplasty, and anticoagulation and antiplatelet therapy are adequate treatment.

CONTRAINDICATIONS TO CAROTID STENTING

There are a number of neurological, anatomical, and clinical features which are considered contraindications to CAS *(21)*. In general, these identify patients who are unlikely to derive significant benefit from CAS or in whom the procedure is likely to be associated with increased risk of cerebral embolization. The neurologic criteria include major functional impairment, significant cognitive impairment, and major stroke within 4 weeks. The anatomical characteristics include inability to achieve safe vascular access, severe tortuosity of the aortic arch, the common carotid artery or the internal carotid artery, intracranial aneurysm or arterio-venous malformation requiring treatment, heavy lesion calcification, visible thrombus in the lesion, total occlusion, and long subtotal occlusion (also termed the string sign) (Table 4). The clinical features include life expectancy less than 5 years, contraindication to aspirin or thienopyridines, and renal dysfunction.

The type of aortic arch has great bearing on the complexity and feasibility of carotid artery stenting. The aortic arch is classified as either type I, II, or III based on the relationship between the arch and the innominate artery: in a type I arch, the origins of the innominate artery, the left common carotid artery, and the left subclavian artery are all located along the same horizontal plane as the superior curvature of the aortic arch. In a type II arch, the innominate artery origin is lower along the aortic arch curvature, and a type III arch is particularly challenging to negotiate during carotid artery stenting, with the innominate artery origin located more than two great vessel diameters below the superior curvature of the aortic arch.

INDICATIONS FOR CAROTID REVASCULARIZATION

In general, no revascularization is recommended for any asymptomatic patient with carotid artery diameter stenosis <60%, or for high surgical risk asymptomatic patients with stenosis <80% *(21)*. CEA is the recommended treatment for low-risk asymptomatic patients with a diameter stenosis between 60 and 99%. This assumes that the risk of perioperative stroke or death is <3% with the CEA *(21)*. That leaves among the asymptomatic patients those high-risk patients with stenosis of 80–99%, and for them the recommendation is CAS with embolic protection performed within a certain research protocol *(21)*.

The threshold for revascularization is lower for patients who have had a stroke or a TIA. Symptomatic patients with a carotid artery diameter stenosis of 50–99% should undergo CEA (as long as the risk of perioperative stroke or death is <6%) *(21)*.

Table 4
Anatomic Relative Contraindications to Carotid Artery Stenting

Inability to achieve vascular access
Severe tortuosity of the aortic arch, common carotid artery, or internal carotid artery
Intracranial aneurysm or arterio-venous malformation requiring treatment
Heavy lesion calcification
Visible thrombus in the lesion
Total occlusion
Long subtotal occlusion (string sign)

An acceptable alternative to CEA is CAS with embolic protection among symptomatic patients with a stenosis of 70–99% *(33)* or those patients with high-risk features and a stenosis of 50–69% under a research protocol *(21)*.

SCREENING FOR CAROTID ARTERY DISEASE

Among asymptomatic patients without a carotid bruit, screening for carotid artery disease is only recommended for some patients before they undergo coronary artery bypass graft (CABG) surgery *(21, 34)*. The patients who should be screened prior to CABG are the ones with age greater than 65 years, left main trunk coronary stenosis, peripheral arterial disease, history of smoking, history of TIA or stroke, or carotid bruit *(21, 35)*. Only patients who are reasonable candidates for a potential carotid revascularization procedure should undergo non-invasive imaging in case a carotid bruit is auscultated. Recently, the US Preventive Services Task Force recommended against screening for asymptomatic carotid artery stenosis in the general adult population *(36)*. Other subspecialty societies have made recommendations which are more liberal, but these are not yet widely accepted in the larger cardiology community *(37, 38)*.

REIMBURSEMENT CONSIDERATIONS FOR CAROTID STENTING

Currently, the Centers for Medicare & Medicaid Services (CMS) reimburse CAS procedures only if the patient is at high risk of adverse outcomes with CEA. In addition, the patient must meet one of the following three criteria: (1) symptomatic carotid artery stenosis of 70–99%, (2) symptomatic stenosis of 50–69% if performed within a clinical trial protocol, or (3) asymptomatic stenosis of 80–99% if performed within a clinical trial protocol.

CONSIDERATIONS FOR TRAINING AND CREDENTIALING

Training and credentialing are important parts of the overall national effort to deliver high-level interventional care with carotid stenting. Training requirements include completion of both a high-level training in a catheter-based field (such as interventional cardiology), as well as a dedicated carotid stenting program. Facilities where CAS programs are approved by the Centers for Medicare & Medicaid Services are required to ensure that all of the physician operators are properly credentialed in CAS. They also need to record CAS outcomes both on an institutional level and on the level of the individual operator and make these data available to national databases. Reimbursement for the CAS procedures is directly tied to fulfilling these criteria.

REFERENCES

1. Bhatt DL, Steg PG, Ohman EM, et al. International prevalence, recognition, and treatment of cardiovascular risk factors in outpatients with atherothrombosis. JAMA 2006;295(2):180–189.
2. Touze E, Mas JL, Rother J, et al. Impact of carotid endarterectomy on medical secondary prevention after a stroke or a transient ischemic attack: results from the Reduction of Atherothrombosis for Continued Health (REACH) registry. Stroke 2006;37(12):2880–2885.
3. Steg PG, Bhatt DL, Wilson PW, et al. One-year cardiovascular event rates in outpatients with atherothrombosis. JAMA 2007;297(11):1197–1206.

4. Beneficial effect of carotid endarterectomy in symptomatic patients with high-grade carotid stenosis. North American Symptomatic Carotid Endarterectomy Trial Collaborators. N Engl J Med 1991;325(7):445–453.

5. Barnett HJ, Taylor DW, Eliasziw M, et al. Benefit of carotid endarterectomy in patients with symptomatic moderate or severe stenosis. North American Symptomatic Carotid Endarterectomy Trial Collaborators. N Engl J Med 1998;339(20):1415–1425.

6. MRC European Carotid Surgery Trial: interim results for symptomatic patients with severe (70–99%) or with mild (0–29%) carotid stenosis. European Carotid Surgery Trialists' Collaborative Group. Lancet 1991;337(8752):1235–1243.

7. Randomised trial of endarterectomy for recently symptomatic carotid stenosis: final results of the MRC European Carotid Surgery Trial (ECST). Lancet 1998; 351(9113):1379–1387.

8. Endarterectomy for asymptomatic carotid artery stenosis. Executive Committee for the Asymptomatic Carotid Atherosclerosis Study. JAMA 1995;273(18):1421–1428.

9. Halliday A, Mansfield A, Marro J, et al. Prevention of disabling and fatal strokes by successful carotid endarterectomy in patients without recent neurological symptoms: randomised controlled trial. Lancet 2004;363(9420):1491–1502.

10. Rothwell PM, Eliasziw M, Gutnikov SA, et al. Analysis of pooled data from the randomised controlled trials of endarterectomy for symptomatic carotid stenosis. Lancet 2003;361(9352): 107–116.

11. Yadav JS, Wholey MH, Kuntz RE, et al. Protected carotid-artery stenting versus endarterectomy in high-risk patients. N Engl J Med 2004;351(15):1493–1501.

12. Mas JL, Chatellier G, Beyssen B, et al. Endarterectomy versus stenting in patients with symptomatic severe carotid stenosis. N Engl J Med 2006;355(16):1660–1671.

13. Naylor AR. SPACE: not the final frontier. Lancet 2006;368(9543):1215–1216.

14. Ringleb PA, Allenberg J, Bruckmann H, et al. 30 day results from the SPACE trial of stent-protected angioplasty versus carotid endarterectomy in symptomatic patients: a randomised non-inferiority trial. Lancet 2006;368(9543):1239–1247.

15. Hobson RW, 2nd. CREST (Carotid Revascularization Endarterectomy versus Stent Trial): background, design, and current status. Semin Vasc Surg 2000;13(2):139–143.

16. Hobson RW, 2nd, Howard VJ, Roubin GS, et al. Carotid artery stenting is associated with increased complications in octogenarians: 30-day stroke and death rates in the CREST lead-in phase. J Vasc Surg 2004;40(6):1106–1111.

17. Featherstone RL, Brown MM, Coward LJ. International carotid stenting study: protocol for a randomised clinical trial comparing carotid stenting with endarterectomy in symptomatic carotid artery stenosis. Cerebrovasc Dis 2004;18(1):69–74.

18. http://www.strokecenter.org/trials/TrialDetail.aspx?tid = 624 accessed on January 29, 2008.

19. http://www.controlled-trials.com accessed on January 29, 2008.

20. http://www.evtoday.com/PDFarticles/0905/EVT0905_F3_Tacit.pdf accessed on February 11th, 2008.

21. Bates ER, Babb JD, Casey DE, Jr., et al. ACCF/SCAI/SVMB/SIR/ASITN 2007 clinical expert consensus document on carotid stenting: a report of the American College of Cardiology Foundation Task Force on Clinical Expert Consensus Documents (ACCF/SCAI/SVMB/SIR/ASITN Clinical Expert Consensus Document Committee on Carotid Stenting). J Am Coll Cardiol 2007; 49(1):126–170.

22. White CJ, Iyer SS, Hopkins LN, Katzen BT, Russell ME. Carotid stenting with distal protection in high surgical risk patients: the BEACH trial 30 day results. Catheter Cardiovasc Interv 2006; 67(4):503–512.

23. Iyer SS, White CJ, Hopkins LN, et al. Carotid artery revascularization in high-surgical-risk patients using the Carotid WALLSTENT and FilterWire EX/EZ: 1-year outcomes in the BEACH Pivotal Group. J Am Coll Cardiol 2008;51(4):427–434.

24. Safian RD, Bresnahan JF, Jaff MR, et al. Protected carotid stenting in high-risk patients with severe carotid artery stenosis. J Am Coll Cardiol 2006;47(12):2384–2389.

25. http://www.clinicaltrials.gov/ct/show/NCT00302237?order = 27 accessed on January 29, 2008.

26. http://www.strokecenter.org/trials/TrialDetail.aspx?tid = 774&printView = true accessed on January 29, 2008.

27. http://www.clinicaltrials.gov/ct/show/NCT00309803?order = 9 accessed on January 29, 2008.

28. http://www.cxvascular.com/News/News.cfm?ccs = 329&cs = 1228 accessed on January 29, 2008.

29. http://www.strokecenter.org/Trials/TrialDetail.aspx?tid = 192 accessed on January 29, 2008.

30. http://www.clinicaltrials.gov/ct/show/NCT00417963?order = 2 accessed on January 29, 2008.
31. Rothwell PM, Eliasziw M, Gutnikov SA, Warlow CP, Barnett HJ. Endarterectomy for symptomatic carotid stenosis in relation to clinical subgroups and timing of surgery. Lancet 2004; 363(9413):915–924.
32. Naylor AR, Mehta Z, Rothwell PM, Bell PR. Carotid artery disease and stroke during coronary artery bypass: a critical review of the literature. Eur J Vasc Endovasc Surg 2002;23(4):283–294.
33. Sacco RL, Adams R, Albers G, et al. Guidelines for prevention of stroke in patients with ischemic stroke or transient ischemic attack: a statement for healthcare professionals from the American Heart Association/American Stroke Association Council on Stroke: co-sponsored by the Council on Cardiovascular Radiology and Intervention: the American Academy of Neurology affirms the value of this guideline. Stroke 2006;37(2):577–617.
34. Goldstein LB, Adams R, Alberts MJ, et al. Primary prevention of ischemic stroke: a guideline from the American Heart Association/American Stroke Association Stroke Council: cosponsored by the Atherosclerotic Peripheral Vascular Disease Interdisciplinary Working Group; Cardiovascular Nursing Council; Clinical Cardiology Council; Nutrition, Physical Activity, and Metabolism Council; and the Quality of Care and Outcomes Research Interdisciplinary Working Group: the American Academy of Neurology affirms the value of this guideline. Stroke 2006;37(6): 1583–1633.
35. Doonan AL, Karha J, Carrigan TP, et al. Presence of carotid and peripheral arterial disease in patients with left main disease. Am J Cardiol 2007;100(7):1087–1089.
36. Screening for carotid artery stenosis: U.S. Preventive Services Task Force recommendation statement. Ann Intern Med 2007;147(12):854–859.
37. Qureshi AI, Alexandrov AV, Tegeler CH, Hobson RW, 2nd, Dennis Baker J, Hopkins LN. Guidelines for screening of extracranial carotid artery disease: a statement for healthcare professionals from the multidisciplinary practice guidelines committee of the American Society of Neuroimaging; cosponsored by the Society of Vascular and Interventional Neurology. J Neuroimaging 2007;17(1):19–47.
38. http://www.vascularweb.org/patients/screenings/SVS_Position_Statement_on_Vascular_Screenings. html accessed on January 29, 2008.

8 Operator Training and Accreditation

Faisal Alquoofi, MD, FRCPC
and Ronak S. Kanani, MD, FRCPC

CONTENTS

ABSTRACT

Carotid artery stenting is of interest to physicians of varied backgrounds and expertise. Although disparate guidelines with important ideological differences exist regarding operator training, they share several important features in common. All professional society guidelines are of the unanimous opinion that patient safety is paramount. There is general agreement that formal training which imparts an adequate depth of cognitive knowledge of the cerebral vasculature and its associated pathophysiologic processes, as well as technical aptitude with cervicocerebral angiography and carotid intervention, including the management of complications, is the cornerstone for the successful care of patients requiring CAS.

Keywords: Carotid intervention; Angiography; Cognitive requirement; Technical skills; Training pathways; Multidisciplinary

From: *Contemporary Cardiology: Carotid Artery Stenting: The Basics*
Edited by: J. Saw, DOI 10.1007/978-1-60327-314-5_8,
© Humana Press, a part of Springer Science+Business Media, LLC 2009

INTRODUCTION

Indications for percutaneous carotid intervention are rapidly emerging as a less invasive alternative to the established procedure of carotid endarterectomy. Specialists from several different disciplines, each with a unique set of skills, expertise, and approach, are involved in the management of carotid disease and currently are, or will be, performing carotid artery stenting (CAS). These disciplines encompass both medical and surgical subspecialties, including vascular surgery, interventional radiology, neurosurgery, and interventional cardiology. In addition, non-interventional physicians, such as neurologists, internists, and noninvasive cardiologists, are interested in the diagnosis and medical management of patients with carotid atherosclerosis.

As a result of this multidisciplinary interest in CAS, various professional subspecialty societies have developed consensus documents that are based on the opinions of investigator experts. These guidelines were meant to serve as training and practice guidelines for each respective society peer group. Two multispecialty consensus groups have produced detailed guidelines for training and credentialing. The Societies of Cardiovascular Angiography and Interventions, Vascular Medicine and Biology, and Vascular Surgery (SCAI/SVMB/SVS) have published guidelines in 2004, which were updated in 2007 *(1)*. Similarly, the American Academy of Neurology, the American Association of Neurological Surgeons, the American Society of Interventional and Therapeutic Neuroradiology, the Congress of Neurological Surgeons, and the Society of Interventional Radiology (AAN/AANS/ASITN/ASNR/CNS/SIR), collectively known as the Neurovascular Coalition (NVC), have also developed training guidelines published in 2005 *(2)*. Both of these guidelines are designed to guide the training and credentialing of members of their respective societies, and the parent organizations do not feel that these guidelines are interchangeable.

The two guidelines both address training pathways and preliminary training for operators interested in CAS. They also discuss the cognitive skills, knowledge base, and technical skills required to safely perform carotid intervention, including outlining the minimum number of diagnostic and therapeutic procedures required. Similarities, as well as several important differences, within these categories exist, which are discussed in detail in the following sections.

TRAINING PATHWAYS

Ideally, training in CAS will be accomplished in accredited training programs specifically designed for each interventional subspecialty. At present, this is not the case, and the SCAI/SVMB/SVS guidelines have suggested alternative training pathways *(1)*. Two pathways have been described for physicians training in carotid intervention. The first occurs within an accredited postgraduate residency or fellowship training program (for example, interventional cardiology, interventional radiology, or vascular surgery) in conjunction with peripheral angioplasty training, including carotid intervention. The second pathway is for operators already in practice. Training occurs in a clinical practice environment. Although the setting for these two pathways differs, the fund of knowledge including the cognitive, clinical, and procedural skills necessary to achieve competency is identical. Upon completion of training, operators from each of the specialties involved should have acquired mastery of the necessary skills to achieve comparable levels of proficiency with carotid intervention.

PRELIMINARY TRAINING

Physicians training in carotid stenting are expected to demonstrate a baseline high level of proficiency in catheter-based intervention. The current guidelines differ with regard to their view of physicians with previous catheter-based experience. The SCAI/SVMB/SVS document recognizes the transferability of previous coronary (a minimum of 300 diagnostic coronary angiograms and 250 coronary interventions) and peripheral (a minimum of 100 diagnostic peripheral angiograms and 50 peripheral interventions) experience *(1)*. In contrast, the NVC guidelines outline a minimum training requirement for all physicians regardless of prior experience. This is in response to the belief that the carotid and intracerebral vasculature are inherently different from other vascular beds and that a learning curve exists for CAS *(2)*. Specific training requirements are outlined below and in Tables 1 and 2.

Table 1
Cognitive Knowledge as Endorsed by SCAI/SVMB/SVS

Diagnostic methods and treatment alternatives

(I) Pathophysiology of carotid artery disease and stroke
   (a) Causes of stroke
      (i) Embolization (cardiac, carotid, aortic, other)
      (ii) Vasculitis
      (iii) Arteriovenous malformation
      (iv) Intracranial bleeding (subdural, epidural)
      (v) Space-occupying lesion
   (b) Causes of carotid artery narrowing
      (i) Atherosclerosis
      (ii) Fibromuscular dysplasia
      (iii) Spontaneous dissection
      (iv) Other
   (c) Atherogenesis (pathogenesis and risk factors)
(II) Clinical manifestations of stroke
   (a) Knowledge of stroke syndromes (classic and atypical)
   (b) Distinction between anterior and posterior circulation events
(III) Natural history of carotid artery disease
(IV) Associated pathology (e.g., coronary and peripheral artery disease)
(V) Diagnosis of stroke and carotid artery disease
   (a) History and physical examination
      (i) Neurologic
      (ii) Non-neurologic (cardiac, other)
   (b) Noninvasive imaging and appropriate use thereof
      (i) Duplex ultrasound
      (ii) MRA
      (iii) CTA
(VI) Angiographic anatomy (arch, extracranial, intracranial, basic collateral circulation, common anatomic variants, and non-atherosclerotic pathologic processes)
(VII) Knowledge of alternative treatment options for carotid stenosis and their results (immediate success, risks, and long-term outcome)
   (a) Pharmacotherapy (e.g., antiplatelet agents, anticoagulation, lipid-lowering agents)

(Continued)

Table 1
(Continued)

Diagnostic methods and treatment alternatives

      (b) Carotid endarterectomy
         (i) Results from major trials (NASCET, ACAS, ECST, ACST)
         (ii) Results in patients with increased surgical risk
      (c) Stent revascularization
         (i) Results with and without distal embolic protection
   (VIII) Case selection
      (a) Indications and contraindications for revascularization to prevent
         stroke
      (b) High-risk criteria for carotid endarterectomy
      (c) High-risk criteria for percutaneous intervention
  (IX) Role of post-procedure follow-up and surveillance

Table 2
Cognitive Knowledge as Endorsed by AAN/AANS/ASITN/ASNR/CNS/SIR

Cognitive elements

(I) A fund of knowledge regarding stroke syndromes and TIA etiologies, evaluation of
    traumatic and/or atherosclerotic neurovascular lesions, and inflammatory conditions of
    the central nervous system
(II) Formal training that imparts an adequate depth of cognitive knowledge of the brain and
    its associated pathophysiological vascular processes, including management of
    complications of endovascular procedures
(III) Diagnostic and therapeutic acumen, including the ability to recognize and manage
    procedural complications
(IV) Ability to recognize clinical intra- or post-procedural neurological symptoms, as well as
    pertinent angiographic findings and the proper cognitive and technical skills to offer
    the most appropriate therapy. This might also entail optimal hemodynamic
    management necessitating sufficient neurointensive skills

COGNITIVE SKILLS AND KNOWLEDGE BASE

There is general agreement in both training guidelines that proficiency in CAS requires competency in the diagnosis, management, and post-procedural care of CAS patients and that CAS involves unique cognitive and clinical management skills compared with those required in other vascular beds. The requisite fundamental knowledge base includes a comprehensive understanding of the risk factors, epidemiology, pathology, pathophysiology, natural history, clinical presentation, and therapeutic alternatives for patients with extracranial carotid artery disease. Thorough understanding of the etiologies and manifestations of the stroke syndromes is of great importance in caring for patients pre- and post-procedurally. Additionally, understanding the accuracy and limitations of carotid duplex ultrasonography, magnetic resonance arteriography, and computed tomographic arteriography is necessary for developing a diagnostic algorithm for carotid artery disease. Similarly, the indications for performance of cerebral arteriography should be clearly understood.

The SCAI has developed a tiered curriculum to address cognitive and technical expertise *(1)*. The first and second tiers of this program address cognitive skills specifically and consist of an intensive, case-based didactic program as well as an online review and self-assessment modules. In comparison, the NVC guidelines *(2)* require a minimum of 6 months of formal neuroscience training in an ACGME (American Council for Graduate Medical Education)-accredited radiology, neuroradiology, neurosurgery, neurology, and/or vascular neurology program. The requisite cognitive knowledge base also includes understanding the stroke syndromes, the pathophysiology of carotid atherosclerosis, the evaluation of traumatic, atherosclerotic, and inflammatory conditions of the central nervous system, and the recognition and management of potential complications of CAS (Table 2). This minimum formal training applies to all practitioners who wish to be credentialed to perform diagnostic cervicocerebral angiography and/or carotid intervention, including practitioners from specialties without dedicated clinical neuroscience training as part of their ACGME-approved residency programs.

TECHNICAL SKILLS

The baseline skill set for operators or trainees interested in CAS must include knowledge of the appropriate use of radiographic contrast agents, including the potential risks and complications associated with them. Operators must also appropriately use x-ray imaging equipment. This includes the ability to obtain digital and subtracted images and the ability to utilize angulated views to optimally examine the cerebrovascular circulation. The safe use of the closed manifold system must be understood. Operators must be facile with the use of guiding catheters, sheaths, guidewires, stents, balloons, and distal embolization protection devices, as well as adjunctive equipment and techniques, such as the use of intravascular snares, embolization coils, and intravascular ultrasound.

The third tier of the aforementioned SCAI curriculum for cognitive and technical expertise with CAS involves case-based learning at regional simulation centers, as well as exposure to live and archived cases. As part of this curriculum, both technical and cognitive expertise will have to be evaluated prior to SCAI certification *(1)*. In comparison, the NVC *(2)* describes no specific curriculum, but instead requires full training in diagnostic neurovascular procedures prior to performing CAS. Both guidelines encompass specific recommendations with regard to the minimum number of diagnostic and therapeutic procedures. This will be discussed further below.

CEREBRAL ANGIOGRAPHY

Competence in the performance and basic interpretation of diagnostic two- and four-vessel cervicocerebral angiography must be achieved in order to perform carotid intervention. Knowledge of both carotid and intracerebral anatomy is required to evaluate stenosis severity, tortuosity, calcification, collateral circulation, aneurysms, and arteriovenous malformations. Anatomic knowledge is also crucial for device delivery, as well as to monitor for procedural complications.

The SCAI/SVMB/SVS guidelines *(1)* specify that in order to achieve and ensure competency in the safe performance of cervicocerebral angiography, interventionalists with proper credentials and demonstrated expertise in noncerebrovascular territories can achieve the required level of technical skill by performing 30 supervised angiograms, half as the primary operator, in a supervised setting. This recommendation acknowledges the transferable nature of basic and advanced catheter skills acquired in other vascular beds.

The NVC guidelines *(2)*, in comparison, recommend a minimum of 100 appropriately supervised cervicocerebral angiograms. This is felt to reflect the American Heart Association requirement of 100 peripheral angiograms prior to independent peripheral intervention.

A learning curve exists regarding image interpretation during cerebral angiography. A similar learning curve exists for appropriate catheter selection and placement. Risk factors for ischemic complications are well recognized and include increased procedural and fluoroscopy times, increased numbers of catheters used, and the performance of arch aortography *(3–5)*. Experience results in decreased complications and fluoroscopy times, which improve in a linear fashion after performing 100 cerebral angiograms *(6)*. Analysis of the trainee learning curve suggests that 200 cerebral angiograms are necessary to ensure physician competence in carotid and intracranial angiography. The importance of training and experience is demonstrated in one 5,000 angiogram retrospective analysis. Fellowship-trained specialists had fewer neurological complications (0.5%) than experienced angiographers (0.6%). Both of these groups had fewer complications than trainees under supervision (2.8%) *(4, 5)*.

CAROTID INTERVENTION

The interventional skills required for carotid stenting are significantly more complex and difficult to master than those for diagnostic cerebral angiography. These skills include, but are not limited to, the following: (1) the proper selection and placement of large sheaths or guiding catheters in often tortuous and calcified carotid arteries; (2) the safe manipulation of guidewires across tight carotid lesions; (3) facility with rapid-exchange, single-operator device delivery systems; (4) proper selection, delivery, and accurate deployment of large self-expanding stents; (5) the correct choice and use of pre- and post-dilation balloons including understanding issues of balloon profile, size, inflation pressure, and inflation time; and (6) the proper selection and use of distal embolic protection devices. In addition to these technical skills, operator judgment and foresight are instrumental in the safe navigation of the target vasculature and to make rational equipment choices. An understanding of potential procedural complications, the ability to anticipate their occurrence, and the skill to avoid and treat them when they occur are paramount. The operator must be capable of recognizing and responding to such angiographic findings as spasm, pseudospasm, residual ulceration, and benign intimal disruption. The operator must also know how to avoid and manage such complications as arterial dissection, stent thrombosis, distal embolization, vessel perforation, and stent malpositioning *(1)*. The pathway to achieving technical competence is designed to address the degree of difficulty and potential risks inherent in this procedure. Prior to undertaking focused training in CAS, the operator is expected to demonstrate a high baseline level of proficiency in a broad base of catheter-based interventions.

According to the SCAI/SVMB/SVS guidelines *(1)*, interventionalists training in CAS must perform a minimum of 25 patient procedures in a supervised setting (trainee scrubbed alongside an experienced operator), 13 of which are as the primary operator (trainee performing the procedure under direct supervision). Meanwhile the NVC guidelines *(2)* outline two training pathways. The first pathway requires a minimum of 25 non-carotid stent procedures, 4 supervised carotid stent procedures, and 16 h of continuing medical education (CME). The second pathway dictates 10 consecutive, supervised CAS procedures with acceptable results as the minimum training requirement. The 16 h of CME includes a didactic program of formal instruction in the cognitive and clinical elements of CAS, along with technical instruction on the procedure and devices utilized. Technical requirements for CAS training are summarized in Tables 3 and 4.

Table 3
Technical Skills as Endorsed by SCAI/SVMB/SVS

Technical requirements for performance of carotid stenting

Minimum numbers of procedures to achieve competence:
(I) Diagnostic cervicocerebral angiograms: 30 (half as primary operator)
(II) Carotid stent procedures: 25 (half as primary operator)
Technical elements for competence in both diagnostic angiography and
   interventional techniques:
  (I) High level of expertise with antiplatelet therapy and procedural
      anticoagulation
  (II) Angiographic skills
    (a) Vascular access skills
    (b) Selection of guidewires and angiographic catheters
    (c) Appropriate manipulation of guidewires and catheters
    (d) Use of "closed system" manifold
    (e) Knowledge of normal angiographic anatomy and common variants
    (f) Knowledge of circle of Willis and typical/atypical collateral pathways
    (g) Proper assessment of aortic arch configuration, as it affects carotid
        intervention
    (h) Familiarity with use of angulated views and appropriate movement of
        the x-ray gantry

Table 4
Technical Skills as Endorsed by AAN/AANS/ASITN/ASNR/CNS/SIR (NVC)

Technical requirements for performance of carotid stenting

(I)   Adequate procedural skill achieved by training in an approved clinical setting,
       supervised by a qualified instructor
(II)   This includes the ability to correctly interpret a cervicocerebral angiogram
(III) Minimum numbers of procedures to achieve competence is 100 diagnostic
       cervicocerebral angiograms
Two training pathways:
(I) 25 non-carotid stent procedures, 4 supervised carotid stent procedures, 16 h of CME
(II) 10 consecutive, successful supervised carotid stent procedures

Industry training programs specific for CAS and distal embolization protection devices exist and are important for device certification, but are not meant to supplant professional society training requirements *(7)*.

MAINTENANCE OF CONTINUING QUALITY OF CARE

As stroke is a potential risk of CAS with significant morbidity, maintenance of certification requires the highest level of competency. Proficiency is maintained by lifelong continuing medical education (CME), as well as by performing regular, successful CAS procedures without complication. Although no minimum case volume requirements have been outlined, the SCAI/SVMB/SVS guidelines *(1)* suggest the ongoing collection of patient and quality data, multidisciplinary rounds to review CAS cases and evaluate outcomes, and comparison of local outcome data with national benchmarks. The NVC guidelines, similarly, suggest the ongoing tracking of outcomes both during and following training and comparison with published standards *(2)*.

ROLE OF SIMULATION

Simulator training has been shown to be of benefit in various medical applications. Although simulator training cannot currently supplant appropriate formal training and clinical experience in cervicocerebral angiography, both current and future trainees may benefit from added training with CAS simulators. A learning curve can be observed when physicians are trained in carotid angiography using virtual reality (VR) simulation. Patel and colleagues instructed 20 interventional cardiologists in carotid angiography and then had the subjects perform 5 serial simulated carotid arteriograms on the VIST (vascular interventional surgical trainer) simulator *(8)*. There were measurable improvements between the first and the fifth procedure, including procedure times, contrast use, fluoroscopy times, and catheter handling errors. In addition, the internal consistency of the VIST simulator and its test–retest reliability were validated with several key procedural metrics. This suggests that simulation is useful in improving operator experience at the initial stages of the learning curve, without risk to patients. Other reports have similarly suggested that simulation is especially well suited for the initial phases of procedural training. Dayal and colleagues, using the VIST simulator to teach CAS to vascular surgeons, observed significant improvement in participants' endovascular techniques. Novice participants perceived a greater benefit from simulator training than did experienced interventionalists *(9)*. In another Study by Dawson et al. *(10)*, the performance of vascular surgery residents performing endovascular procedures was evaluated using a high-fidelity endovascular procedure simulator (SimSuite). This study showed an improvement in resident performance with the use of the SimSuite without direct risk to patients.

SUMMARY

CAS is an important and rapidly changing area of medicine of interest to physicians of varied backgrounds and expertise. Although disparate guidelines with important ideological differences exist regarding operator training, they share several important features in common. Given the potential for significant neurologic morbidity, all professional society guidelines are of the unanimous opinion that patient safety is paramount. There is general agreement that formal training which imparts an adequate

depth of cognitive knowledge of the cerebral vasculature and its associated pathophysiologic processes, as well as technical aptitude with cervicocerebral angiography and
carotid intervention, including the management of complications, is the cornerstone for
the successful care of patients requiring CAS. Although the specific training volumes
vary, there is agreement that defined, formal training and experience in both the
cognitive and technical aspects of CAS are essential for adequate operator training.
Similarly, there is general agreement that outcomes of CAS procedures should be
tracked and evaluated prospectively in comparison to national databases *(11–15)*.
All societies endorse the principles of training and quality assurance espoused in the
multi-society Quality Improvement Guidelines for the Performance of Carotid Angioplasty and Stent Placement *(16)*, which include a defined training pathway for any
qualified practitioner for carotid stent training. Such training should ensure that CAS
operators, regardless of their specific background, will provide patients with the most
technically skilled and safe procedure possible.

REFERENCES

1. ACCF/SCAI/SVMB/SIR/ASITN 2007 Clinical Expert Consensus Document on Carotid Stenting. JACC 2007;49(1):2007:126–170.
2. Connors JJ III, Sacks D, Furlan AJ, Selman WR, Russell EJ, Stieg PE, Hadley MN. For the
   NeuroVascular Coalition Writing Group. Radiology 2005;234:26–34.
3. Davies KN, Humphrey PR. Complications of cerebral angiography in patients with symptomatic
   carotid territory ischemia screened by carotid ultrasound. J Neurol Neurosurg Psychiatry
   1993;56:9647–9672.
4. Mani RL, Eisenberg RL. Complications of catheter cerebral arteriography: analysis of 5000
   procedures. II. Relation of complication rates to clinical and arteriographic diagnoses. AJR Am
   J Roentgenol 1978;131:867–869.
5. McIvor J, Steiner TJ, Perkins GD, et al. Neurological morbidity of arch angiography in cerebrovascular disease. The influence of contrast medium and the radiologist. Br J Radiol
   1987;60:117–122.
6. Dion JE, Gates PC, Fox AJ, et al. Clinical events following neuroangiography: a prospective
   study. Stroke 1987;18:997–1004.
7. White CJ. Training and certification for carotid stenting: is the fox guarding the hen house?
   Catheter Cardiovasc Interv 2005;66:50–51.
8. Patel AD, Gallagher AG, Nicholson WJ, Cates CU. Learning curves and reliability measures for
   virtual reality simulation in the performance of carotid angiography. J Am Coll Cardiol
   2006;47:1796–1802.
9. Dayal R, Faries PL, Lin SC, et al. Computer simulation as a component of catheter-based
   training. J Vasc Surg 2004;40:1112–1117.
10. Dawson D, Meyer J, RCIS, et al. Training with simulation improves residents' endovascular
    procedure skills. J Vasc Surg 2007;45:149–154.
11. Executive Committee for the Asymptomatic Carotid Atherosclerosis Study. Endarterectomy for
    asymptomatic carotid artery stenosis. JAMA 1995;273:1421–1428.
12. Cooperative Study between the ASNR, ASITN, and SCVIR. Quality improvement guidelines for
    adult diagnostic neuroangiography. AJNR Am J Neuroradiol 2000;21:146–150.
13. Standard for the performance of diagnostic cervicocerebral angiography in adults. Res. 5-1999.
    American College of Radiology Standards 2000–2001. Reston VA: ACR, 2000;415–426.
14. Gomez CR, Kinkel P, Masdeu JC, et al. American Academy of Neurology guidelines for
    credentialing in neuroimaging. Report from the task force on updating guidelines for credential-
    ing in neuroimaging. Neurology 1997;49:1734–1737.
15. Higashida RT, Hopkins LN, Berenstein A, et al. Program requirements for residency/fellowship
    education in neuroendovascular surgery/interventional Neuroradiology: a special report on grad-
    uate medical education. AJNR Am J Neuroradiol 2000;21:1153–1159.
16. Bakshi R, Alexandrov AV, Gomez CR, Masdeu JC. Neuroimaging curriculum for neurology
    trainees: report from the Neuroimaging Section of the AAN. J Neuroimaging 2003;13:215–217.

IV TECHNICAL APPROACH OF CAROTID ARTERY STENTING

9 Vascular Access: Femoral, Radial, Brachial, and Direct Carotid Approach

Robert H. Boone, MD and Ravish Sachar, MD

CONTENTS

ABSTRACT

Vascular access is the cornerstone of all endovascular procedures. Common femoral artery puncture is the most common route of access and, when performed properly, permits successful carotid stent deployment in over 98% of cases. However, access site complications are the most frequent cause of morbidity, and their incidence can be reduced with proper technique. Furthermore, radial and brachial approaches may occasionally be required, or may offer an increased chance of procedure success. Current technology has allowed the development of better equipment which in turn has meant that direct carotid puncture is rarely (if ever) required.

Keywords: Vascular access; Femoral artery; Radial artery; Brachial artery; Carotid artery

INTRODUCTION

Successful carotid stenting is a complex process with multiple steps. As outlined in other chapters, adequate positioning of the guide or sheath in the common carotid artery is critical to wire advancement and successful delivery of embolic

From: *Contemporary Cardiology: Carotid Artery Stenting: The Basics*
Edited by: J. Saw, DOI 10.1007/978-1-60327-314-5_9,
© Humana Press, a part of Springer Science+Business Media, LLC 2009

protection devices. Careful choice of vascular access site can greatly increase the chance of successful guide position. However, vascular access problems are the leading cause of procedural morbidity with all endovascular procedures. Complications include hematoma, retroperitoneal bleeding, arteriovenous fistula, arterial aneurysm/pseudoaneurysm, and arterial dissection. With care and attention to proper technique, the incidence of these complications can be significantly reduced, and procedure success improved.

Historically, arterial access was performed via cut-down procedures allowing direct visualization of the arterial wall which facilitated safe puncture and ensured adequate hemostasis, but recovery times were long and procedures required more anesthesia. However, modern technology has made percutaneous arterial access routine and has limited cut-down techniques to procedures requiring introduction of larger devices (i.e., transcatheter heart valve implantation) and treatment for complications of percutaneous arterial access. In this chapter we outline the indications/contraindications, methods, and complications associated with percutaneous access of the femoral, radial, and brachial arteries and refer the reader to the wide variety of vascular surgery textbooks for further information on cut-down techniques.

GENERAL PRINCIPLES

The general technique for percutaneous arterial access is that developed by Seldinger *(1)* (Fig. 1). After skin preparation (cleaning/shaving) and the application of local anesthetic, a hollow bore needle is advanced through the skin, underlying fascia, and arterial wall to sit within the arterial lumen.

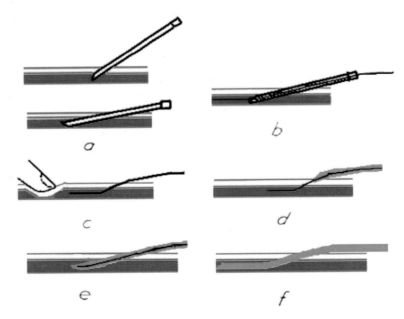

Fig. 1. The Seldinger technique: (**a**) The artery punctured with hollow bore puncture needle, and the needle tip tilted upward. (**b**) The flexible wire inserted. (**c**) The needle withdrawn and the artery compressed. (**d**) The sheath/catheter threaded onto the wire. (**e**) The sheath/catheter inserted into the artery. (**f**) The wire withdrawn. Adapted from Seldinger *(1)*.

A flexible J-tipped wire is advanced through the hollow bore needle into the arterial lumen, and the wire tip is advanced a reasonable distance proximal to the arterial puncture site. The hollow bore needle is removed while the wire is maintained within the arterial lumen. Subsequently a dilator and sheath are placed over the wire and advanced into the arterial lumen. The wire and dilator are withdrawn while leaving in place the sheath with back bleed valve and side port. The sheath is aspirated, flushed, and may then be connected to a pressurized flush system to avoid clot formation. The flush solution should always be heparinized saline (10 units/1 mL normal saline), and with carotid procedures in particular, it is critical to be vigilant in ensuring clot does not form at the sheath tip.

While the process is straightforward, several issues should be highlighted to avoid complications. A key issue is that of hemostasis. This is primarily achieved by compression of the arterial puncture site against an underlying bony structure. Therefore, it is important to landmark precisely and puncture in a location that will ensure compression against an underlying bony structure. Another factor is the nature of arterial puncture. Puncture of the back wall should be avoided as hemostasis becomes more difficult to achieve. Furthermore, puncture should be into the arterial apex and not into the side wall. Such off-center punctures increase the risk of dissection and limit the effectiveness of closure techniques. Finally, overlying vascular structures need to be avoided. Puncture through a vein into an artery will greatly increase the chance of arteriovenous fistulae formation.

FEMORAL ACCESS

The majority of carotid interventions are successfully performed using percutaneous common femoral artery (CFA) cannulation. The right CFA is most commonly used as this permits easy catheter and table manipulation with the operator standing on the patient's right side.

Indications/Contraindications

Most operators would agree that the CFA is the route of choice for carotid procedures. Its large size, easy accessibility, and routine use in other endovascular procedures make it an ideal choice. Occasionally the CFA cannot be used. For example, in patients with severe peripheral vascular disease the iliofemoral system may be so diffusely diseased that cannulation of this system is impossible. Prior aortofemoral bypass is not a contraindication for percutaneous CFA access, and graft material can often be accessed directly *(2)*. It is our practice not to access bypass grafts that are less than 1 year old. Prior trauma with distorted underlying anatomy may make CFA cannulation more difficult. Other potential contraindications for CFA access include overlying infection and morbid obesity.

Methods

The method for percutaneous access of the CFA consists of locating landmarks, skin preparation/local anesthetic, puncture/sheath placement, and closure.

Landmarks

A thorough understanding of the femoral triangle is paramount to successful CFA puncture. The femoral triangle consists of the inguinal ligament superiorly, the medial border of sartorius muscle laterally, and the lateral border of adductor longus muscle medially. The contents of the triangle from medial to lateral are femoral vein, common femoral artery, and femoral nerve. The inguinal ligament is difficult to palpate but runs in a direct line from the easily appreciated anterior superior iliac spine of the ilium to the pubic tubercle of the pubic bone. It serves to separate the structures of the pelvis from that of the lower limb, and care must be taken to ensure puncture of the artery occurs below the inguinal ligament in order to avoid the potential complication of retroperitoneal bleeding that occurs more frequently with high punctures. The common femoral artery continues from the external iliac artery after it passes through the inguinal ligament. It splits to become the profunda femoris and the superficial femoral artery. Puncture of either of these branches (i.e., too low) has been associated with increased risk of complications including pseudoaneurysm and arteriovenous fistulae *(3, 4)*. The landmarks discussed are presented in Fig. 2.

PUNCTURE

Prior to skin puncture, the site must be shaved and cleaned with an antiseptic solution. We advocate cleaning a circular area 10 cm in diameter centered around the proposed puncture site. Both groins should be prepped. Local anesthetic (1% lidocaine without epinephrine) is delivered via a single puncture technique using a 21-gauge needle. We suggest raising a small skin bleb and subsequent advancement of the needle (maintaining slight negative pressure) on the medial side of the artery with injection of 5 mL on needle withdrawal. Rather than withdraw completely out of the skin, we recommend re-angulation of the needle with advancement (maintaining negative pressure) on the lateral side of the artery and injection on needle withdrawal.

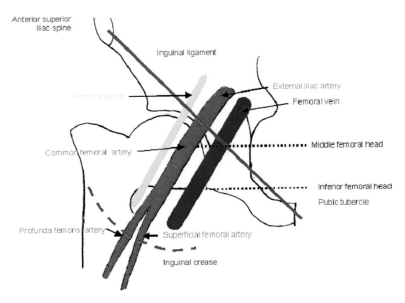

Fig. 2. Diagrammatic representation of the femoral triangle. Note the inguinal crease is below the level of the inguinal ligament, and the femoral bifurcation occurs above the inguinal crease. The common femoral artery overlies the femoral head.

Ideal puncture occurs when the needle is placed within the CFA at the level of the femoral head *(1, 5, 6)*. There are several landmarking techniques used to ensure ideal puncture. Historically, many operators punctured 1–2 cm below the inguinal crease. However, a variety of studies have shown that the inguinal crease is distal to the bifurcation of the CFA in approximately 70% of subjects *(5–7)*, and thus it is no longer recommended as a landmark. The maximal femoral pulse was over the CFA in 92.7% of limbs. More recently many authors have advocated the use of fluoroscopy as a method to identify the common femoral head which may be used as a landmark for puncture *(5, 8, 9)*. We advocate the identification of the point of maximal impulse below the inguinal ligament. Once this point has been identified, we suggest placing a radio-opaque instrument on the skin (i.e., hemostat) and confirming the skin puncture site is over the lower half of the common femoral head. Puncturing at a 45° angle with the skin at this point should ensure puncture within CFA as it overlies the femoral head (Fig. 3).

We use an 18-gauge puncture needle, a 0.035″ J guidewire, and 6 French sheath/dilator. When advancing the guidewire up the iliofemoral system, it is important to ensure movement is free and easy. If there is difficulty with advancement at the needle tip, the guidewire should be removed and the needle slightly repositioned to ensure vigorous pulsatile flow. If there is further difficulty with wire advancement,

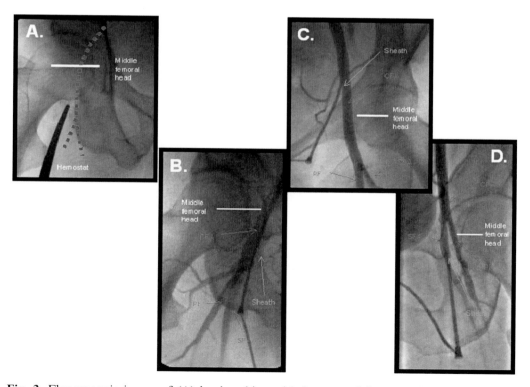

Fig. 3. Fluoroscopic image of (**A**) landmarking with hemostat lying on skin projecting over inferior border of femoral head. Angiographic images of (**B**) near-ideal femoral puncture with the sheath entering the common femoral artery (CFA) at the inferior border of the femoral head, (**C**) a puncture that is too high entering the CFA above the femoral head, and (**D**) puncture that is too low entering the superficial femoral artery (SFA) below the femoral head (note high bifurcation of CFA). Note: PF, profunda femoris.

the needle should be withdrawn, the groin compressed, landmarks reassessed, and a second puncture attempted. Third-time punctures are not indicated and rarely successful, and if necessary should be an indication to attempt femoral access on the alternate leg. If there is resistance to guidewire passage after several centimeters, the likely cause is atherosclerotic iliofemoral disease. In this case, fluoroscopy is often useful to define calcification and wire position. We suggest careful removal of the puncture needle while maintaining wire position. After wiping the wire with wet gauze, 5 or 6 Fr dilator can be advanced up the wire to near the area of resistance and a small amount of contrast injected under fluoroscopy to determine the cause of resistance. Possible causes include tortuosity, stenosis, or dissection, which may be overcome with use of a floppy steerable (Wholey Hi-Torque Floppy Guidewire^{TM}, Covidien, Hazelwood, MO) or hydrophilic (Glidewire^{TM}, Terumo, Somerset, NJ) guidewire. If these wires can be successfully navigated to the aorta, we suggest the placement of a long, flexible sheath to ensure easy catheter delivery and manipulation.

HEMOSTASIS

Hemostasis following sheath removal may be obtained in a variety of ways. Manual compression was used historically, and continues to be the most reliable option when other methods fail. The use of mechanical clamp devices has increased dramatically in recent years, and a randomized trial by Pracyk et al. *(10)* showed that hemostasis achieved with the use of a mechanical clamp rather than hand pressure significantly reduced ultrasound-defined femoral vascular pathology. It is our default practice to mechanically clamp all patients. However, newer technology has made percutaneous closure increasingly commonplace.

CLOSURE

There are a wide variety of closure devices. These include Angio-Seal^{TM} (St. Jude Medical, St. Paul, MN), StarClose^{TM} (SC) (Abbott Vascular, Abbott Park, IL), and Perclose ProGlide (Abbott Vascular, Abbott Park, IL). All devices are deployed over a wire that is placed through the sheath prior to removal. The Angio-Seal device is a collagen plug, StarClose is a nitinol clip deployed onto the arterial wall, and Perclose utilizes a suture-mediated closure system. In comparison to manual closure, all these devices offer the potential advantages of reduced rates of complications, reduced time to hemostasis and ambulation, improved patient comfort, and cost-effectiveness. They are also easy to use with a short learning curve and have a high rate of deployment success. A meta-analysis of the effectiveness of these devices has shown them to be effective in achieving hemostasis and may do so with a lower rate of complication in comparison with manual compression *(11)*. However, the majority of studies included in this analysis were non-randomized and therefore potentially subject to bias. More recently Deuling et al. *(12)* reported the results of a randomized trial of manual compression, Angio-Seal, and StarClose. They found the safety profile similar to manual compression: StarClose was more often unsuccessfully deployed (or not deployed) than Angio-Seal, and patient comfort and early ambulation were improved with device closure. The latest data from over 200,000 procedures collected through the American College of Cardiology – National Cardiovascular Data Registry support the concept that vascular closure devices are associated with a lower incidence of vascular complications *(13)*. For further information, interested readers are referred to recently published reviews of device closures by Dauerman et al. *(14)* or Madigan et al. *(15)*.

Complications

Despite the huge number of endovascular procedures performed via the femoral artery daily, there remains the potential for access site complications. Potential complications (and their incidence) are hematoma (2–7%) *(16, 17)*, pseudoaneurysm (0.3–6%) *(17–19)*, arteriovenous fistula (0.02–0.6%) *(17, 18)*, infection (0.03%), dissection (0.18%), ischemia (0.07%) *(17)*, and retroperitoneal hematoma (0.2–0.7%) *(13, 17, 20)*. Factors associated with higher risk of complications can be grouped into patient factors, procedural factors, and drug factors. These are outlined in Table 1. Puncture site and method of vascular closure are the two factors which can be influenced by the procedural operator.

Table 1
Risk Factors for Vascular Complications with Femoral Access

Patient factors	Procedure factors	Drug factors
Female gender	Level of puncture site	Thrombolytics
Older	Larger arterial sheath	GP IIb/IIIa inhibitor use
Hypertension	Prolonged sheath time	Over-anticoagulation
Obesity	Intra-aortic balloon pump	
Low weight	Concomitant venous sheath	
Renal failure	Need for repeat intervention	
Low platelet count	Manual compression	

RADIAL ACCESS

Radial artery access should be considered for all patients with contraindications to femoral access. However, with increasing experience, it can become a routine access site, especially for right internal carotid artery lesions. Radial access for carotid interventions works best with right radial access for right internal carotid revascularization. Left internal carotid artery revascularization via the right radial approach is possible, but with lower success rates *(21)*. Treatment of either internal carotid artery via the left radial artery is challenging as it requires introduction of equipment into the aorta and then a sharp angle back into either common carotid artery. Without backup at the point of maximal angulation within the aorta, the risk of prolapse is increased.

Indications/Contraindications

The three indications for radial access are (i) contraindications to femoral access, (ii) a need for early ambulation or mobility such as someone with severe back pain, and (iii) concern over bleeding complications with a femoral access given the lower rate of bleeding complications with radial approaches *(22–24)*. Contraindications to radial access include need for catheters greater than 6 Fr, hemodialysis fistula within the arm of access, and a failed modified Allen's test *(25)*, *(8)*.

The radial artery is not an "end artery" and therefore structures distal to the puncture site are perfused from an alternate arterial blood supply. This intact distal territory means occlusion of the radial artery is well tolerated. The hand receives a dual blood supply from the radial and ulnar arteries, which then form a loop in the deep and superficial palmar arches (Fig. 4). Prior to accessing the radial artery, the patency of this loop needs to be established by the modified Allen's test. An oxygen saturation probe is placed on the thumb while the radial artery is compressed. The patency of the palmar arch (ulnar artery) is demonstrated by arterial waveform (reduced amplitude or delayed waveform permitted) and oxygen saturations of >90% after 2 min of observation (Fig. 5). The radial artery can be accessed only if palmar arch patency can be observed.

Methods

Landmarks: The radial artery can be palpated just proximal to the wrist, but should be punctured 1–2 cm proximal to the radial styloid. This avoids having to puncture through the heavily fibrous flexor retinaculum.

*Puncture:*Site preparation is as for the femoral approach. Positioning is important. The arm should be abducted to 90° and supported on a table raised to a comfortable height for the operator. A small volume of local anesthetic (1–2 mL) is

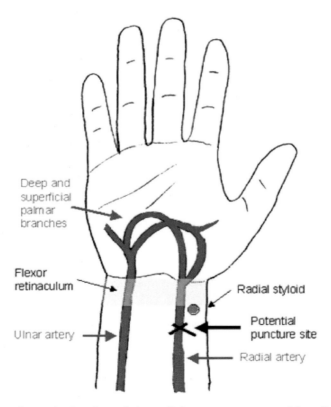

Fig. 4. Diagrammatic representation of the radial artery anatomy with collateral circulation (palmar arch) from the ulnar artery. Note the preferred cannulation site is 1–2 cm proximal to the radial styloid. Adapted from Baim and Simon *(8)*.

Oximetry wave form: pre-compression	Oximetry wave form: maintained radial artery compression	

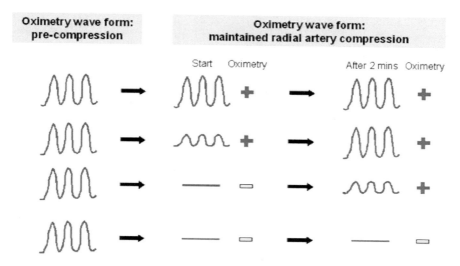

Fig. 5. Assessment of palmar arch patency using the modified Allen's test. Pulse oximetry probe on the thumb while the radial artery is compressed. An arterial waveform (even delayed in appearance and with reduced amplitude) and saturation of >90% confirm palmar arch patency. Adapted from Baim and Simon *(8)*.

administered via a 25-gauge needle infusing a small skin bleb. Care must be taken not to puncture the radial artery with local anesthetic as it may put the artery into spasm and preclude further access.

Puncture is accomplished in a similar manner to that of the femoral artery, but equipment is smaller. We use a 4 cm 21-gauge micropuncture needle, a 0.018″ guidewire, and 5 Fr 23 cm hydrophilic sheath with a tapered introducer. Following arterial puncture, care must be taken in advancing the wire gently within the relatively small artery. Resistance may be a sign of sub-intimal location or significant tortuosity where further advancement may end with arterial perforation or rupture. Over the wire placement of small, hollow bore plastic dilator may allow angiography of the distal artery to determine the nature of resistance. We have an assistant continuously drop normal saline onto the sheath as it passes through the skin to permit easier advancement and minimize the chance of spasm. In order to further minimize spasm, we give a vasodilator cocktail of 100–200 mcg nitroglycerin and 1.25–2.5 mg verapamil directly into the sheath following placement. In a similar fashion we give 2,500–5,000 units of unfractionated heparin directly into the sheath following the vasodilator cocktail. Alternatively, the heparin may be given intravenously. We mix both solutions in approximately 5 cc of normal saline within a 10 cc syringe and aspirate approximately 5 cc of blood into the syringe prior to injection in an effort to minimize the "sting" associated with acidity of both solutions.

Once the sheath is in place, the arm is adducted to lie close to the patient but typically is rested within an arm board.

Hemostasis: Radial sheaths can be removed immediately following the procedure within the catheterization laboratory. The artery is superficial and easily compressed, and closure devices are not used. However, there are a variety of commercially available compression devices that are usually placed prior to transfer out of the laboratory, i.e., RadiStop™ (Radi Medical Systems, Inc., Uppsala, Sweden),

HemoBand (HemoBand Corporation, Portland, OR), and TR Band™ (Terumo, Somerset, NJ). Occlusive pressure should be applied for approximately 180 min following carotid interventions, but patients may mobilize with compression devices in place.

Complications

Major complications following radial access procedures are rare *(23, 26, 27)*. Radial artery occlusion is the most common potential complication and was reported to occur in 5% of patients in the randomized access trial of Kiemeneij et al. *(23)*. Importantly, at 3 months, only 3% of the study population continued to have radial artery occlusion, and no patients had any functional impairment. All patients had demonstrated palmar arch patency prior to enrolling in the trial. Furthermore, incidence of occlusion has decreased with periprocedural heparin use *(28, 29)*. Forearm hematomas are possible and must be carefully assessed to ensure compartment syndrome does not ensue. If hematomas occur, bleeding can often be controlled with placement of a second occlusion device proximal to the original device. Other more rare complications include arterial rupture on sheath removal after a prolonged case which required immediate compression and emergent vascular surgery for repair *(8)*, access site infections, and sterile abscesses *(30)*.

BRACHIAL ACCESS

Historically, brachial access was the dominant technical approach for cardiac catheterization. Traditionally this was accomplished by a cut-down technique permitting direct arterial and venous puncture. However, with the advent of percutaneous techniques, cut-down approaches are rarely performed. We describe a percutaneous brachial approach and recommend a standard cardiac catheterization textbook (i.e., *Grossman's Cardiac Catheterization, Angiography, and Intervention (8)*) for further information on cut-down techniques.

Indications/Contraindications

The indications for a brachial approach are similar to those listed for a radial approach; however, brachial access allows for the use of larger catheters (i.e., up to 8 Fr). Furthermore, in patients who have contraindications to femoral access, and do not have a patent palmar arch, percutaneous brachial access may be the next best option. Unlike the radial approach, access can be on the ipsilateral or contralateral side to the planned carotid intervention. The contralateral approach can be facilitated by using a flexible tip catheter (Morph® Vascular Access Catheter; BioCardia, San Francisco, CA) to access the contralateral common carotid. As such catheters are currently available in 8 Fr sizes only, they cannot be used via the radial approach. Development of smaller flexible tip guide catheters in the future may allow contralateral carotid interventions via the radial approach.

Relative contraindications to brachial access include absence of a brachial pulse, presence of an arteriovenous fistula, overlying soft tissue infection, severe ipsilateral axillary or subclavian vascular disease, and an inability to supinate the hand or extend the elbow.

Methods

Landmarks: The anatomy of the antecubital fossa is presented in Fig. 6 Key components are the humeral epicondyles, biceps tendon, bicipital aponeurosis (a fibrous sheath underlying the antecubital skin crease), and the median nerve (lying just medial to brachial artery). Positioning involves the hand in supination and the arm fully extended at the elbow. The artery is palpated within the antecubital fossa, and the planned puncture site is 2 cm above the antecubital skin folds, slightly superior to the level of the humeral epicondyles and medial to the biceps tendon.

Puncture: The patient's arm should be positioned in a manner similar to that for radial access, with full supination of the hand and arm fully extended at the elbow. Skin prep and application of local anesthetic is as described for the femoral and radial approaches. We suggest using a 25-gauge needle for application of local anesthetic, with care being taken to avoid trauma to the median nerve. For puncture we suggest using a 21-gauge needle, a special 0.021″ heavy-duty J-tipped guidewire, and a 6 Fr sheath. The techniques for wire advancement and sheath placement are the same as for femoral access. We do not generally give vasodilator cocktails for a brachial approach, nor do we routinely give heparin. As with all access procedures, care must be taken with aspiration and flushing to ensure there is no clot buildup within the sheath.

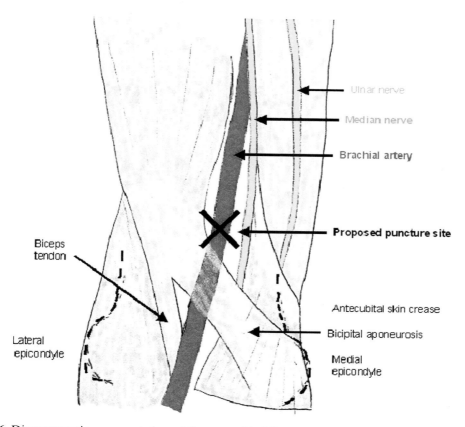

Fig. 6. Diagrammatic representation of the antecubital fossa on the right arm. The artery is best punctured 1–2 cm above the antecubital skin crease medial to the bicipital aponeurosis. Note the median nerve just medial to the brachial artery. Humeral epicondyles are represented by the *dashed lines.*

Hemostasis: Manual compression for 15 minutes is the hemostasis technique of choice with brachial punctures. Alternatively, Baim and Simon *(8)* describe a technique where proximal control is obtained using a blood pressure cuff while a gauze dressing and clear intravenous infusion pressure bag inflated to above systolic pressure is placed over the puncture site. The blood pressure cuff is then deflated allowing the IV bag to maintain hemostasis, which is gradually released over 20–25 min.

Complications

Little is published about the incidence of complications using a percutaneous brachial approach. In a series of 1,579 angioplasty cases performed via either brachial or femoral approaches, Johnson et al. *(31)* found the incidence of peripheral vascular complications to be 1.6% in the brachial access group. More recently, in their randomized access trial, Kiemeneij et al. *(23)* found that the incidence of hematoma associated with ≥2 mmol/L drop in hemoglobin was 1%, while pseudoaneurysm occurred in 1.3% of those having a procedure with brachial access. More recently, Hildick-Smith and colleagues *(32)* reported on complications in 55 patients having had coronary angiography via a brachial approach between 1997 and 2000 in a lab where femoral approach was standard. They found 5.5% of patients had major complications [which included pseudoaneurysm requiring surgery (1.8%), hematoma requiring surgery (1.8%), and hematoma with median nerve compression and dysfunction for 1 month (1.8%)]. Another 31% of patients had minor complications [need for repeat coronary angiography via alternative approach (18%), weakness of radial pulse < 24 h (3.6%), brachial artery dissection without clinical sequelae (3.6%), brachial artery spasm terminating procedure (1.8%), and wound oozing (5.4%)]. They sensibly concluded that complications are unacceptably frequent when percutaneous brachial access procedures are performed by operators not routinely using a brachial approach.

DIRECT CAROTID ACCESS

With the advancement of endovascular technology, catheters have become available in a variety of preshaped forms, and balloons and stents have become more flexible and deliverable. This has greatly increased the success of intubating the aortic origin of the carotid vessels and delivering wires, embolic protection, balloons, and stents to the carotid vessels from the arm or common femoral approaches. Therefore, the need for direct carotid punctures has decreased and is no longer routinely performed.

Indications/Contraindications

The great vessels may arise from the aortic arch in extremely acute angles. In situations like this, anatomical factors may guide catheter engagement of the carotid arteries or hinder embolic protection, balloon, or stent delivery. Therefore, direct carotid puncture may be the only option for an endovascular procedure. The presence of extensive atherosclerotic disease within the common carotid artery is a contraindication to this approach as puncture with a plaque has high incidence of embolism and stroke. Like other percutaneous approaches, relative contraindications include overlying soft tissue infection using one of the access points described above.

Methods

Landmarking: Figure 7 is a diagrammatic representation of direct carotid access. The key landmarks are the medial border of the sternocleidomastoid muscle, clavicle, and thyroid cartilage. Patient positioning is important. The procedure is most easily accomplished when the head is hyperextended, rotated somewhat laterally, with the ipsilateral shoulder slightly elevated. Ideally, puncture should be as low in the neck as possible, and Diethrich et al. *(33)* suggested 2 cm above the clavicle is a reasonable location to provide enough length of common carotid into which the sheath maybe placed below the carotid bifurcation.

Anesthesia: For direct carotid puncture, it is important that the patient not move or talk. This is relatively easy to achieve with more distal access, but for direct puncture of the neck, it may be best for patients to receive general anesthesia and be intubated for ventilatory support *(33)*. The downside to general anesthesia is the need for intubation, the complex logistics of ensuring availability of an anesthesiologist, and the inability to immediately assess neurologic status following the procedure. If general anesthesia is considered, choice of a short-acting, rapidly reversible agent is preferred given the need for extubation and neurologic assessment immediately following the procedure and before the patient is transferred out of the interventional room *(34)*. Cervical block and local anesthesia have also been successfully used *(35, 36)*.

Puncture: Patient positioning and anesthesia have been described above. Skin prep is the same as previously described. For equipment we suggest using an 18-gauge puncture needle and a 0.035″ J-tipped hydrophilic guidewire with puncture

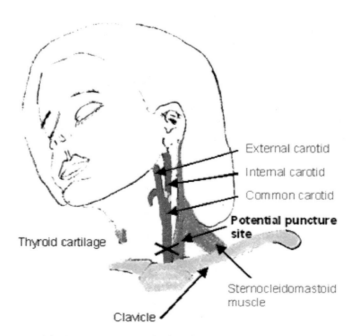

Fig. 7. Common carotid artery represented with the patient's head hyperextended and rotated laterally with the shoulder on the treatment side slightly elevated. Puncture should be 1–2 cm above the clavicle just medial to the sternocleidomastoid muscle and well below the carotid bifurcation. Adapted from Diethrich et al. *(33)*.

and wire insertion as previously described. It is important to emphasize the crucial need for slow and careful wire advancement to ensure there is no disruption of atherosclerotic material or advancement within a sub-intimal channel. Furthermore, we suggest the wire be advanced under fluoroscopic guidance to sit within the external carotid artery prior to needle removal and placement of the sheath. For sheaths, we suggest using a 7 Fr 6 cm sheath with dilator in the usual fashion. Again, because of the concern over embolization, we insert the sheath with fluoroscopic guidance positioned so that the distal end is 2 cm proximal to the carotid bifurcation. Flush and aspiration must be done with extra care, and we give 3,000–5,000 units of heparin through the sheath to aid with thrombus prevention.

Hemostasis: Following procedural completion, our first step for achievement of hemostasis is measurement of an activated clotting time (ACT). We prefer to have the ACT in the range of <150 s prior to sheath removal and administer protamine sulfate as required. The sheath is then removed and manual pressure is held over the puncture site for 15 min. Anesthesia is maintained until the puncture is completely sealed. We attempt to prevent hypertension during manual pressure to prevent hematoma formation. Likewise, it is important to try to avoid coughing and retching with extubation as this can also contribute to hematoma formation. In fact, we suggest manual pressure to be applied until after the patient is extubated.

Complications

As with other percutaneous techniques, the potential complications are hematoma, pseudoaneurysm, and arteriovenous fistula with sheath removal. Early experience by Diethrich and colleagues showed an 11% vascular complication rate, and they favored a transfemoral approach as technology evolved. They highlighted the importance of coordinating sheath removal with anesthesia to minimize the chance of coughing, retching, and hypertension which can result in hematoma formation and potential neurologic sequelae (33). As discussed above, there is also an increased risk of embolic events related to the puncture with direct carotid access. Although Diethrich and colleagues only started systemic anticoagulation after their first 38 patients, they continued to have neurologic sequelae in 10.9% of their first 110 patients. It is unclear if this could have been reduced with embolic protection devices (33).

SUMMARY

Modern endovascular technology permits percutaneous access to the arterial system from a variety of locations to enable carotid stenting. Common femoral arterial access is performed most routinely and is the preferred access site, but vascular complications can occur. With attention to procedural details, and possibly with increased use of closure devices, the incidence of these complications can be reduced. Radial access is associated with a lower incidence of vascular complications, but sheath sizes are smaller and engagement of guide catheters can be more difficult. Brachial access allows greater sheath size, but operators who are not adept with this approach may have a higher incidence of vascular complications. Direct carotid puncture permits access to the carotid vessels when impossible by other routes, but it is more technically challenging and is associated with a higher incidence of vascular complications and adverse neurologic sequelae. Despite the choice of access sites, 98% of carotid procedures can be successfully completed with modern equipment using a percutaneous transfemoral approach.

REFERENCES

1. Seldinger S. Catheter replacement of the needle in percutaneous arteriography: A new technique. Acta Radiologica 1953;39:368–376.
2. Rosenfield K, Babb JD, Cates CU, et al. Clinical competence statement on carotid stenting: training and credentialing for carotid stenting – multispecialty consensus recommendations: a report of the SCAI/SVMB/SVS Writing Committee to develop a clinical competence statement on carotid interventions. J Am Coll Cardiol 2005;45:165–174.
3. Fransson SG, Nylander E. Vascular injury following cardiac catheterization, coronary angiography, and coronary angioplasty. Eur Heart J 1994;15:232–235.
4. Kim D, Orron DE, Skillman JJ, et al. Role of superficial femoral artery puncture in the development of pseudoaneurysm and arteriovenous fistula complicating percutaneous transfemoral cardiac catheterization.[see comment]. Catheter Cardiovasc Diagn 1992;25:91–97.
5. Garrett PD, Eckart RE, Bauch TD, Thompson CM, Stajduhar KC. Fluoroscopic localization of the femoral head as a landmark for common femoral artery cannulation. Catheter Cardiovasc Interv 2005;65:205–207.
6. Grier D, Hartnell G. Percutaneous femoral artery puncture: practice and anatomy.[see comment]. Br J Radiol 1990;63:602–604.
7. Lechner G, Jantsch H, Waneck R, Kretschmer G. The relationship between the common femoral artery, the inguinal crease, and the inguinal ligament: a guide to accurate angiographic puncture. Cardiovasc Interven Radiol 1988;11:165–69.
8. Baim DS, Wahr D, George B, et al. Randomized trial of a distal embolic protection device during percutaneous intervention of saphenous vein aorto-coronary bypass grafts. Circulation 2002; 105:1285–1290.
9. Schnyder G, Sawhney N, Whisenant B, Tsimikas S, Turi ZG. Common femoral artery anatomy is influenced by demographics and comorbidity: implications for cardiac and peripheral invasive studies. Catheter Cardiovasc Interven 2001;53:289–295.
10. Pracyk JB, Wall TC, Longabaugh JP, et al. A randomized trial of vascular hemostasis techniques to reduce femoral vascular complications after coronary intervention. Am J Cardiol 1998;81: 970–976.
11. Vaitkus PT. A meta-analysis of percutaneous vascular closure devices after diagnostic catheterization and percutaneous coronary intervention. J Invasive Cardiol 2004;16:243–246.
12. Deuling JHH, Vermeulen RP, Anthonio RA, et al. Closure of the femoral artery after cardiac catheterization: a comparison of Angio-Seal, StarClose, and manual compression.[see comment]. Catheter Cardiovasc Interven 2008;71:518–523.
13. Yusuf S, Zhao F, Mehta SR, Chrolavicius S, Tognoni G, Fox KK. Effects of clopidogrel in addition to aspirin in patients with acute coronary syndromes without ST-segment elevation. N Engl J Med 2001;345:494–502.
14. Dauerman HL, Applegate RJ, Cohen DJ. Vascular closure devices: the second decade. J Am Coll Cardiol 2007;50:1617–1626.
15. Madigan JB, Ratnam LA, Belli AM. Arterial closure devices. A review. J Cardiovasc Surg 2007;48:607–624.
16. Berry C, Kelly J, Cobbe SM, Eteiba H. Comparison of femoral bleeding complications after coronary angiography versus percutaneous coronary intervention. Am J Cardiol 2004;94: 361–363.
17. Tavris DR, Dey S, Albrecht-Gallauresi B, et al. Risk of local adverse events following cardiac catheterization by hemostasis device use – phase II. J Invasive Cardiol 2005;17:644–650.
18. Ohlow MA, Secknus MA, von Korn H, et al. Incidence and outcome of femoral vascular complications among 18,165 patients undergoing cardiac catheterisation. Int J Cardiol July 2008 (epub).
19. Webber GW, Jang J, Gustavson S, Olin JW. Contemporary management of postcatheterization pseudoaneurysms. Circulation 2007;115:2666–2674.
20. Farouque HM, Tremmel JA, Raissi Shabari F, et al. Risk factors for the development of retroperitoneal hematoma after percutaneous coronary intervention in the era of glycoprotein IIb/IIIa inhibitors and vascular closure devices. J Am Coll Cardiol 2005;45:363–368.

21. Folmar J, Sachar R, Mann T. Transradial approach for carotid artery stenting: a feasibility study. Catheter Cardiovasc Interv 2007;69:355–361.
22. Choussat R, Black A, Bossi I, Fajadet J, Marco J. Vascular complications and clinical outcome after coronary angioplasty with platelet IIb/IIIa receptor blockade. Comparison of transradial vs transfemoral arterial access. Eur Heart J 2000;21:662–667.
23. Kiemeneij F, Laarman GJ, Odekerken D, Slagboom T, Van Der Wieken R. A randomized comparison of percutaneous transluminal coronary angioplasty by the radial, brachial, and femoral approaches: the access study. J Am Coll Cardiol 1997;29:1269–1275.
24. Mann T, Cubeddu G, Bowen J, et al. Stenting in acute coronary syndromes: a comparison of radial versus femoral access site. J Am Coll Cardiol 1998;32:572–576.
25. Hovagim A, Katz R, Poppers P. Pulse oximetry for evaluation of radial and ulnar arterial blood flow. J Cardiothorac Anaesth 1989;3:27–30.
26. Archbold RA, Robinson NM, Schilling RJ. Radial artery access for coronary angiography and percutaneous coronary intervention. Br Med J 2004;329:443–446.
27. Bazemore E, Mann JT, 3rd. Problems and complications of the transradial approach for coronary interventions: a review. J Invasive Cardiol 2005;17:156–159.
28. Nagai S, Abe S, Sato T, et al. Ultrasonic assessment of vascular complications in coronary angiography and angioplasty after transradial approach. Am J Cardiol 1999;83:180–186.
29. Spaulding C, Lefevre T, Funck F, et al. Left radial approach for coronary angiography: results of a prospective study. Catheter Cardiovasc Diagn 1996;39:365–370.
30. Kozak M, Adams DR, Ioffreda MD, et al. Sterile inflammation associated with transradial catheterization and hydrophilic sheaths. Catheter Cardiovasc Interven 2003;59:207–213.
31. Johnson LW, Esente P, Giambartolomei A, et al. Peripheral vascular complications of coronary angioplasty by the femoral and brachial techniques. Catheter Cardiovasc Diagn 1994;31:165–172.
32. Hildick-Smith DJ, Khan ZI, Shapiro LM, Petch MC. Occasional-operator percutaneous brachial coronary angiography: first, do no arm. Catheter Cardiovasc Interven 2002;57:161–165; discussion 166.
33. Diethrich EB, Marx P, Wrasper R, Reid DB. Percutaneous techniques for endoluminal carotid interventions. J Endovasc Surg 1996;3:182–202.
34. Kharrazi MR. Anesthesia for carotid stent procedures. J Endovasc Surg 1996;3:211–216.
35. Bergeron P, Chambran P, Benichou H, Alessandri C. Recurrent carotid disease: will stents be an alternative to surgery? J Endovasc Surg 1996;3:76–79.
36. Alessandri C, Bergeron P. Local anesthesia in carotid angioplasty. J Endovasc Surg 1996;3:31–34.

10 Aortic Arch and Cerebrovascular Anatomy and Angiography

Jacqueline Saw, MD, FRCPC
and Simon Walsh, MD

CONTENTS

ABSTRACT

A thorough understanding of the cerebrovascular anatomy is essential to help operators perform carotid stenting safely and successfully. A complete pre-procedural angiography to assess the great vessels and carotid arteries anatomy helps operators to strategize and select their equipment. We will review the cerebrovascular anatomy and the technical aspects of diagnostic carotid angiography.

Keywords: Carotid artery; Middle cerebral artery; Anterior cerebral artery; Posterior cerebral artery; Vertebral artery

INTRODUCTION

A thorough understanding of the cerebrovascular anatomy is essential for carotid interventionalists to enable carotid artery angiography and stenting to be performed safely and successfully. Performing a complete pre-procedural angiography to assess the great vessels and carotid arteries anatomy (including the collateral circulation) allows operators to strategize their approach to carotid artery stenting (CAS) with respect to equipment choice and techniques necessary to complete the procedure in a safe and expedient manner. This chapter is divided into two main sections: a review of the cerebrovascular anatomy and technical aspects of diagnostic carotid angiography.

From: *Contemporary Cardiology: Carotid Artery Stenting: The Basics*
Edited by: J. Saw, DOI 10.1007/978-1-60327-314-5_10,
© Humana Press, a part of Springer Science+Business Media, LLC 2009

GREAT VESSEL AND CEREBROVASCULAR ANATOMY

The Aortic Arch

The adult aortic arch normally gives rise to the innominate (right brachiocephalic) artery, the left common carotid artery (LCCA) and the left subclavian artery (Fig. 1). However, this great vessel branching pattern is seen in only 65% of the population. There are several arch anatomic variations, the most common variant (in ~27% of cases) is either a common origin of the innominate and LCCA or the LCCA arising distinctly as a branch of the innominate (Fig. 2). This configuration is often referred

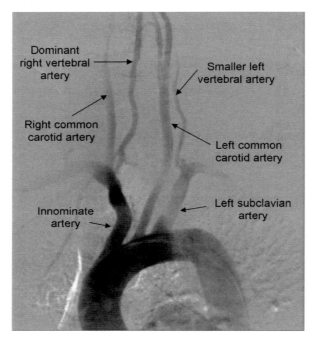

Fig. 1. Normal aortic arch branch pattern.

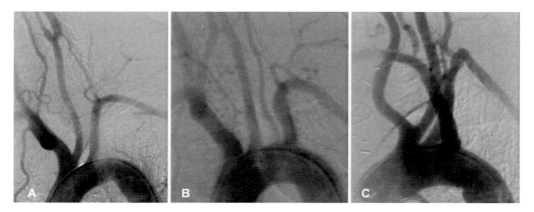

Fig. 2. Aortic arch variants: (**A**) bovine aortic arch with the left common carotid artery branching off from the innominate artery, (**B**) separate origin of the left vertebral artery from the aortic arch, (**C**) common carotid trunk and separate origin of the right subclavian artery distally from the aortic arch.

to as a "bovine arch", although this terminology is actually a misnomer. The actual true bovine arch described in cows is a single brachiocephalic trunk off the aortic arch, which then splits into (a) right subclavian artery, (b) common carotid trunk and (c) left subclavian artery *(1–2)*.

Other less common variations include a separate origin of the left vertebral artery directly from the arch between the LCCA and the left subclavian artery (occurs in ~6%), and the right subclavian artery arising from the arch distal to the left subclavian artery and then passing behind the oesophagus (~1%). Much more rare variants include a common origin of the LCCA and left subclavian artery (two brachiocephalic trunks), separate origins of the right subclavian artery (proximally) and the right common carotid artery (RCCA), single arch vessel, a common carotid trunk and a common subclavian trunk, and right-sided aortic arch *(3)*.

Assessment of the aortic arch anatomy is crucial for CAS. In addition to providing information on calcification, aneurysmal dilatation, atheroma and normal anatomic variations, the operator must also determine the classification of the aortic arch that is present. With increasing age, the aorta tends to unfold and elongate, with the great vessels origin being displaced caudally. This creates a steeper aortic arch over time and spreads the origins of the great vessels as well as altering their angle of take-off relative to the top of the arch. The aortic arch is classified into three categories: types I, II and III (Figs. 3 and 4). This classification is most commonly based upon the

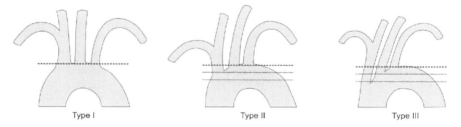

Fig. 3. Classification of the aortic arch into types I, II and III.

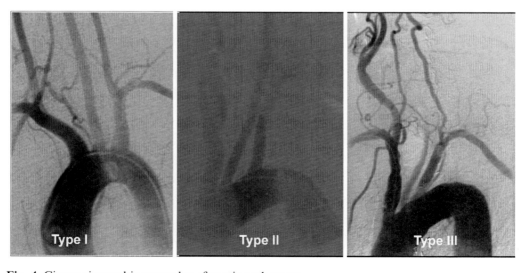

Fig. 4. Cineangiographic examples of aortic arch types.

degree of inferior displacement of the great vessels from the top curvature of the arch. The widest diameter of the proximal portion of the LCCA is used as the reference diameter, and the apex of the aortic arch is taken as the point of reference. If all the great vessels arise within one reference LCCA diameter of the arch apex, then the arch is classified as type I. If all the great vessels arise within two reference LCCA diameters, then the arch is type 2. Finally if all the great vessels arise more than two reference LCCA diameters from the arch, it is classified as type III.

An alternative method of classifying the arch has also been proposed. The type I aortic arch can also be characterized by the three great vessels originating in the same horizontal plane as the outer curvature of the aortic arch. In the type II aortic arch, the innominate artery originates between the horizontal planes of the outer and inner curvatures of the aortic arch. In the type III aortic arch, the innominate artery originates below the horizontal plane of the inner curvature of the aortic arch *(4)*.

For carotid intervention, the steeper the arch and in particular the more inferior the origin of the target artery (in type II or III aortic arches, especially when accessing the innominate from a femoral route), the greater the difficulty in gaining access to the target vessel.

The Subclavian Arteries

In most individuals, the right subclavian artery arises from the innominate artery. The left subclavian artery typically has a separate origin and is the most distal branch of the great vessels from the ascending aorta. The origin of the left subclavian artery is usually posterior to the LCCA, approximately at the level of the fourth thoracic vertebra (T4). The subclavian arteries are divided into three parts: the first part extends from the ostium of the vessel to the medial border of the anterior scalene muscle, the second part passes behind the muscle and the third part extends from the lateral border of the scalene to the lateral border of the first rib. Beyond this, the vessel becomes the axillary artery. Variations in subclavian artery origins are discussed previously and are much more frequently seen with the right subclavian artery.

The subclavian arteries give rise to four main branches. These are the vertebral artery, the thyrocervical trunk, the internal mammary artery and the costocervical artery. The vertebral arteries are usually the first branches of the subclavian arteries. The thyrocervical trunk is usually a short vessel that arises from the superior portion of the first part of the subclavian artery. The internal mammary artery arises inferiorly from the subclavian artery, approximately opposite to the origin of the thyrocervical trunk. The costocervical artery is usually the smallest and most distal of the branches of the subclavian artery *(5)*.

The Anterior Circulation

Common Carotid Arteries (CCA)

The RCCA usually arises from the innominate artery, which then continues as the right subclavian artery. Typically this bifurcation occurs behind the sternoclavicular joint. The LCCA originates within the thorax from the aortic arch between the innominate and left subclavian arteries. Variations in the origin of the RCCA are unusual, whilst it is frequent for the LCCA to arise off the innominate artery.

The common carotid arteries typically do not give rise to any branches proximal to the carotid bifurcation of the internal and external carotid arteries. Rarely, the ascending pharyngeal, superior or inferior thyroid arteries may arise from the CCA. This is often associated with a higher carotid bifurcation. Normally the bifurcation of the internal and external carotid arteries lies at the C4–C5 level. However, in ~40% of patients the bifurcation is higher, whilst it is lower in ~10% *(5)*.

EXTERNAL CAROTID ARTERY (ECA)

This vessel is responsible for supplying the structures of the neck, face, scalp, maxilla and tongue outside the skull. The branches are variable in both location and number, but the most common order of origin is superior thyroid, lingual, facial, ascending pharyngeal, occipital, posterior auricular, maxillary and superficial temporal arteries (from proximal to distal) (Fig. 5).

The ECA also gives rise to more distal branches that supply the dura of the basal and lateral brain surfaces, of the middle and anterior cranial fossa, as well as the posterior fossa dura. When there is critical stenosis of the ipsilateral internal carotid artery (ICA), the ECA can give rise to intracranial blood supply via collaterals and reverse flow in the ophthalmic artery. In addition, following ipsilateral vertebral artery occlusion, the occipital branch of the ECA may provide flow to the terminal segment of the vertebral artery via intramuscular collaterals.

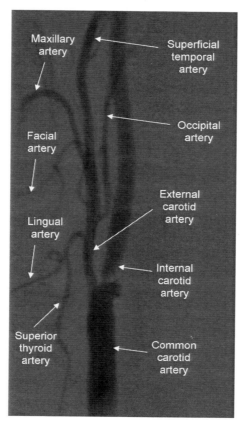

Fig. 5. Branching of the common carotid artery into the internal carotid artery (with an ostial lesion in this example) and external carotid artery (with its major branches labelled).

The ECA may become compromised by carotid stenting. However, there is an extensive collateralization of the distal portions of the bilateral ECA systems (via multiple muscular communicators). Therefore, closure of a single ECA rarely results in significant symptoms. If the origins of both ECA are compromised the patient may experience jaw claudication for a few weeks after the procedure, although this usually resolves with no specific management *(5)*.

INTERNAL CAROTID ARTERY (ICA)

The ICA supplies blood to the anterior cerebral hemispheres, as well as the ipsilateral eye, nose and forehead. After bifurcation from the ECA, the ICA runs posterolateral to the ECA. There are several nomenclature classification systems to describe the ICA, and traditionally it is common to divide the ICA into five main segments (cervical, petrous, cavernous, clinoid and supraclinoid segments) (Fig. 6). A more recent classification by Bouthillier *(6)* divides the ICA into seven segments based on the angiographic appearance: cervical segment (C1), petrous segment (C2), lacerum segment (C3), cavernous segment (C4), clinoid segment (C5), ophthalmic segment (C6) and communicating segment (C7). The traditional petrous portion would encompass the C2 and C3 segments, and the supraclinoid portion would encompass the C6 and C7 segments of this new nomenclature.

From its origin at the C4–C5 bifurcation, the cervical ICA (C1) begins with a fusiform dilated carotid sinus and passes up the neck into the skull base without giving off any branches. The proximal cervical portion of the ICA tends to have

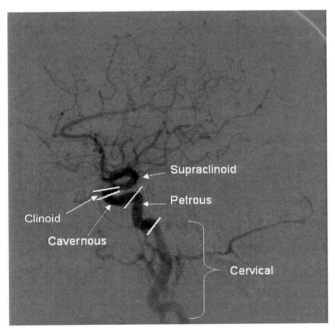

Fig. 6. Internal carotid artery classification: cervical segment (C1), petrous segment (C2), lacerum segment (C3), cavernous segment (C4), clinoid segment (C5), ophthalmic segment (C6), and communicating segment (C7). The traditional petrous portion would encompass the C2 and C3 segments, and the supraclinoid portion would encompass the C6 and C7 segments of the new Bouthillier nomenclature *(6)*.

only gentle curvatures; however, the mid- to distal segment may be tortuous, kinked or looped, which creates difficulties for CAS (including passage of filter embolic protection devices) (see Fig. 12 in Chapter 11). The most common site for atheroma is at the origin of the ICA or in the proximal portion of the cervical segment.

The petrous segment (C2) of the ICA starts when it enters the petrous temporal bone of the skull base. It then travels through the carotid canal beginning with the vertical segment, followed by the genu, and into the horizontal segment. The vertical segment is ~1 cm long, which then turns at the genu into the horizontal segment. The horizontal segment is ~2 cm in length, with a course that is anterior and medial towards the petrous apex, and then ends at the foramen lacerum. The petrous ICA may give off two small branches (although not usually visualized by angiography): the caroticotympanic artery and the artery of the pterygoid canal (the vidian artery). These small arteries may become important as they can provide collateral flow from the ECA when the ICA is occluded.

The lacerum segment (C3) is a very short segment that begins above the foramen lacerum and runs extradural being surrounded by periosteum and fibrocartilage. It ends at the petrolingual ligament of the sphenoid bone. There are usually no branches, although the vidian artery sometimes arises from this segment.

The ICA then continues as the cavernous segment (C4) that runs in the S-shaped cavernous sinus, starting from the petrolingual ligament to the proximal dural ring. In this tortuous segment, the ICA runs between the layers of dura mater that make up the wall of the cavernous sinus. Thus, this segment is relatively inflexible and tortuous, which often poses challenges to interventionalists performing intracranial intervention by restricting equipment access. The cavernous ICA gives off the meningohypophyseal trunk, the artery of the inferior cavernous sinus (inferolateral trunk) and small capsular arteries that supply the wall of the cavernous sinus. The meningohypophyseal trunk supplies the dura, tentorium and inferior pituitary, whilst the inferolateral trunk supplies the cranial nerves.

The clinoid segment (C5) is a short segment that begins after the cavernous sinus at the proximal dural ring and extends to the distal dural ring. Above this point, the ICA enters the dura into the subarachnoid space. Thus, the supraclinoid segment is intradural. The clinoid segment usually has no branches, although the ophthalmic artery sometimes arises from this segment.

The ophthalmic segment (C6) starts from the distal dural ring and extends to the origin of the posterior communicating artery (PCOM). This segment gives off the ophthalmic artery and the superior hypophyseal artery. The ophthalmic artery enters the optic cavity via the optic canal and supplies the retina. Occlusion of this vessel leads to monocular blindness, whilst transient ischemia results in the symptom of amaurosis fugax. Distal branches of the ophthalmic artery anastomose with distal branches of the maxillary artery, and thus can give rise to ECA to ICA collaterals when the ICA is occluded.

The communicating segment (C7) is the terminal segment which starts at the origin of the PCOM and ends at the carotid terminus, which bifurcates into the anterior cerebral artery (ACA) and middle cerebral artery (MCA). The fourth important branch from this segment is the anterior choroidal artery, which arises 2–4 mm after the PCOM posteriorly. The PCOM (when present) joins the anterior circulation (of the ICA) to the posterior circulation (vertebrobasilar system), by connecting to the posterior cerebral artery (PCA) at the junction between the P1 and

P2 segments. This is an important collateral component of the Circle of Willis. When the PCOM is the major contributor to the PCA P1 segment, then the PCA is termed foetal *(3, 5)*. Numerous perforating arteries can arise from the PCOM that can supply the thalamus, hypothalamus, subthalamus, internal capsule, optic chiasm, optic tract and pituitary stalk. This vessel is also a common site for aneurysms. The anterior choroidal artery provides arterial supply to several important structures. These include the temporal lobe, internal capsule, thalamus, lateral geniculate body, cerebral peduncle and optic tract. Anterior choroidal artery infarction is catastrophic, resulting in a dense contralateral haemiparesis affecting the face, arm and leg. In addition, there can also be contralateral hemisensory loss and contralateral haemianopia if the lateral geniculate body is involved.

MIDDLE CEREBRAL ARTERY (MCA)

The MCA supplies most of the temporal lobe, anterolateral frontal lobe, insula and parietal lobe. Complete occlusion of the MCA is usually an embolic phenomenon. This will lead to a contralateral hemiplegia that is associated with a homonymous hemianopia on the same side as the weakness (contralateral to the MCA occlusion). Angiographically, the MCA is divided into four segments: the M1 or sphenoidal segment, the M2 or insular segment, the M3 or opercular segment and the M4 or cortical segment (Fig. 7). In this classification, anatomical location rather than branches define the segments of the MCA.

The M1 segment starts at the carotid terminus, followed by a proximal horizontal segment which terminates at the sylvian fissure. It gives rise to lenticulostriate perforators that supply the internal capsule, the body and part of the head of the caudate nucleus and the globus pallidus. Angioplasty within this segment can compromise the perforators and cause ischemia of the internal capsule. Infarction in the distribution of the M1 segment leads to a contralateral haemiplegia and is associated with a high mortality rate *(3)*. The M1 segment also divides into the superior and inferior subdivisions, and emboli often lodge at this bifurcation *(5)*.

The M2 segment starts at the superior turn of the insula and ends at the circular sulcus of the insula (hairpin). M2 occlusion results in a contralateral hemiparesis that affects the face and arm more severely than the leg. Contralateral homonymous hemianopia is also seen and is often associated with visual neglect towards the hemianopic field. Broca's aphasia (motor), Wernicke's aphasia (receptive) and apraxia in both upper extremities can also occur with M2 occlusion in the dominant hemisphere *(3)*. Non-dominant hemisphere occlusion leads to neglect, confusion and delirium.

The M3 segment starts at the circular sulcus of insula and extends to the lateral convexity. Beyond this continues the M4 or cortical segment, which supplies the lateral cortical surface. Together, the M3 and M4 segments supply the lateral two-thirds of the cerebral hemispheres. Distal embolic events in the M3 and M4 territories result in very specific neurological deficits. These are highly variable according to the location of the occlusion.

ANTERIOR CEREBRAL ARTERY (ACA)

The ACA supplies the medial surface of the cerebral cortex (frontal and parietal lobes) and the anterior portions of the corpus callosum, basal ganglia and internal capsule. It arises from the bifurcation of the ICA at the carotid terminus and joins its counterpart (the contralateral ACA) via the anterior communicating artery

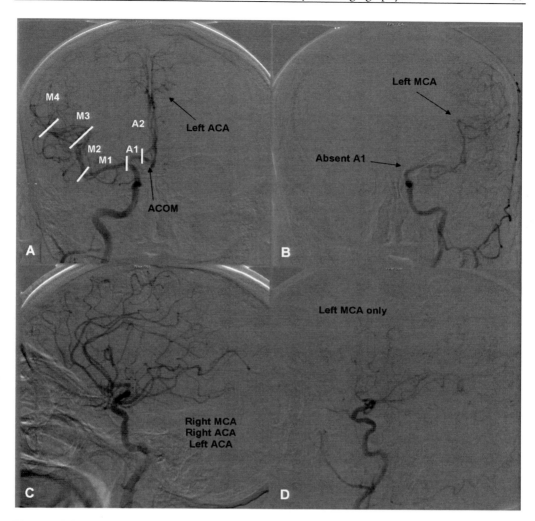

Fig. 7. Right and left internal carotid artery angiograms in the posteroanterior (**A** and **B**) and lateral (**C** and **D**) projections of the same patient, showing the middle cerebral artery (MCA) and anterior cerebral artery (ACA) classifications. (**A**) The right internal carotid artery bifurcates into the right ACA and MCA, and the right ACA supplies the left ACA via the anterior communicating artery (ACOM). (**B**) This patient has an incomplete Circle of Willis with absent left A1 segment, and posterior communicating arteries (PCOM) are also not visualized. (**C**) Lateral projection showing filling of the right MCA, right ACA and left ACA via ACOM. (**D**) Lateral projection showing filling of the left MCA only.

(ACOM), thus completing the anterior portion of the Circle of Willis. However, the ACOM can be atretic or absent, in which case crossover filling between the hemispheres will not be visualized. Furthermore, in about 7–10% of cases, the A1 segment of the ACA is hypoplastic or absent (Fig. 7). Occlusion of the ACA leads to contralateral weakness in the lower limb as well as sensory deficits such as poor touch localization with bilateral stimuli. Bilateral occlusion of the ACAs will compromise flow to the frontal lobe and lead to a "locked-in" syndrome or akinetic mutism.

The ACA is divided into five segments, A1–A5 (Figs. 7 and 8). The A1 segment runs from the origin of the ACA to the ACOM. Perforators from the A1 segment

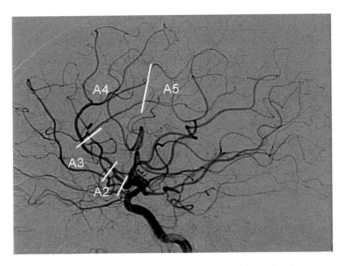

Fig. 8. Anterior cerebral artery classification (see text for explanation).

supply the septal region and hypothalamus. The A2 segment of the ACA runs superiorly and posteriorly around the rostrum of the corpus callosum. This segment also supplies the hypothalamus. The recurrent artery of Heubner arises from the A2 segment. This vessel supplies the anterior caudate nucleus, the anterior putamen, the globus pallidus and the anterior limb of the internal capsule. Infarction of the recurrent artery of Heubner may cause mild weakness in the contralateral limb, dysarthria and patients frequently experience profound apathy with difficulty initiating movement *(3)*.

The A2 segment ends at the junction of the rostrum and genu of the corpus callosum. The A3 segment begins from the corpus callosum genu to where the ACA turns sharply posterior above the genu. The A4 segment is the anterior segment located in the corpus callosum, and the A5 segment is the posterior segment in the corpus callosum. The A4 and A5 segments are divided by an imaginary line just posterior to the coronal suture *(7)*. However, these definitions are difficult to remember, and most clinicians refer to the latter segments (A3–A5) simply as distal ACA segments.

The distal branches of the ACA give rise to numerous cortical branches (Fig. 9). These include the orbitofrontal artery (supplies the orbital gyri, olfactory bulb and olfactory tract), frontopolar artery (supplies the edge of the subfrontal sulcus, the inferior portion of the cingulated gyri and the anterior portion of the superior frontal gyrus) and the callosomarginal artery (supplies the anterior two-thirds of the medial cerebral hemispheres). Finally, in about 75% of cases, the pericallosal branch of the ACA anastomoses with the terminal branches of the PCA.

The Posterior Circulation

VERTEBRAL ARTERIES

The vertebral artery is usually the first branch arising from the proximal segment of the subclavian artery. The left vertebral artery can also arise directly from the aortic arch (usually between the left common carotid and left subclavian arteries). Less frequently, the left vertebral artery can arise from the LCCA. Variations of the

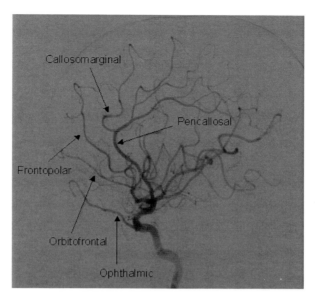

Fig. 9. Distal branches of the anterior cerebral artery.

origin of the right vertebral artery are less common, although this vessel can originate from the RCCA, the innominate artery or the aortic arch. In up to 3% of cases, either vertebral artery can arise from the thyrocervical or costocervical trunk *(5)*. Finally, the vertebral arteries may terminate at the posterior inferior cerebellar artery (PICA) origin and not contribute to basilar artery flow. Inequality in the diameter between the two vertebral arteries is also common, with one vessel being dominant (Fig. 1) in the majority of people (usually the left side in ∼60% of cases). In more extreme examples, the non-dominant vertebral artery can be atretic or even absent.

The vertebral artery can be divided into four or five segments (Fig. 10). The initial portion of the vessel typically has no branches. The V1 segment starts at the origin of the vertebral artery and classically ends when it enters the C6 transverse foramen (in ∼90% of cases; the remainder of the times V1 can enter the transverse foramen from C3 to C7). The V2 portion comprises the segment of the vertebral artery that runs within the intervertebral foramina until it exits the transverse foramen of C2 (or atlas). In the four-segment classification, V3 is defined as the extracranial segment of the vertebral artery between exiting C2 and entering the foramen magnum at the base of the skull, and V4 is the intracranial segment between the dura mater till it joins the contralateral vertebral artery to become the basilar artery at the base of the medulla oblongata.

Branches from the intervertebral segment include the meningeal, muscular and radicular arteries (that enter the spinal canal and provide collateral flow to the anterior and posterior spinal arteries). The horizontal segment of V3 gives rise to meningeal branches and flow to the medulla and the posterior surface of the spinal cord. The intracranial segment gives rise to the anterior spinal and posterior inferior cerebellar arteries. The anterior spinal arteries supply the pyramids, medial lemniscus, interolivary bundles, hypothalamic nuclei, posterior longitudinal fasciculus and the anterior two-thirds of the spinal cord.

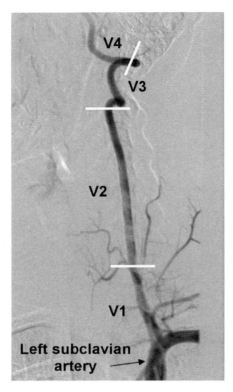

Fig. 10. Left vertebral artery angiogram showing the different segments from V1 to V4 (see text for explanation).

The posterior inferior cerebellar artery (PICA) is the largest branch of the vertebral artery and supplies the lower medulla, tonsils, vermis, fourth ventricle as well as the inferolateral cerebellum. The anterior inferior cerebellar artery (AICA) is a branch off the basilar artery. The distal AICA and PICA form an anastomosis at the lateral part of the cerebellum. Occasionally, when the AICA is very dominant, the PICA can be absent (in ~20% of cases unilaterally absent and in 1% of cases bilaterally absent), or vice versa. In about 1% of cases, the vertebral artery terminates at the PICA.

The clinical consequences of unilateral vertebral artery occlusion are variable and can be relatively benign. Occlusion resulting in PICA territory ischemia results in Wallenberg's syndrome (with ipsilateral nystagmus, Horner's syndrome, reduced corneal reflex and loss of pain and temperature sensation on the face, and contralateral loss of pain and temperature sensation on the body and extremities).

Basilar Artery

The basilar artery is a short vessel that is formed by the convergence of the two vertebral arteries. It lies in the median groove of the pons and terminates as it bifurcates into the posterior cerebral arteries (PCA) (Figs. 11 and 12). Paired branches of the basilar artery provide blood supply to the brain stem, cerebellum and cerebral cortex. The major branches are the anterior inferior cerebellar artery (AICA), the pontine perforators, the internal auditory artery, the superior

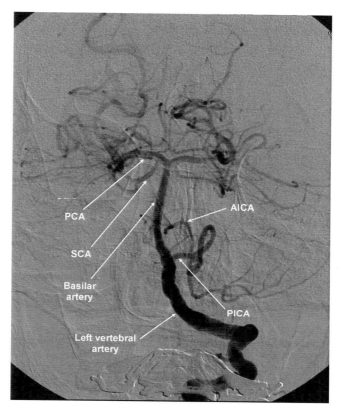

Fig. 11. Left vertebral artery angiogram showing the intracerebral branches in the posteroanterior projection: posterior inferior cerebellar artery (PICA), anterior inferior cerebellar artery (AICA), superior cerebellar artery (SCA) and posterior cerebral artery (PCA).

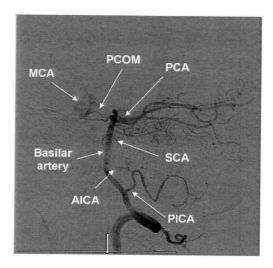

Fig. 12. Left vertebral artery angiogram showing the intracerebral branches in the lateral projection: posterior inferior cerebellar artery (PICA), anterior inferior cerebellar artery (AICA), superior cerebellar artery (SCA), posterior cerebral artery (PCA), posterior communicating artery (PCOM) and middle cerebral artery (MCA).

cerebellar artery (SCA) and the PCA. The pontine perforators are small vessels that arise at right angles on either side of the basilar artery, supplying the pons and adjacent brain. Percutaneous intervention of the basilar artery can lead to closure of these pontine perforators with catastrophic pontine infarction. The AICA supplies the pons, medulla, cerebellum, as well as the glossopharyngeal and vagal nerves. The SCA supplies the pons, as well as the deep cerebellar nuclei. Distally, the SCA connects with the terminal branches of both the inferior cerebellar arteries (AICA and PICA). Basilar artery occlusion results in variable clinical sequelae, since the larger cerebellar arteries can bypass a blocked basilar artery via the anastomoses described previously, and the anterior circulation may also provide flow through the PCOM.

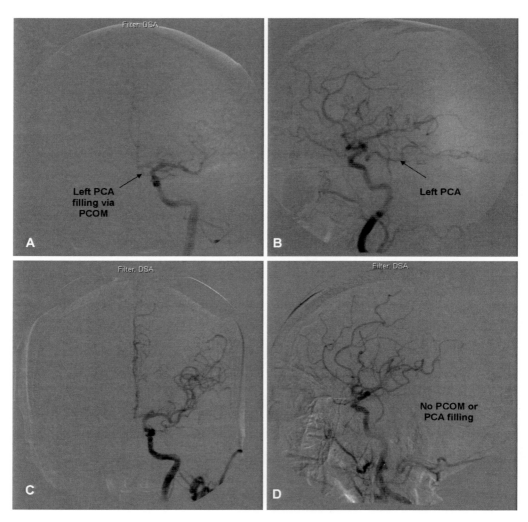

Fig. 13. Intracerebral angiograms of a patient with a left posterior communicating artery (PCOM) filling the left posterior cerebral artery (PCA) via injection of the left carotid artery in the (**A**) posteroanterior projection and (**B**) lateral projection. In comparison, this other patient does not have an angiographically visible left PCOM as shown in the (**C**) posteroanterior projection and (**D**) lateral projection.

Posterior Cerebral Artery (PCA)

The PCA is divided into four segments, P1–P4. The P1 segment begins at the origin of the PCA and ends at the PCOM origin. The P1 segment usually supplies thalamic perforators to the thalamus and subthalamic nuclei. The PCOM joins the PCA to the distal ICA (Fig. 13). The PCOM varies in length and diameter and is unilaterally absent in about one-third of autopsy cases *(8)*. The variation in PCOM size tends to diminish with age, being larger in diameter in children. In the adult configuration, the P1 segment has a larger diameter than the PCOM. In about 30% of cases, the PCOM is of the same calibre or larger than the PCA. A fetal-type PCA is used to describe cases where the P1 segment is hypoplastic or absent, in which case the ICA contributes the predominant blood supply to the PCA *(9)* (Fig. 14). This is clinically important to note since posterior circulation strokes may arise from occlusion of the anterior circulation in this foetal-type physiology.

The P2 segment begins after the origin of PCOM to its major branch, the lateral posterior choroidal artery, which supplies the posterior thalamus. The P3 and P4 segments are distal PCA segments whose branches supply cortical regions such as the undersurface of the temporal lobe, the posterior third of the interhemispheric surface, occipital lobe, visual cortex and the corpus callosum.

Circle of Willis

The Circle of Willis is the major collateral pathway of the brain. Anteriorly, it is composed of the two ICA, which gives off the two ACA that are joined by the ACOM. The anterior circulation communicates with the posterior circulation via the two PCOM arteries, which connect the distal ICA with the PCA, completing the loop (Fig. 15). However, a complete ring is only found in up to 50% of patients *(3)*.

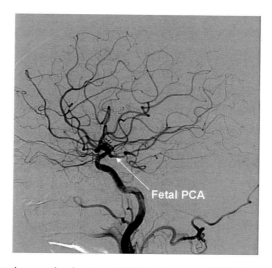

Fig. 14. Fetal-type posterior cerebral artery (PCA) where the PCOM segment is larger in calibre compared to the P1 segment.

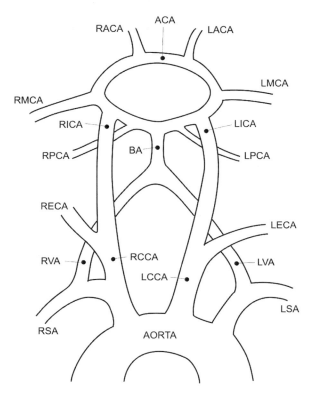

Fig. 15. Schematic diagram of the Circle of Willis showing connection between the anterior and posterior circulation via the anterior communicating and posterior communicating arteries.

GREAT VESSEL AND CEREBROVASCULAR ANGIOGRAPHY

Basic Principles

All images are acquired with digital subtraction angiography (DSA) in order to provide high-quality images, where the overlying bony structures are removed from the image. Whilst non-invasive imaging modalities such as Doppler assessment, CT angiography or MR angiography will provide valuable information for the clinician, DSA of the extracranial and intracranial vessels remains the gold standard for assessment prior to intervention. DSA will provide high-resolution imaging that distinguishes between critical lesions and complete occlusions as well as allowing detailed plaque assessment to evaluate the presence of ulceration, thrombus or calcification. These images will also provide information on lesion length and reference vessel diameter to enable selection of the correct stent size. Finally, specific anatomical characteristics such as the presence of marked tortuosity will alert the operator to the need for alternative strategies to facilitate a successful intervention.

Arterial Access

When there is no contraindication, access via the femoral artery is the preferred route of access for diagnostic and interventional procedures in the carotid or vertebral arteries. This is because access to the neck vessels can be quite challenging from brachial or radial approaches. However, on occasion, these approaches may be required. Direct carotid puncture has also been described, although, with the development of embolic protection devices and the evolution of contemporary carotid stenting practice, this technique is no longer performed in the vast majority of institutions. This is due to the inherent risks with direct carotid puncture. These include carotid dissection, thrombosis, neck haematoma, tracheal compression, stent deformation, and the need for general anaesthesia *(5)*.

In general, we rarely perform isolated diagnostic carotid angiography without proceeding on to carotid stenting. Therefore, a 5 or 6 Fr sheath is usually placed in the femoral artery and the access sheath is later up-sized to facilitate the intervention. Our practice is to perform diagnostic angiography through 5 Fr catheters. These smaller calibre catheters allow adequate vessel opacification, whilst decreasing the risk of manipulation with larger sized catheters. Some operators recommend 4 Fr catheters for diagnostic procedures; however, these require very forceful contrast injection for adequate images.

Anticoagulation, Catheter Preparation and Contrast Agents

Heparin is routinely administered to all patients for diagnostic extracranial and intracranial angiography. We usually administer a smaller dose for the diagnostic images (50 IU/kg). If proceeding on to intervention, an activated clotting time (ACT) is checked prior to engaging the guide in the carotid artery. Additional heparin is then administered as necessary to produce a target ACT of 250–300 s *(10)*.

Utmost caution is taken to prevent introduction of air into the cerebral vasculature. All catheters are suctioned and flushed to remove any air bubbles prior to diagnostic imaging. The contrast syringe is kept relatively free of blood in order to minimize the risk of thrombus formation in the syringe and catheter. In addition, the contrast syringe is orientated at an angle (>30°) during injections to prevent the introduction of air into the system.

We use an iso-osmolar contrast agent during image acquisition (e.g., Iodixanol; Visipaque, GE Healthcare, Buckinghamshire, UK). This is generally well tolerated, associated with less discomfort during injection, has a low rate of adverse reaction, and has a good renal safety profile.

Aortic Arch Angiography

An aortic arch angiogram is routinely performed first. This will allow the operator to classify the aortic arch and will also demonstrate any proximal stenosis in the great vessels. The aortic arch angiogram will help the operator in selecting the equipment and strategy for the interventional procedure. With larger image intensifiers, it is also possible to visualize the carotid bifurcation during the aortogram.

To obtain the images, a 5 Fr pigtail catheter is advanced to the ascending aorta just proximal to the innominate artery. The image intensifier is positioned in the LAO 45–60° projection. This angle opens out the arch and separates the origins of the great vessels. If the image intensifier is of sufficient size, the carotid bifurcation is often separated sufficiently to provide useful diagnostic images. Ideally, prior to image acquisition, the patient's head is turned to the right. However, if the patient is prepared for a carotid intervention, the head may be immobilized for the arch angiogram. The contrast injector is then programmed to inject at 600 psi. Typically a total of 30 cc (15 cc/s for 2 s) contrast will provide adequate DSA images in smaller patients. For larger patients, a higher volume may be required (40 cc injected at 20 cc/s over 2 s will usually suffice). As with all imaging using DSA, the patient must not move. Therefore, the patient is instructed to hold still, hold their breath, and not swallow.

Selective Carotid Angiography

Depending on the aortic arch classification, a variety of different catheters may be utilized for selective carotid angiography. For the majority of patients (those with type I, II or even some with type III arches) a 5 Fr diagnostic JR4 catheter will allow access to the carotids. For more difficult cases, reverse-curve catheters may be required to permit selective vessel engagement. These include the VTK (Cook Inc.) and Simmons (Cook Inc.) catheters, which are discussed below. In general, they carry more risks of dislodging embolic material or creating dissections at the origins of the great vessels as they are manipulated along the superior surface of the arch, and thus should only be used by more experienced interventionalists.

Usually, the carotid artery that is not selected for intervention (on the basis of clinical indication and non-invasive information) is imaged first. Imaging the target vessel second permits the use of exchange wires and the delivery of the interventional guides seamlessly during the procedure. The JR4 catheter is advanced to the aortic arch over a standard 0.035″ guidewire. The guidewire is then removed and the entire system is flushed carefully to remove any air bubbles. The origin of the vessel of interest is then selectively engaged (usually by counterclockwise rotation). A roadmap image is constructed usually in an ipsilateral 20–30° view, although angles can vary according to individual anatomy. A stiff angled Glidewire® (Terumo Medical Coporation, Somerset, NJ) is then advanced into the mid- or distal segment of the common carotid artery. The diagnostic catheter is tracked carefully over this wire. At this point the operator should take care to ensure that the guidewire does not "drift" higher up the vessel whilst the catheter is advanced. Finally the wire is removed and the entire system is meticulously flushed to ensure that there is no air in the system.

Selective acquisitions of cineangiograms are then performed with DSA focusing on the carotid bifurcation, the commonest site of severe lesions. The image should be centred at the level of the mandible. A standard imaging sequence will be an ipsilateral 30° view of the carotid bifurcation (RAO for the right carotid and LAO for the left) followed by a left lateral view (LAO 90° for both vessels). However, these angulations are simply a guide. Whilst good separation of the internal and external carotid arteries will often be achieved, individual anatomy is highly variable. Therefore, the operator must ensure that the lesion has been well demonstrated with no vessel overlap with angiographic views to achieve this aim (Fig. 16). Other views that are helpful are PA (posteroanterior), contralateral 30° and ipsilateral 60° views with caudal or cranial angulations. Finally, as with all DSA images, the patient is again instructed to hold still, hold their breath and not to swallow.

After obtaining satisfactory images of the extracranial carotid arteries, the operator progresses on to intracerebral angiography. This provides important information about the flow to the cerebral circulation as well as collateral supply. Furthermore, baseline images will allow the operator to identify abnormalities after intervention in case of embolization. These images are obtained first in a modified PA cranial view. The operator should adjust the angulation of the image intensifier from PA to slight LAO or RAO projections to ensure that the suture lines in the

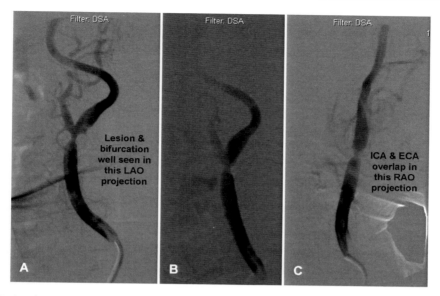

Fig. 16. Angiograms of the extracranial left carotid artery showing the bifurcation into the internal and external carotid arteries in various projections. The best view for this patient is 30° left anterior oblique projection (**A**), which shows the lesion to be most severe, compared to the lateral (**B**) and right anterior oblique (**C**) projections.

skull overlap. Then cranial angulation is applied (usually 10–20°) to bring the upper orbital margins in line with the base of the skull. These manoeuvres will provide optimal imaging of the anterior and middle cerebral arteries with minimal bony overlap. Next, a left lateral image is obtained. When intracerebral images are being acquired, the patients are told not to blink in addition to the usual instructions of holding still, stopping breathing and not swallowing.

Vertebral Angiography

In general, it is not necessary to assess the vertebral arteries when planning carotid intervention. Occasionally patients will have posterior circulation symptoms and will require assessment of the vertebral system. Very rarely, if there is bilateral carotid occlusion, vertebral stenosis may result in anterior circulation symptoms.

The vertebral arteries are of a smaller calibre than the common carotid arteries. As discussed previously, one is often non-dominant and may be very small. In general non-selective vertebral angiography will provide adequate images. Furthermore, this approach will minimize the risk of traumatizing the vertebral artery. In addition, vertebral artery stenosis typically involves the origin of the vessel, and direct engagement with a catheter may cause pressure dampening and possible dissection. In the majority of patients, it is possible to advance a 5 Fr JR4 catheter over a standard 0.035″ guidewire into the innominate or left subclavian artery close to the vertebral origin. In order to maximize vertebral filling, a blood pressure cuff is inflated on the ipsilateral arm. The pressure in the cuff should just exceed systolic pressure in order to temporarily occlude blood flow distally to the arm. Typically, a contralateral 30° view will adequately demonstrate the origin and main vessel (LAO 30° for right vertebral origin, and RAO 30° for left vertebral origin). The intracranial images are then acquired in the PA (with 20–30° cranial) and left lateral projections. At times, a PA caudal projection (~30° caudal) is necessary with the patient's mouth open to visualize the vertebrobasilar junction without bony interference. If direct catheter engagement is required to adequately visualize the intracranial vertebral vessels, a 5 Fr angle taper Glidecath® (Terumo) may be used to selectively engage the vertebral origin with minimal trauma.

Reverse-Curve Diagnostic Catheters

When VTK or Simmons catheters are required to engage vessels, careful manipulation is required to minimize the risk of complications. The VTK catheter should be advanced into the descending aorta over a 0.035" guidewire. After the guidewire is withdrawn, the catheter is meticulously flushed. The catheter should then be turned counterclockwise to orientate the tip in an upwards direction (towards the ostia of the great vessels). These are then engaged in turn from distal to proximal (left subclavian, left common carotid and then innominate arteries). Images can be acquired as needed. A separate maneuvre is required to engage the right common carotid. After the catheter has been pushed around the arch to engage the ostium of the innominate, it is gently retracted. This will straighten the catheter's secondary curve and thus lift the tip upwards towards the right CCA. Often, this maneuvre alone will allow the operator to engage the required vessel. However, in more difficult cases it may be necessary to obtain a roadmap image, advance a stiff-angled Glidewire® into the vessel and then advance the catheter over the wire.

In order to disengage the VTK catheter, the operator should advance it into the ascending aorta whilst rotating clockwise. This points the tip downwards and away from the origins of the great vessels. The 0.035" guidewire should always be reintroduced to straighten the catheter, and then both are withdrawn together.

Complications of Cerebrovascular Angiography

When the technique first emerged, there was a 1–1.5% risk of a neurological complication associated with carotid angiography. These risks include transient ischemic attacks (0.5%), minor strokes (0.5%), major strokes (0.8%) and death (0.3%) *(11)*. However, as operator experience improved, together with routine anticoagulation and antiplatelet therapy and improved equipment, the risk of a neurological complication with carotid angiography has diminished in contemporary series *(4, 11–13)*. The risk of stroke with diagnostic carotid and cerebral angiography is ~0.5% and the risk of death is very low *(11)*.

As with any invasive procedure that requires an arterial access, carotid angiography carries a risk of access site injury, pseudoaneurysm, access site or retroperitoneal bleeding, the need for blood transfusion, contrast nephropathy, allergic reactions to contrast and cholesterol embolization. In general, the risk of any access site complication is ~1% during procedures carried out via the femoral artery.

CONCLUSIONS

Extracranial and intracranial carotid angiography remains the gold standard to evaluate the anatomy of the supra-aortic and intracerebral vasculatures. The operator should have detailed knowledge of the cerebral vascular anatomy. A comprehensive diagnostic carotid angiography with intracerebral evaluation should be performed prior to carotid artery stenting. In the hands of experienced interventionalists who take utmost precautions, carotid angiography can be done safely with very low complications.

REFERENCES

1. Layton KF, Kallmes DF, Cloft HJ, Lindell EP, Cox VS. Bovine aortic arch variant in humans: clarification of a common misnomer. Am J Neuroradiol 2006;27:1541–1542.
2. Buerkel DM, Gurm HS. The human bovine arch – a common misnomer. Catheter Cardiovasc Interv 2007;70:162.
3. Cho L, Mukherjee D. Basic cerebral anatomy for the carotid interventionalist: the intracranial and extracranial vessels. Catheter Cardiovsc Interv 2006;68:104–111.
4. American Society of Interventional & Therapeutic Neuroradiology, Society for Cardiovascular Angiography and Interventions, Society for Vascular Medicine and Biology, Society of Interventional Radiology, Bates ER, Babb JD, Casey DE et al. ACCF/SCAI/SVMB/SIR/ASITN 2007 Clinical Expert Consensus Document on Carotid Stenting: A Report of the American College of Cardiology Foundation Task Force on Clinical Expert Consensus Documents (ACCF/SCAI/SVMB/SIR/ASITN Clinical Expert Consensus Document Committee on Carotid Stenting). J Am Coll Cardiol 2007;49;126–170.
5. Saw J, Exaire JE, Lee DS, Yadav JS. Handbook of Complex Percutaneous Carotid Intervention. Humana Press Inc, New York; 2007.
6. Bouthillier A, van Loveren H, Keller J. Segments of the internal carotid artery: a new classification. Neurosurgery 1996;38(3):425–432.
7. Perlmutter D, Rhoton AL. Microsurgical anatomy of the distal anterior cerebral artery. J. Neurosurg 1978;49:204–228.
8. Wells CE. The cerebral circulation. The clinical significance of current concepts. Arch Neurol 1960;3:319–331.
9. Fleur van Raamt A, P.T.M. Mali W, Jan van Laar P, van der Graaf Y. The fetal variant of the circle of Willis and its influence on the cerebral collateral circulation. Cerebrovas Dis 2006;22:217–224.
10. Saw J, Bajzer C, Casserly IP, et al. Evaluating the optimal activated clotting time during carotid artery stenting. Am J Cardiol 2006;97:1657–1660.
11. Fayed AM, White CJ, Ramee SR, Jenkins JS, Collins TJ. Carotid and cerebral angiography performed by cardiologists: cerebrovascular complications. Catheter Cardiovasc Interv. 2002;55:277–280.
12. Leonardi M, Cenni P, Simonetti L, Raffi L, Battaglia S. Retrospective study of complications arising during cerebral and spinal diagnostic angiography from 1998 to 2003. Interven Neuroradiol 2005;11:213–221.
13. Morgan JH 3rd, Johnson JH, Brown RB, Harvey RL, Rizzoni WE, Tyson CS, Robinson SJ, Solis MM. Initial experience with routine selective carotid arteriography by vascular surgeons. Am Surg. 2006;72:684–686.

11

Extracranial Carotid Stent Interventional Approach

Jacqueline Saw, MD, FRCPC

CONTENTS

ABSTRACT

Carotid artery stenting (CAS) techniques and equipment have dramatically improved over the past two decades. Modern-day CAS can be performed safely with good technical success rates. Nevertheless, the CAS procedure can be challenging and warrants meticulous techniques as the resultant complications can be debilitating and life threatening. We detailed a basic step-by-step technical approach to guide operators through this challenging procedure.

Keywords Carotid stenting; Angioplasty; Telescoping; Emboli protection device

INTRODUCTION

Since the inception of carotid angioplasty over two decades ago, techniques and equipment for carotid artery stenting (CAS) have radically improved. Equipment with lower profile (e.g., smaller outer diameter sheaths with large inner lumen, 0.014″ system balloon catheters and stent catheters) and targeted to carotid arteries (e.g., emboli protection devices, self-expanding stents) have evolved dramatically, leading to improved technical success and procedural safety. Nevertheless, CAS is a challenging procedure which should be performed by experienced endovascular specialists with good interventional techniques. Since the complications associated with CAS can potentially be devastating and debilitating, meticulous techniques should be exercised to prevent these neurological events.

From: *Contemporary Cardiology: Carotid Artery Stenting: The Basics*
Edited by: J. Saw, DOI 10.1007/978-1-60327-314-5_11,
© Humana Press, a part of Springer Science+Business Media, LLC 2009

With a conscientious approach, CAS can be safely performed with a low 30-day death or stroke (major or minor) event rate of 2–4% with modern-day equipment *(1–3)*. Other CAS-related complications are tabulated in Chapter 14, and patients should be educated about these risks prior to embarking on the procedure. Furthermore, baseline evaluation of patients should confirm that patients meet accepted indications and lack contraindications as outlined in Chapter 7. Pre-procedural preparations and medication use (including antiplatelet and antithrombotic agents) are discussed in Chapter 6. This chapter will guide the readers through a step-by-step approach to CAS.

CAROTID ARTERY STENTING PROCEDURE

Arterial Access

The femoral artery is the preferred access site for CAS. If there is significant lower extremity peripheral arterial disease, the brachial artery or radial artery may be utilized. In such cases, the contralateral arm is typically used (e.g., left brachial artery access for right carotid artery), which would facilitate guide engagement (see Chapter 9). In modern-day practice, direct carotid arterial puncture is rarely used due to higher complication rates (e.g., carotid dissection, thrombosis, neck hematoma). Equipment improvements over the past decade have enabled over 98% technical success with CAS through the femoral approach.

The modified Seldinger technique is utilized to obtain arterial access with a 5 Fr or 6 Fr short sheath. After diagnostic carotid angiography, this sheath can be exchanged to a long 6 Fr sheath (e.g., Shuttle® or Destination® sheaths) or a short 8 Fr sheath (for use with 8 Fr guides) depending on the CAS approach selected.

Anticoagulation

After gaining arterial access, intravenous heparin (50–100 units/kg) is administered to achieve an optimal activated clotting time between 250 and 300 s *(4)*. Alternatively, bivalirudin 0.75 mg/kg bolus followed by 1.75 mg/kg/h infusion may be used *(5)*; although this regimen has been established with percutaneous coronary intervention, it has not been formally tested with CAS. The routine use of GP IIb/IIIa inhibitors is avoided because of potentially higher intracranial hemorrhage and stroke events *(6)*. However, it may be used in bailout situations (cerebral embolization during CAS), patients presenting with large thrombotic acute stroke, or patients where emboli protection devices could not be used *(7)*.

Baseline Diagnostic Carotid and Cerebral Angiography

Detailed diagnostic carotid and cerebral angiography is typically performed as part of the CAS procedure to illustrate the cerebrovascular anatomy prior to stenting. This helps operators plan their interventional approach and select the appropriate equipment according to anticipated challenges. It is routine to start with a thoracic aortogram using a 5 Fr pigtail at 30–60° LAO (left anterior oblique) projection to evaluate the arch anatomy and the proximal segments of the great vessels.

Selective bilateral carotid angiography is then performed with 5 Fr diagnostic catheters, with simple curved catheters (Fig. 1) such as JR4 or angle taper

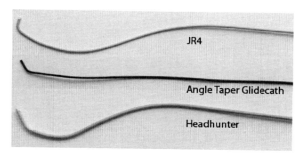

Fig. 1. Commonly used simple curved diagnostic catheters.

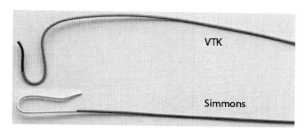

Fig. 2. Examples of reverse-curved carotid diagnostic catheters.

Glidecath® (Terumo Medical Corporation, Somerset, NJ) for patients with type I or II aortic arches. With type III arches, complex curved catheters (Fig. 2) are frequently necessary, such as VTK catheter (Cook Medical Inc., Bloomington, IN) or Simmons catheters (Cook Medical Inc., Bloomington, IN). In patients with a bovine arch, it is often challenging to engage the left common carotid artery (CCA) with catheters prolapsing into the ascending aorta, thus the VTK catheter is often necessary. In more challenging arches, more complex catheters like the Simmons catheters may be required. These complex or reverse-curved catheters need to be reformed in the aorta prior to engaging the CCA, with the VTK being simpler to reform (Fig. 3) compared to the Simmons. Several techniques of reforming the

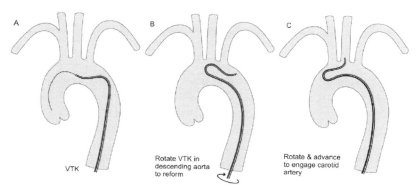

Fig. 3. Reforming the VTK catheter in the descending aorta. (**A**) VTK catheter is advanced over a guidewire to the descending aorta. (**B**) Guidewire is removed and the VTK catheter is rotated to reform in the descending aorta. (**C**) VTK catheter is advanced and rotated to engage the carotid artery.

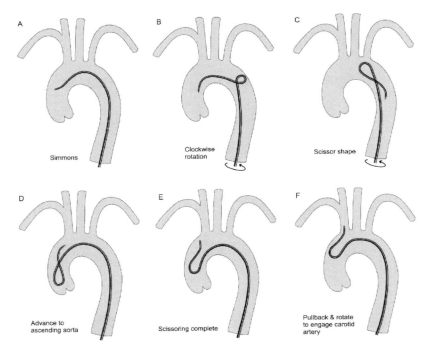

Fig. 4. The "scissor" technique to reform Simmons catheter: (**A**) advance Simmons over the wire into the transverse aorta; (**B**) rapidly rotate catheter clockwise to form a loop with the knee of the catheter at the peak of the aortic arch; (**C**) continue clockwise rotation until catheter "scissors" as the tip flips from the transverse arch into the descending aorta; (**D**) this "scissored" catheter is advanced into the ascending aorta and then rotated to open up the scissored configuration.

Simmons catheters have been described: quick aortic turn or scissoring technique (Fig. 4), left subclavian artery technique (Fig. 5), and the aortic valve method (Fig. 6) *(8)*. However, we favor reforming the Simmons catheter in the distal abdominal aorta at the iliac artery bifurcation, which has the least likelihood of disrupting atherosclerotic plaque in the aortic arch. With this technique from the femoral approach, the Simmons catheter is first advanced over a wire into the contralateral iliac artery; it is then pushed with its "duck-bill" configuration in a retrograde fashion into the abdominal aorta and up to the aortic arch pre-formed (Fig. 7).

Vertebral angiography is usually not performed prior to CAS, unless the operator suspects symptomatic vertebral stenosis or need to fully assess the collateral Circle of Willis circulation (particularly if emboli protection with occlusion balloon is intended). Obviously, safe and vigilant angiographic techniques should be practiced, with careful catheter manipulation and contrast injection to avoid air and atherothrombotic embolism.

Several characteristics on the arch and carotid angiography should warn the operators of increased procedural complexities: presence of a steep type III arch, stenosis of ostial or proximal segments of the innominate or common carotid arteries, bovine aortic arch, tortuous carotid arteries (e.g., cervical carotid artery loops), disease in the origin of the external carotid artery, and heavily calcified carotid artery target lesion.

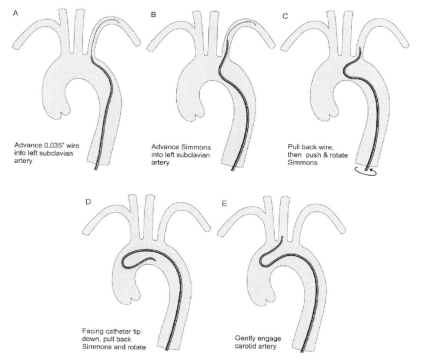

Fig. 5. The left subclavian technique to reform Simmons catheter: (**A**) advance the 0.035″ guidewire into the left subclavian artery; (**B**) track the Simmons catheter into the left subclavian artery until the secondary curve is just proximal to the ostium of the subclavian artery; (**C**) pull back the wire and then simultaneously push and rotate the catheter into the ascending aorta; (**D**) configure the catheter tip to face down and then pull catheter back and rotate; (**E**) this maneuver will engage the left carotid or innominate artery.

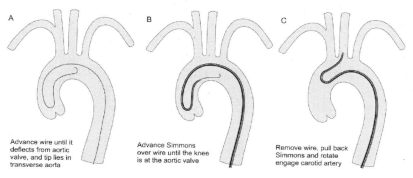

Fig. 6. The aortic valve technique to reform Simmons catheter: (**A**) advance wire (preferably removal core wire) until it deflects off the aortic valve with the tip in the transverse aorta; (**B**) advance the Simmons catheter over the wire until the knee is on the aortic valve; (**C**) the wire is removed and the catheter is then rotated and pulled back to engage the innominate or left carotid artery.

Sheath or Guide Approach

With knowledge of the cerebrovascular anatomy, operators can anticipate challenges and strategize their interventional approach. First, the operator has to select the equipment to engage the CCA. This is done via one of two

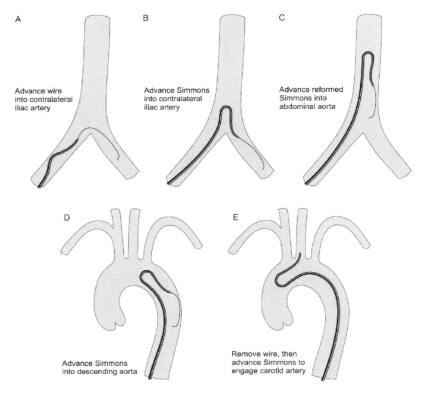

Fig. 7. Reforming the Simmons catheter in the iliac artery: (**A**) advance the wire into the contral-ateral iliac artery, (**B**) followed by advancing the tip of the Simmons catheter into the contralateral common iliac artery, (**C**) the reformed Simmons catheter is then advanced into the abdominal aorta, (**D**) and further advanced over the wire into the descending thoracic aorta, (**E**) the wire is then removed and the Simmons catheter torqued and advanced to engage the carotid artery.

approaches, either using a long sheath or a guide catheter. The choice of either approach depends on the perceived technical difficulty of the CAS procedure (Table 1). The sheath approach is typically used when the case is perceived to be straightforward (e.g., type I aortic arch without significant tortuosity of the carotid artery or calcification). If the operator is concerned about any challenges (e.g., type III arch, heavy calcification, or tortuous carotid artery), then a guide should be used instead.

Sheath Approach

Several commercial long sheaths are available and suitable for placement into the CCA. We typically favor a 6 Fr 90 cm long sheath, such as the Flexor® Shuttle® sheath (Cook Medical Inc., Bloomington, IN). The Flexor® line of sheaths also includes a Shuttle Select™ system (Cook Medical Inc., Bloomington, IN) that incorporates a specially designed Slip-Cath® catheter together with the Shuttle® sheath, which has a unique transition for improved trackability and minimizes the need for device exchanges. Other available long sheaths include the Pinnacle® Destination® sheath (Terumo Medical Corporation, Somerset, NJ) and the Super

Table 1
Sheath Versus Guide Catheter Approach

Sheath approach	Guide catheter approach
Smaller arterial access (6–7 Fr)	Larger arterial access (8–9 Fr)
Requires over-the-wire exchange: diagnostic catheter to engage common carotid artery, then exchange with sheath/dilator (except Shuttle Select™)	Easier access: engage common carotid artery using a 5 Fr catheter telescoped within the 8 Fr guide, then advance guide over 5 Fr catheter
Sheath dilator allows smooth transition and better tracking into carotid artery, lower chance of scrapping plaque debris	Abrupt transition at the tip may scrape plaque debris, despite telescoping setup
Sheath may kink with steep type III arch	Lower potential of kinking
No torque control	Good torque control
Less support for advancing equipment	More support for tortuous vessels, calcified lesions, and challenging aortic arch
Difficult to advance sheath higher in the carotid artery without reinserting the dilator	Easier to advance guide higher in the carotid artery during the procedure

Arrow-Flex® Carotid Access Sheath (Arrow International). Sometimes a 7 Fr diameter sheath is necessary (e.g., for delivery of certain monorail carotid stent catheters).

Given that most long sheaths are not prepackaged with a catheter, operators usually have to select a 5 Fr diagnostic catheter (e.g., JR4 or VTK depending on arch anatomy) to engage the innominate or left CCA. Under roadmap guidance, a 0.035″ stiff-angled Glidewire® (Terumo Medical Corporation, Somerset, NJ) is then advanced into one of the main branches of the external carotid artery (ECA), and the diagnostic catheter is tracked into the ECA. A long stiff Amplatz wire is used to replace the Glidewire®. The diagnostic catheter is then exchanged for the sheath and its dilator carefully under fluoroscopy. Operators should be aware that although the sheath typically has a radio-opaque tip, the dilator does not. Thus, care should be taken not to advance the dilator too distally into the ECA. The sheath should be parked at the distal CCA, about 2–5 cm from the bifurcation of the carotid artery (or below the target lesion if present in the CCA). Once in position, the dilator and Amplatz wire are removed, and the Tuohy-Borst adapter loosened to expel blood and potential debris.

An alternative approach is to telescope a 5 Fr diagnostic catheter within the long sheath (once the sheath had been advanced into the abdominal aorta over its dilator), which would minimize catheter exchange. After the diagnostic catheter is used to engage the origin of the innominate or left CCA, a 0.035″ stiff-angled Glidewire® is then advanced into one of the main branches of the ECA, and the diagnostic catheter is tracked into the ECA. The sheath can then be advanced over the diagnostic catheter into the distal CCA. However, in this approach, the discrepancy in catheter and sheath diameters results in a gap (as opposed to the smooth transition of the dilator and its sheath) that reduces trackability and may also scrap atherosclerotic debris. The Shuttle Select™ system is a nice alternative in this regard.

GUIDE APPROACH

Several commercially available 100 cm length guide catheters may be used for CAS (Fig. 8). Typically an 8 Fr guide is used, although sometimes a 9 Fr guide is needed (e.g., for certain monorail carotid stents). We almost always choose an 8 Fr H1 guide (Cook Medical Inc, Bloomington, IN), using the telescoping technique to advance the guide catheter into the CCA. In order to telescope the diagnostic catheter within the guide, a longer 125 cm length diagnostic catheter is necessary. We typically use a 5 Fr 125 cm length diagnostic JR4 or VTK catheter to telescope within the guide (Fig. 9). After the 5 Fr diagnostic catheter is used to engage the innominate or left CCA, a 0.035″ stiff-angled Glidewire® is advanced into the ECA under roadmap guidance. If the ostial ECA has a significant stenosis (Fig. 10), the Glidewire® may be parked in the distal CCA. The diagnostic catheter is then advanced over the Glidewire® into the distal CCA, followed by tracking along the guide catheter into the distal CCA, with a counterclock torque when going across the great vessel origin (Fig. 11). The diagnostic catheter and Glidewire® are then removed, and the Tuohy-Borst adapter loosened to expel blood that may contain atherosclerotic debris from catheter manipulation. If there is significant tortuosity in the CCA (Fig. 12), then the guide catheter should be parked proximal to the tortuous segment.

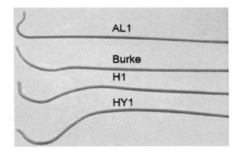

Fig. 8. Commonly used carotid guide catheters.

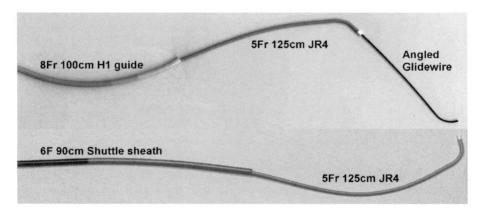

Fig. 9. Telescoping a 5 Fr 125 cm JR4 inside an 8 Fr 100 cm H1 guide (top panel), and telescoping a 5 Fr 125 cm JR4 inside a 6 Fr 90 cm Shuttle sheath (*bottom panel*).

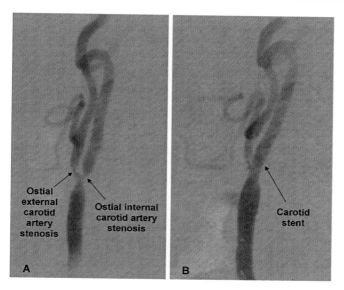

Fig. 10. Cineangiograms showing (**A**) ostial external carotid lesion prior to stenting and (**B**) following stent placement across the external carotid artery.

DIRECT GUIDE APPROACH

In quite infrequent cases, a type III arch may be so challenging that the guide catheter cannot be advanced beyond the origin of the CCA. In these cases, the procedure probably should be abandoned and the patient be referred for surgical endarterectomy. However, if the surgical alternative is not possible, experienced operators may proceed with a good support guide engaging only the origin of the CCA. An 8 Fr AL1 guide may be used in such cases; the AL1 guide may also be altered with a paperclip and a blow-dryer to eliminate the primary curve and soften the secondary curve, to facilitate engagement of the great vessel. If more support is needed, an additional 0.014″ buddy guidewire (e.g., Ironman, Balance Heavy Weight) can be placed in the ECA (Fig. 13). Alternatively, a 0.035″ stiff Amplatz wire may be placed in the ECA, but this will require a 9 Fr guide catheter.

Emboli Protection Device

Once the guide or sheath is in the distal CCA, an emboli protection device (EPD) is used to cross the internal carotid artery (ICA) lesion. Two classes of EPD are available for use, filter EPD and balloon occlusion devices (see Chapter 12). The filter EPDs are generally preferred for CAS as they are easier to use; moreover, some patients may not tolerate temporary ipsilateral occlusion to cerebral blood flow (especially those with contralateral stenosis or incomplete Circle of Willis). Nevertheless, there are niche indications for balloon occlusion devices, such as critically severe stenosis (that limits filter EPD passage), bulky atherosclerotic plaques, and tortuous carotid arteries.

FILTER EPD

The filter EPD 0.014″ guidewire tip is shaped to accommodate the severity and angle of the stenosis. If the carotid stenosis is severe (≥90%), we find that having both a primary and secondary curve helps advance the filter across the lesion. The

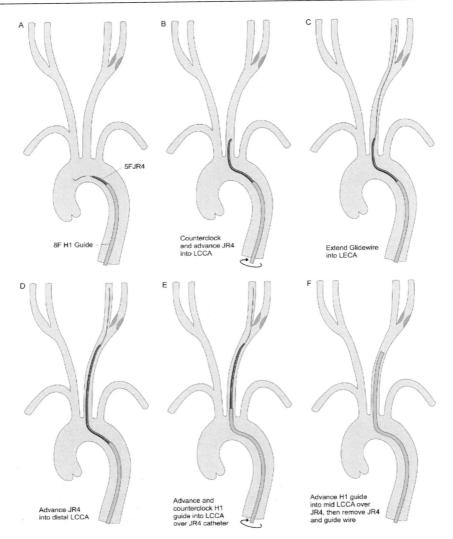

Fig. 11. Schematic representation of guide access for carotid artery stenting: **(A)** Telescoping setup with a 5 Fr JR4 inside an 8 Fr H1 guide is advanced over a guidewire into the aortic arch. **(B)** The JR4 catheter is rotated counterclockwise to engage the left common carotid artery (LCCA). **(C)** A stiff-angled Glidewire® is advanced into the left external carotid artery (LECA) under roadmap guidance. **(D)** The JR4 catheter is advanced into the distal LCCA, and **(E)** the H1 guide is then tracked along the JR4 with a counterclockwise turn as it advances across the origin of the CCA. **(F)** The H1 guide is advanced into the distal LCCA, and the Glidewire® and JR4 are then removed.

distance from the primary curve to the secondary curve should roughly equate the diameter of the CCA. The filter EPD is then slowly advanced across the stenosis; as this portion of the procedure is not protected, operators should be careful not to dislodge emboli or dissect ruptured plaque. The floppy tip of the guidewire is advanced to the petrous portion of the ICA, and the filter basket is then deployed proximal to the petrous bone in the straight portion of the cervical ICA (Fig. 14). However, if there is severe tortuosity in the cervical ICA (e.g., significant 180–360°

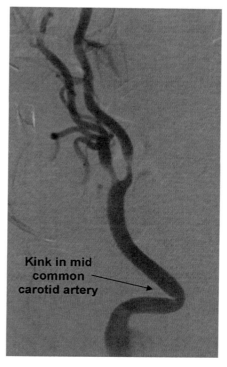

Fig. 12. Cineangiogram showing significant tortuousity in the mid-common carotid artery, which impedes advancement of guide catheters.

loops), the filter EPD may have to be deployed more proximally, typically just before the loops (Fig. 15). Although the method of filter deployment differs depending on the device used, it typically involves unsheathing of the delivery catheter which constrains the filter device. After deployment, an angiogram should be performed to ensure that the basket is well apposed to the vessel wall. Typically a 6–7 mm filter EPD diameter will achieve good apposition in that segment.

BALLOON OCCLUSION EPD

Placement of a balloon occlusion EPD is quite different from a filter EPD. We will limit our discussion to the GuardWire® (Medtronic, Inc., Minneapolis, MN) system since this is the only balloon occlusion EPD that is FDA approved. The GuardWire™ is first advanced across the carotid lesion to at least 2–3 cm distally, preferably at the pre-petrous cervical ICA particularly if the vessel is large. The GuardWire™ balloon is then inflated to the desired diameter to occlude the ICA. To inflate the balloon, the GuardWire™ is attached to the EZ Adapter and the knob is turned to open the Microseal. The EZ Flator inflation device is then rotated to inflate the balloon to the desired pressure. The Microseal is sealed off with the EZ Adapter to keep the balloon inflated, and the adapter is then disconnected to allow the GuardWire™ to serve as a conventional angioplasty wire. Contrast is then injected to confirm complete occlusion of blood flow. Once the carotid stent is deployed and post-dilatation performed, the Export® catheter is advanced to the

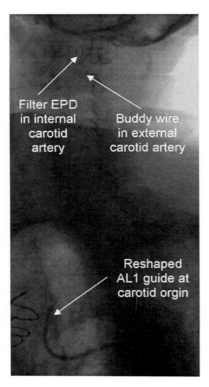

Fig. 13. Direct guide approach with reshaped AL1 guide at the origin of the left common carotid artery, a buddy wire in the external carotid artery, and a filter emboli protection device (EPD) in the internal carotid artery.

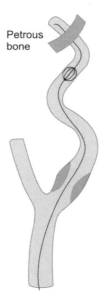

Fig. 14. The filter emboli protection device (EPD) should be deployed in the straight portion of the cervical internal carotid artery, just before the petrous bone of the skull.

GuardWire™ balloon, and blood is suctioned to retrieve liberated debris suspended in the stagnant blood column. The EZ Adapter is then reattached to open up the Microseal, and the GuardWire™ balloon is then deflated and removed.

About 5% of patients will not tolerate temporary cerebral blood flow occlusion by the GuardWire™, particularly those with contralateral occlusion or poor collateral circulation (9). Such intolerance may manifest as decrease in level of consciousness, complete loss of consciousness, seizure, or neurological deficit. In these patients, the GuardWire™ balloon has to be deflated multiple times (with aspiration prior to each deflation) during the procedure, usually between pre-dilatation and stenting. In about 1% of cases, patients are completely intolerant of the balloon occlusion, in which case this EPD should be abandoned in favor of a filter EPD. Therefore, it is important that four-vessel cerebral angiography (i.e., carotid and vertebral angiography) be performed prior to the use of the GuardWire™ to assess the Circle of Willis.

In addition, flushing of the carotid artery prior to aspiration is generally not recommended, as this may divert suspended emboli toward the ECA. This can be detrimental when there are ECA to ICA collaterals via the ophthalmic artery, ascending pharyngeal or internal maxillary arteries, which could result in cerebral and retinal embolization (10, 11). Similarly, emboli may be diverted to the posterior circulation if there are collaterals between the ECA and the vertebral artery.

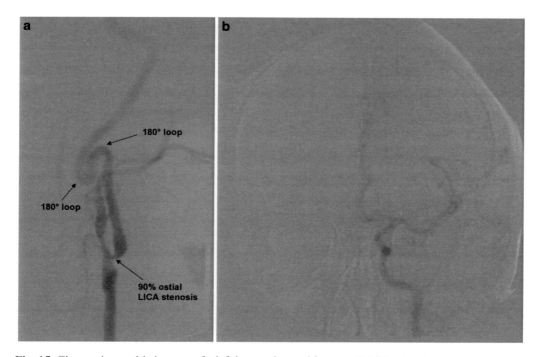

Fig. 15. Cineangiographic images of a left internal carotid artery (LICA) stenting: (**A**) severe 90% ostial LICA lesion with two 180° loops at the mid-segment of the cervical LICA, (**B**) baseline intracranial circulation of the LICA, (**C**) placement of the filter emboli protection device which had to be placed proximal to the tortuous loops (instead of the usual location just before the petrous bone), (**D**) after placement of stent from distal left common carotid artery into the LICA, (**E**) intracranial angiography post-stenting.

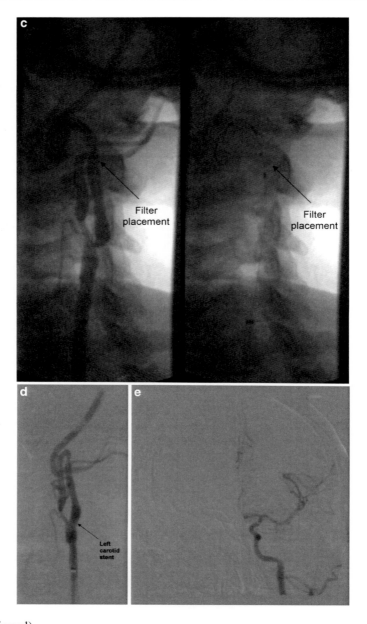

Fig. 15. (continued)

Balloon Pre-dilatation

After the EPD is successfully deployed, balloon pre-dilatation of the carotid stenosis is generally performed using a 0.014″ coronary angioplasty balloon, especially for severe lesions and calcified lesions. Any commercially available coronary balloons can be used for this purpose [e.g., Maverick™ (Boston Scientific), Cross-Sail™ (Guidant Corp.)]. The size of the balloon depends on the severity of the calcification. Generally a 4 mm diameter balloon that is 20 mm in length can be used. However, heavily calcified lesions may require starting with a smaller diameter balloon (1.5 or 2.0 mm diameters). At times, the lesion is so critically severe that pre-dilatation with a 1.5 mm balloon is necessary prior to crossing with a filter EPD (an alternative strategy would be to use a balloon occlusion EPD in these scenarios). These coronary balloons can be inflated to 6–8 atm for ~5 s. If significant bradycardia or hypotension occurs during pre-dilatation, atropine (0.6–1 mg) may be administered, especially prior to repeat balloon dilatation (e.g., post-dilatation).

Stent Placement

In modern-day CAS, balloon-expandable stents are no longer used (except for ostial CCA lesions) because of stent deformation since the extracranial carotid is a superficial artery *(12)*. Self-expanding nitinol or stainless steel stents are now routinely used for the extracranial carotid artery, and many are now commercially available and FDA approved (see Chapter 12). The AccuLink™ stent and AccuNet™ device (Guidant Corporation, Santa Clara, CA), the Xact® and EmboShield™ system (Abbott Vascular Devices, Redwood City, CA), the Precise™ stent and AngioGuard XP™ (Cordis Corporation, Warren, NJ), the Protégé® stents and SPIDER™ filter EPD (ev3 Inc., Plymouth, MN), the Nexstent® stent and Filterwire EZ™ (Boston Scientific, Natick, MA), and the Exponent® stent and GuardWire™ device (Medtronic, Inc., Minneapolis, MN) systems are currently FDA approved at mid-2008.

The length of stent required depends on the lesion length (usually 20–40 mm), with avoidance of unnecessary long lengths. As most carotid stenoses involve the ostium of the ICA, the majority of stent placements (~80%) have to extend from the distal CCA to the proximal ICA. In these cases, the diameter of the stent should match the distal CCA (most commonly using an 8 mm diameter straight stent or a 7–10 mm tapered stent). For non-tapered stents, overexpansion of the ICA with stents >8 mm should be avoided, as it may cause dissection and intramural hematoma. Overall, a stent-to-artery ratio of 1.1:1 to 1.4:1 for the ICA is considered appropriate. For patients with a large size mismatch between the ICA and CCA, tapered stents (e.g., AccuLink™, Xact®, Protégé®, Nexstent®) are preferred which may provide more homogeneous radial force and mechanical stress on the arterial walls. Although tapered stents appear appealing in these cases, there are no comparative studies between tapered and straight stents. In terms of stent positioning, operators should ensure that the stent crosses the ECA into the CCA entirely, without leaving an edge of the stent struts "hanging" in the CCA, as this may obstruct balloon and retrieval catheters advancement after stent deployment (Fig. 16).

Less frequently, the stenosis is beyond the ostial segment of the ICA such that the carotid stent can be placed completely in the proximal ICA, without crossing into the CCA. In these cases, operators should avoid starting the stent right at the ostium of the ICA, which may result in an unfavorable angle into the ICA for subsequent catheter advancements (Fig. 16). Generally, a 7 mm diameter stent can be used for placement of stent exclusively in the ICA.

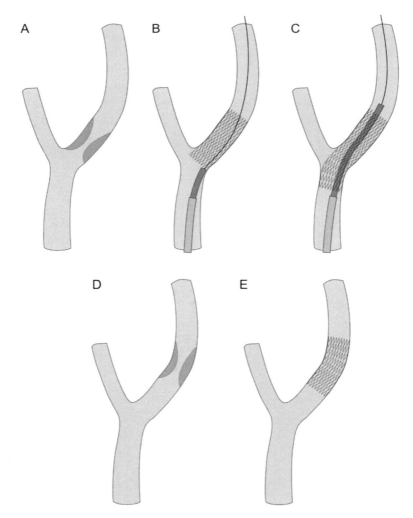

Fig. 16. For ostial or proximal internal carotid artery (ICA) lesion (**A**), placement of a stent covering only the ICA with the stent edge "floating" at the ostium of the ICA (**B**) can obstruct catheter movements with catheter tip snagged by the proximal stent edge. It is best to place the stent from the distal common carotid artery (CCA) into the ICA (**C**) for these ostial or proximal lesions. For mid-ICA lesion (**D**), the stent can be positioned completely in the ICA without crossing into the CCA (**E**).

Once the operator has advanced the stent into the desired location, a helpful step to prevent inadvertent forward "jumping" of stent during deployment is to advance the stent slightly distal to the stenosis, then pulling back to the desired position prior to deployment. This helps to release the stored energy from longitudinal compression of the delivery system inner core, which is built up during advancement of the stent into the carotid artery. The self-expanding stent is slowly unsheathed for deployment, during which repositioning is sometimes necessary especially if the stent "jumps" forward.

Balloon Post-dilatation

After satisfactory stent deployment, if there is significant residual stenosis, post-dilatation of the stent can be performed with a 5.0–6.0 mm diameter by 20 mm length peripheral balloon [e.g., Amiia™ (Cordis Corporation, Miami, FL), Viatrac™ (Guidant, Indianapolis, IN)] to 6–8 atm for ~5 s. Because of the high risk of distal embolization during this portion of the procedure, post-dilatation may be omitted if there is only mild residual stenosis, especially in symptomatic patients, or those with bulky atherosclerotic or non-calcified plaques. High-pressure inflations are to be avoided because of the risk of carotid dissection, perforation, and distal embolization. The post-dilatation balloon should not protrude outside the stented region to minimize the risk of edge dissection. A residual stenosis of up to 20% is considered as an acceptable result. The perception is that self-expanding stents will progressively expand to its intended diameter over time, and thus operators should not aim for pristine 0% residual stenosis because of the risk of embolization. The use of a non-compliant balloon is not generally recommended, unless the lesion is heavily calcified and the residual stenosis is >20% following standard post-dilatation.

Besides distal embolization, post-dilatation is also the stage where activation of the carotid sinus reflex most frequently occurs, especially if the lesion is situated in the carotid bulb. Thus, operators should be particularly vigilant during this portion of the procedure, watching closely for any change in neurological status. Atropine can be administered for significant bradycardia and hypotension. Prophylactic atropine administration is typically not required as this reflex is usually transient. Intravenous dopamine is sometimes necessary for prolonged or profound bradycardia and hypotension.

After inflation of the post-dilatation balloon, a careful and gentle injection of contrast for a cineangiogram is recommended to evaluate for slow flow or no reflow. Slow flow has been demonstrated in ~10% of CAS procedures especially following post-dilatation and is associated with higher peri-procedural stroke events (13). In these situations, patients often show signs of neurological ischemic compromisation due to embolic debris clogging up the filter EPD. Thus, operators have to reestablish cerebral flow very promptly. To manage slow flow, the stagnant column of blood proximal to the deployed filter has to be suctioned without delay, using either an aspiration catheter [e.g., Export® aspiration catheter (Medtronic Inc., Minneapolis, MN), Pronto extraction catheter (Vascular Solutions, Minneapolis, MN)] or a 5 Fr 125 cm multipurpose catheter. Approximately 40–100 cc of blood should be suctioned, and then the operator can immediately proceed to retrieve the filter EPD.

Retrieval of EPD

During retrieval of the filter EPD, the operator may occasionally encounter difficulties in advancing the retrieval catheter to the deployed filter. This is usually encountered at the stented segments, which may be due to inadequate expansion of stents, position of stents (e.g., protrusion of stent edges), exposed stent struts (especially with open cell stents or with calcified lesions causing strut protrusions), or angulated and tortuous vessel segments. Several maneuvers can be attempted to advance the retrieval catheters in these cases (see Table 2), including changing head positions, rotating the retrieval catheters and/or guide catheters, and further post-dilatations.

Table 2
Maneuvers to Facilitate Filter Emboli Protection Device Retrieval

Techniques to help advance retrieval catheters across carotid stent

- Re-advance retrieval catheters with different torque rotations
- Change orientation of the guide catheter tip by rotation
- Rotate patient's head (turn left or right, flex or extend) to alter carotid artery orientation
- Reshape the retrieval catheter tip or use a different retrieval catheter
- Post-dilate the stent to enlarge lumen and alter stent configuration
- Use a buddy wire to increase support and to straighten the carotid artery

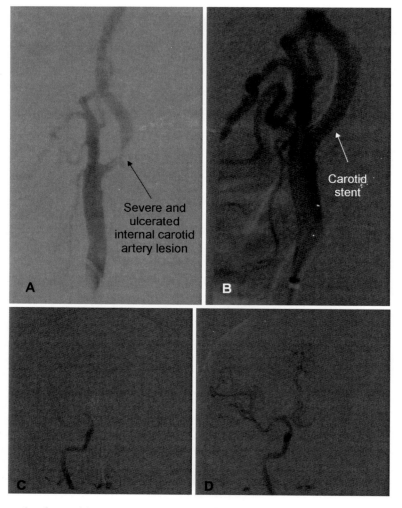

Fig. 17. Example of carotid artery stenosis pre- and post-stenting: (**A**) severe and ulcerated right internal carotid artery stenosis, (**B**) after stenting of the right internal carotid artery, (**C**) intracranial angiography pre-stenting, (**D**) intracranial angiography post-stenting.

Final Carotid and Cerebral Angiography

After removal of the EPD, repeat angiography of the carotid bifurcation and the intracranial circulation should be performed (Figs. 17, 18, and 19). This allows the operators to assess for cerebral flow, collateral circulation, and distal embolization (which may sometimes be subtle). Patients are also examined for neurological deficit at this stage. If a large embolization to the M1 or M2 middle cerebral artery territory has occurred, operators would need to promptly establish patency via a mechanical approach. This can be achieved by crossing the embolus with a 0.014″ 300 cm length coronary wire, followed by advancing and deploying a coronary angioplasty balloon or a snare device *(14)*. In refractory cases, transcatheter intra-arterial tPA or GP IIb/IIIa inhibitors can be administered via a catheter just proximal to the embolus. On the other hand, small distal embolizations beyond the M2 segment are generally tolerated, causing only transient ischemic symptoms, and thus they generally can be treated conservatively.

POST-PROCEDURAL MONITORING

Procedural and post-procedural monitoring of the hemodynamic and neurological status is detailed in Chapter 15. In summary, patients are closely monitored in a telemetry ward overnight. Blood pressure, heart rate, and neurochecks are routinely assessed q15min for 4 h, then q1h for 4 h, then q4h overnight. It is common for patients to have prolonged hypotension post-procedure due to the prolonged vasodilatory response to the carotid baroreceptor reflex. Patients are typically asymptomatic with mild hypotension. However, if the patient is symptomatic or if the systolic pressure is persistently <80 mmHg despite saline infusion, oral

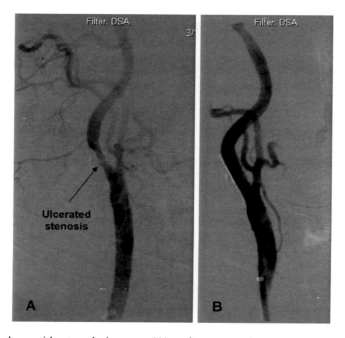

Fig. 18. Ulcerated carotid artery lesion pre- (**A**) and post-stenting (**B**).

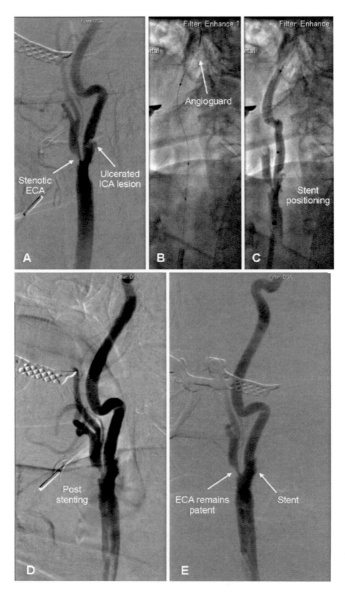

Fig. 19. Complex carotid stenting with tortuous internal carotid artery (ICA) distal to the proximal ulcerated lesion, and severe disease involving the ostium of the external carotid artery (ECA). (**A**) Baseline, (**B**) Angioguard filter emboli protection device was able to be maneuvered distal to the tortuous segment and deployed in the pre-petrous segment, (**C**) stent positioning, (**D**) and (**E**) different angiographic views post-stenting showing that the ECA remained patent.

pseudoephedrine (30–60 mg q4h prn) can be administered. Infrequently, intravenous vasoconstrictor support (e.g., dopamine, norepinephrine) may be required. At the opposite spectrum, patients with underlying systemic hypertension may have significant blood pressure elevation post-procedure. In these cases, blood pressures would need to be tightly controlled with systolic pressures <140 mmHg to prevent the development of hyperperfusion syndrome. Intravenous beta-blockers or infusion with nitroglycerin may be necessary, especially if hyperperfusion occurs.

CONTRALATERAL CAROTID STENOSIS

For patients with significant bilateral carotid stenosis where bilateral CAS is required, it is usually recommended to stage the contralateral procedure several days to 1 month apart. There are small case series which suggest that simultaneous bilateral CAS may be safe *(15, 16)*. However, this approach may unnecessarily expose patients to higher risks of cerebral hyperperfusion, hemodynamic compromisation, and ischemic complications. Thus, unless the patient requires urgent non-carotid surgeries (e.g., coronary bypass surgery), a staged approach is preferred.

CONCLUSION

Carotid stenting techniques and equipment have dramatically improved over the past two decades. Thus, modern-day CAS can be performed safely with good technical success rates. Nevertheless, the CAS procedure can be challenging and warrants meticulous techniques as the resultant complications can be debilitating and life threatening. We have detailed a basic step-by-step approach to guide operators through this procedure and provided anecdotes to potential problems that may arise during carotid stenting.

REFERENCES

1. Yadav JS, Wholey MH, Kuntz RE, et al. Protected carotid-artery stenting versus endarterectomy in high-risk patients. N Engl J Med 2004;351:1493–1501.
2. Kastrup A, Groschel K, Kraph H, Brehm B, Dichgans J, Schulz J. Early outcome of carotid angioplasty and stenting with and without cerebral protection devices. A systematic review of the literature. Stroke 2003;34:813–819.
3. Wholey MH, Al-Mubarek N. Updated review of the global carotid artery stent registry. Catheter Cardiovasc Interv 2003;60:259–266.
4. Saw J, Casserly I, Sachar R, et al. Evaluating the optimal activated clotting time during percutaneous carotid interventions. Cathet Cardiovasc Interv 2004;62:91.
5. Folmar J, Sachar R, Mann T. Transradial approach for carotid artery stenting: a feasibility study. Catheter Cardiovasc Interv 2007;69:355–361.
6. Wholey MH, Eles G, Toursakissian B, Bailey S, Jarmolowski C, Tan WA. Evaluation of glycoprotein IIb/IIIa inhibitors in carotid angioplasty and stenting. J Endovasc Ther 2003;10:33–41.
7. Kopp CW, Steiner S, Nasel C, et al. Abciximab reduces monocyte tissue factor in carotid angioplasty and stenting. Stroke 2003;34:2560–2567.
8. SMith DC, Simmons CR. The quick aortic turn: a rapid method for reforming the simmons sidewinder catheter. Radiology 1985:247–248.
9. Henry M, Polydorou A, Henry I, Hugel M. Carotid angioplasty under cerebral protection with the PercuSurge GuardWire System. Catheter Cardiovasc Interv 2004;61:293–305.
10. Al-Mubarak N, Roubin G, Vitek J, Iyer S, New G, Leon M. Effect of the distal-balloon protection system on microembolization during carotid stenting. Circulation 2001;104:1999–2002.
11. Wilentz JR, Chati Z, Krafft V, Amor M. Retinal embolization during carotid angioplasty and stenting: mechanisms and role of cerebral protection systems. Catheter Cardiovasc Interv 2002;56:320–327.
12. Mathur A, Dorros G, Iyer SS, Vitek JJ, Yadav SS, Roubin GS. Palmaz stent compression in patients following carotid artery stenting. Cathet Cardiovasc Diagn 1997;41:137–140.

13. Casserly IP, Abou-Chebl A, Fathi RB, et al. Slow-flow phenomenon during carotid artery intervention with embolic protection devices: predictors and clinical outcome. J Am Coll Cardiol 2005;46:1466–1472.
14. Yadav JS. Technical aspects of carotid stenting. EuroPCR. Version 3 ed. Paris, 2003:1–18.
15. Chen MS, Bhatt DL, Mukherjee D, et al. Feasibility of simultaneous bilateral carotid artery stenting. Catheter Cardiovasc Interv 2004;61:437–442.
16. Al-Mubarak N, Roubin GS, Vitek JJ, Gomez CR. Simultaneous bilateral carotid stenting for restenosis after endarterectomy. Cathet Cardiovasc Diagn 1998;45:11–15.

12

Equipment for Extracranial Carotid Artery Stenting

Peter Ruchin, MD
and Jacqueline Saw, MD, FRCPC

CONTENTS

ABSTRACT

Since the first carotid angioplasty in 1980, more steerable hydrophilic guidewires, low-profile embolic protection devices, balloons, and stents have meant lower complication rates and better outcomes. Sound knowledge of options and a judicious choice of interventional equipment are paramount to ensuring a safe and efficacious procedure.

Keywords Equipment; Balloon; Guidewire; Emboli protection device; Nitinol; Stainless steel; Self-expanding stents; Balloon-expandable stents

INTRODUCTION

The early carotid angioplasty experience was fraught with a high incidence of technical failure and unacceptable procedural morbidity and mortality. Much of this early failure was due to the lack of modern-day equipment to facilitate the procedure. Since the first carotid angioplasty in 1980, more steerable hydrophilic guidewires, low-profile embolic protection devices, balloons, and stents have meant

From: *Contemporary Cardiology: Carotid Artery Stenting: The Basics*
Edited by: J. Saw, DOI 10.1007/978-1-60327-314-5_12,
© Humana Press, a part of Springer Science+Business Media, LLC 2009

lower complication rates and better outcomes. Further improvements with hydrophilic sheaths and reduction of the outer lumen diameters of catheters have resulted in reduced complications related to arterial access. The significant progress in supra-aortic intervention was predominantly aided by technological advances in design and manufacture, together with meticulous operator techniques. Sound knowledge of options and a judicious choice of interventional equipment are paramount to ensuring a safe and efficacious procedure.

GUIDEWIRES

0.014″ or 0.018″ Guidewires

We will only briefly review these 0.014″ or 0.018″ guidewires, as they are not commonly used in extracranial carotid stenting. The relatively infrequent circumstances they are used include when a buddy wire support is needed, when pre-dilatation is needed before crossing with a filter embolic protection device (EPD), when intracranial rescue is needed, or if the EPD Spider™ (ev3, North Plymouth, MN, USA) system is used (which runs over a standard 0.014″ guidewire). These wires are generally well known to coronary interventionalists, as they are essentially coronary guidewires (Table 1). A standard wire of choice with adequate support and good maneuverability is the Hi-Torque Balance Middleweight Universal (Abbott Vascular, Santa Clara, CA, USA) wire which has a polytetrafluoroethylene (PTFE)-coated, stainless steel proximal shaft to allow smoother shaft passage. Other similar wires include the Hi-Torque Floppy II (Abbott Vascular, Santa Clara, CA, USA), IQ wire (Boston Scientific, Natick, MA, USA), and the Wizdom wire (Cordis, Miami, FL, USA). If extra support is required, then choices include the Balance Heavyweight (Abbott Vascular, Santa Clara, CA, USA) or Grand Slam wire (Abbott Vascular, Santa Clara, CA, USA). The use of more robust and supportive wires must be weighed against the risk of trauma to the carotid vasculature and plaque disruption.

In tortuous carotid arteries, a hydrophilic coated wire may be more desirable to advance into the distal carotid vasculature, especially if intracranial rescue is needed for distal embolization. Choices here include, but are not limited to, the Whisper MS and Whisper Extra Support wires (Abbott Vascular, Santa Clara, CA, USA). However, these hydrophilic wires are prone to migrate distally and can cause distal perforation if not vigilantly guarded. Furthermore, they may inadvertently disrupt carotid plaques and cause sub-intimal dissections. And thus, they are rarely used during extracranial CAS and should only be used with extreme care in the intracranial circulation.

0.035″ Peripheral Guidewires

The use of 0.035″ peripheral wires is necessary in several steps of the CAS procedure, including traversing peripheral vasculature which is frequently diseased, to facilitate catheter intubation of the common carotid artery (CCA), and for wiring and anchoring the external carotid artery (ECA) in order to advance sheaths or catheters to the CCA. Commonly used guidewires include both hydrophilic and non-hydrophilic wires (see Table 2).

FLEXIBLE PERIPHERAL WIRES

To allow catheter access to the great vessels, a flexible, soft-tipped workhorse peripheral wire is typically used, such as a Wholey Hi-Torque Floppy wire

Table 1
Examples of Commonly Used Coronary 0.014″ Guidewires

Guidewire	Manufacturer	Characteristics	Compatibility and length
Uncoated wire			
Hi-Torque Balance Middleweight Universal	Abbott Vascular	PTFE-coated shaft Straight or J tip 3 cm radiopaque tip	0.014″ 190 or 300 cm DOC® compatible
Hi-Torque Floppy II	Abbott Vascular	PTFE-coated shaft Shapeable ribbon 2 cm radiopaque tip	0.014″ 190 cm DOC® compatible
IQ	Boston Scientific	Silicone-coated shaft Straight or J tip 2 cm radiopaque tip	0.014″ 185 or 300 cm
Wizdom	Cordis	PTFE-coated shaft Straight or J tip Soft or supersoft tip 3 cm radiopaque tip	0.014″ 180 or 300 cm
Extra-support wires			
Balance Heavyweight	Abbott Vascular	PTFE-coated shaft Firm wire body Soft, straight, or J tip 4.5 cm radiopaque tip	0.014″ 190 or 300 cm DOC® compatible
Grand Slam	Abbott Vascular	Firm wire body Soft, straight tip 3 cm radiopaque tip	0.014″ 180 or 300 cm
Hydrophilic-coated wires			
Whisper MS	Abbott Vascular	Polymer cover with hydrophilic coating Straight or J tip 3 cm radiopaque tip Medium wire body support	0.014″ 190 or 300 cm
Whisper Extra-Support	Abbott Vascular	Polymer cover with hydrophilic coating Straight or J tip 3 cm radiopaque tip High tensile steel core	0.014″ 190 or 300 cm
Pilot 50,150, or 200 (variable shaft weight)	Abbott Vascular	Polymer cover with hydrophilic coating Straight or J tip 3 cm radiopaque tip	0.014″ 190 or 300 cm

Table 2
Commonly Used Peripheral Guidewires

Guidewire	Manufacturer	Characteristics	Compatibility and length
Flexible guidewires			
Wholey Hi-Torque Floppy	Mallinckrodt	Flexible atraumatic tip Teflon coating	0.035″ 260 cm
Magic Torque™	Boston Scientific	3 cm shapeable tip Hydrophilic coating	0.035″ 260 cm
Hydrophilic guidewire			
Glidewire®	Terumo Medical	Lubricious coating Angled, straight, or J tip Stiff shaft, nitinol core	0.035″ 260 cm
Stiff guidewires			
Amplatz Super Stiff™	Boston Scientific	1, 3.5, 6 cm straight tip or J tip (3 mm) Stiff shaft, PTFE coated	0.035″ 260 cm
Amplatz Extra Stiff	Cook Inc.	Shapeable straight tip or J tip (3 mm) PTFE coated	0.035″ 260 cm or 0.038″ 300 cm

(Mallinckrodt, Hazelwood, MO, USA) or Magic Torque™ (Boston Scientific, Natick, MA, USA) wire. The Wholey wire has a flexible atraumatic tip, a gold radiopaque tip for visualization, and a Teflon coating to reduce friction. And it comes in 145, 175, and 260 cm lengths. The Magic Torque™ wire has a 3 cm shapeable tip, hydrophilic coating on the distal 10 cm, and PTFE coating on the distal 11–50 cm. There are also four platinum radiopaque markers spaced 1 cm apart at the distal end. The Magic Torque™ comes in 180 and 260 cm lengths.

HYDROPHILIC PERIPHERAL WIRES

To advance into the CCA and the ECA, 0.035″ hydrophilic wires are preferred as they are more steerable and easier to advance into these vessels. We typically use a stiff support hydrophilic wire for this purpose, which provides sufficient body to allow passage of both guiding catheters and sheaths. The 260 cm stiff shaft, angle-tipped Glidewire® (Terumo Medical Corporation, Somerset, NJ, USA) is our hydrophilic workhorse wire of choice. This wire has a lubricious coating, allowing smooth passage, and a superelastic nitinol core to prevent wire kinking, yet providing flexibility. The stiff shaft aids by straightening out the CCA and the ECA to facilitate catheter tracking.

STIFF PERIPHERAL WIRES

Stiff guidewires are essential in carotid stenting as they allow tracking and exchange of sheaths and guiding catheters. The most commonly used are the Amplatz Extra Stiff (Cook Incorporated, Bloomington, IN, USA) and the Amplatz Super Stiff™ (Boston Scientific, Natick, MA, USA). Both are available in 260 cm lengths and both are PTFE coated. The Super Stiff™ has three different length straight tips (1, 3.5, and 6 cm) which can be manually shaped; it also comes in a pre-shaped J tip (3 mm curve). The Extra Stiff is also available in a 300 cm length, 0.038″ version for extra support and also available in a pre-shaped J tip (3 mm curve) configuration.

CATHETERS AND SHEATHS

Carotid angiography can be successfully performed in the great majority of cases simply by choosing the appropriate catheters (see Table 2). We prefer 5 Fr catheter systems, although 4 Fr is also suitable, especially if the anatomy is not complex and catheter stability is not an issue. The most important factor in the selection of catheters is based upon the patient's aortic arch configuration and whether there are any vessel origin anomalies.

Diagnostic Catheters: Types I and II Aortic Arch

In patients with a Type I aortic arch, the use of a standard Judkin's right catheter (JR4) is successful in the majority of cases. Other available catheters include the angle taper Glidecath® (Terumo Medical Corporation, Somerset, NJ, USA), the Berenstein (Boston Scientific, Natick, MA, USA), and the Headhunter (Cook, Bloomington, IN, USA) (see Fig. 1). We suggest using a 5 Fr catheter system routinely as a diagnostic, although a 4 Fr system is an alternative. Should the JR4 catheter not be suitable for intubation, a reverse-curve catheter is our next choice (see section on reshaping of reverse curve catheters in Chapter 11). Our preference

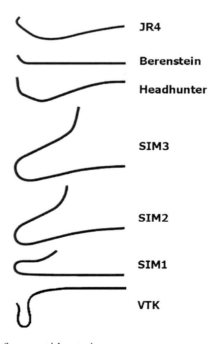

Fig. 1. Diagnostic catheters for carotid arteries.

for such catheter is the VTK catheter (Cook, Bloomington, IN, USA). The standard catheter length for these catheters is 100 cm, but a 125 cm catheter is required should one be employing the telescoping technique.

Diagnostic Catheters: Type III Aortic Arch

With more challenging aortic arch morphology the use of reverse-curve catheters is recommended. If the VTK catheter is not successful, then a Simmons-shaped catheter (I, II, or III length post-curve) would be our next choice (see Fig. 1). As mentioned for Type I and II arches, these catheters are usually 100 cm catheters, and a 125 cm length is required if the telescoping technique is to be employed.

Guide Catheters

The choice of guide catheters varies between operators and institutions, depending on multiple factors including operator preference, familiarity, and cost (see Fig. 2). Of importance is the fact that they must be 8 Fr with an internal luminal diameter of 0.088″ to enable smooth passage of the self-expanding stents used. Our preference is the Headhunter (H1) guide catheter (Cordis, Miami, FL, USA) which has a smooth secondary curve and a more angulated primary curve. Other 8 Fr guide catheters choices include, but are not limited to, a multipurpose guide, a Headhunter Yadav HY1 guide (Cordis, Miami, FL, USA), and a Burke (Modified Cerebral) guide (Cordis, Miami, FL, USA). With a steep Type III aortic arch or a true challenging bovine arch, a direct guide approach positioned at the ostium of the CCA can be achieved using an Amplatz left 1 (AL1) 8 Fr guide catheter.

Sheaths

The alternative to guide catheters is the use of long sheaths (see Fig. 3) with suitable internal diameters to allow passage of 5 Fr telescoping catheters and self-expanding stents. Our guide of choice is a 6 Fr 90 cm Flexor® Shuttle® sheath (Cook, Bloomington, IN, USA), which has an internal diameter of 0.087″ that is equivalent to an 8 Fr guiding catheter. The 7 Fr size has an internal diameter of 0.113″ and is equivalent to a 10 Fr guide catheter, but this larger size is not usually required. The sheath approach has several useful features for carotid stenting. Because of its very nature, a sheath maximizes internal diameter while minimizing the external diameter

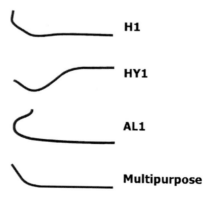

Fig. 2. Commonly used guide catheters for carotid arteries.

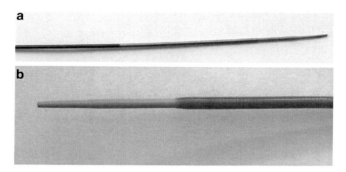

Fig. 3. Commonly used carotid sheaths: (**A**) Flexor® Shuttle® sheath (Cook, Bloomington, IN, USA), (**B**) Pinnacle® Destination® sheath (Terumo Medical Corporation, Somerset, NJ, USA).

at the arterial puncture site. This is important in reducing peri-procedural arterial access bleeding. Additionally this sheath has a lubricious coating for easy trackability and a soft, radiopaque tip to enhance visibility and minimize trauma to the CCA.

Another commonly used sheath is the Pinnacle® Destination® sheath (Terumo Medical Corporation, Somerset, NJ, USA), which has excellent flexibility and trackability. It is available in straight, multipurpose, and various other shapes. The proximal end is available in either a cross-cut or a Tuohy-Borst valve option. Size options include 6 or 7 Fr internal diameter and a standard 90 cm length. The dilator is 0.038″ wire compatible and the sheath is braided with three areas being radiopaque (the sheath, the dilator, and a gold tip marker) to allow for more precise positioning. The internal lumen is PTFE coated with a nylon exterior which also has a hydrophilic coating, both minimizing friction for equipment and sheath delivery, respectively. The tip is designed to be atraumatic and is much softer than the shaft. This system also has smooth wire–dilator and dilator–sheath transitions, which allow easy advancement through the arteriotomy to the target vessel position.

Another option is the Arrow Interventional Carotid Access Set (Arrow International), which comprises a 90 cm long sheath with a 7 Fr internal diameter. The Super Arrow-Flex® sheath also comes in various sizes from 4 Fr to 11 Fr, up to 100 cm in length and 0.035″–0.038″ compatible. The sheath is hydrophilic, and its tip is straight and radiopaque. The coil wire construction of this sheath minimizes the potential for sheath kinking and is favored for complex vessel tortuosity and calcification.

ANGIOPLASTY BALLOONS

Pre-dilatation Balloons

The use of pre-dilatation in carotid stenting is commonly performed and follows crossing the stenosis with an EPD. Coronary 0.014″-compatible monorail balloons are typically used as they are low profile, easy to pass, and are familiar to operators in the cardiac catheterization laboratory. Most commonly a 4.0 mm diameter by 20 mm length balloon is used and inflated to 6–8 atm for ~5 s. Larger diameter balloons are reserved for cases where there is difficulty tracking the stent after routine pre-dilatation. Longer balloons are only required for long lesions or sometimes for in-stent restenosis to avoid the "melon seeding" phenomenon. Rarely, the EPD is too bulky to cross a critically severe lesion, in which case a 0.014″ coronary guidewire is used to first cross the lesion. This allows pre-dilatation with a small

1.5 or 2.0 mm diameter balloon, prior to crossing the lesion with the EPD again. Commonly used pre-dilatation balloons include the Maverick[2TM] (Boston Scientific, Natick, MA, USA), Sprinter[TM] (Medtronic, Minneapolis, MN, USA), and CrossSail[TM] (Guidant, Indianapolis, IN, USA) balloons.

Post-dilatation Balloons

Post-dilatation is a high-risk step in percutaneous carotid revascularization due to the high embolic load that may be showered upstream as demonstrated on transcranial Doppler studies. However, this step is important with self-expanding stent deployment to ensure adequate deployment of the stent and reduce the occurrence of both in-stent restenosis and the potential, however low, for acute thrombosis. Aggressive post-dilatation is not usually required and small residual stenoses of up to 20% are acceptable. Peripheral arterial balloons which are 0.014" or 0.18" guidewire compatible are generally used for this step and are inflated to low nominal pressures of 6–8 atm. Lengths of 20 mm usually suffice and diameters used range from 5 to 6 mm in 0.5 mm increments. Again, inflation times are kept brief (~5 s). Most balloons used are semi-compliant, with non-compliant balloons reserved for heavily calcified lesions. Examples of semi-compliant balloons include Gazzelle[TM] (Boston Scientific, Natick, MA, USA), Amiia[TM] (Cordis, Miami, FL, USA), and Viatrac[TM] (Guidant, Indianapolis, IN, USA). The Titan[TM] (Cordis, Miami, FL, USA) balloon is an example of a non-compliant peripheral balloon.

CAROTID STENTS AND EPD

The early use of balloon-expandable, generic-built stents in the carotid artery came with several limitations. The early balloon-expandable stainless steel stents not only suffered problems with regard to distal plaque embolization (partially due to design and the lack of EPD use) but also did not withstand the external superficial forces in the neck. Due to movements and local muscular contractions, significant restenoses occurred due to stent compressions and fractures. With the advent of self-expanding nitinol and stainless steel stents, balloon-expandable devices now only have a limited role, mainly at the ostium of the CCA, where significant radial strength is required for aorto-ostial lesions.

Contemporary carotid stenting tends to favor the use of self-expanding nitinol stents, which are constructed of a nickel–titanium alloy. These nitinol stents are preferred as they have minimal foreshortening, are more flexible, and conform better to vessel curvature. However, one self-expanding stainless steel (cobalt–chromium alloy) stent is still used, namely the Wallstent® (Boston Scientific, Natick, MA, USA). Stainless steel self-expanding stents tend to have reduced radial force, are more rigid, and do not conform to the vessel wall as readily as their nitinol counterparts. Additionally the operator must be aware that the stainless steel stents can foreshorten by up to 20%, which must be taken into account both when choosing stent length and during placement and deployment. Due to the reduced radial force, this stent usually has to be oversized, and generally a 10 mm diameter × 20 mm length works well for most carotid bifurcations.

Emboli protection devices can be divided into filter and balloon occlusion devices. The balloon occlusion devices can be further classified as proximal and distal occlusion devices. The prototypical filter EPD is constructed of a guidewire with an integrated filter basket, although some devices have a detached guidewire and filter basket system. When the filter EPDs are deployed, blood flows antegrade through the filter pores, and the filter membrane traps embolic debris that are larger than the pores. These devices do not interrupt antegrade blood flow, and thus, angiography can be performed when filters are deployed to allow visualization of equipment placement. Once deployed, the filter guidewire functions as a conventional angioplasty guidewire accommodating balloon and stent equipment. Despite their disadvantages of high crossing profiles and missing emboli smaller than the pores, they remain the favored EPD during CAS because of their simplicity of use. The only FDA-approved balloon occlusion EPD is the Percusurge® GuardWire™ (Medtronic, Minneapolis, MN, USA), which is a distal balloon occlusion device. It is more cumbersome to deploy technically compared to the filter EPD and may not be tolerated by all patients. Table 3 details the advantages and disadvantages of filter versus distal balloon occlusion EPD.

Several specially designed carotid self-expanding stents are now commercially available and FDA approved (Table 4). These are described in more detail with their intended EPD (Table 5), which were generally approved together with their stents as a system for use during CAS.

Open Versus Closed Strut Stent Design and Rationale

There has been significant debate about the benefits and limitations of open versus closed-cell stent design (Fig. 4). The literature has yet to demonstrate a significant

Table 3
Filter EPD Versus Guardwire® Distal Balloon Occlusion EPD

	Filter devices	*Guardwire® occlusion device*
Apposition to vessel wall	Good apposition if filter matches vessel size, but incomplete apposition if filter too large or small	Good apposition if balloon size (2.5–5 or 3–6 mm) matches vessel size
Crossing Profile	Bulky and large crossing profile	Small crossing profile 0.014″
Ease of use	Easy to use	More cumbersome, requires aspiration and fast operation
Emboli protection	Captures emboli larger than the pore size of the filter	Theoretically captures all emboli with occlusion balloon and aspiration catheter
Embolic potential	Potentially higher embolic risk during filter crossing and filter retrieval	Low embolic risk during wire crossing and retrieval. May embolize if inadequate aspiration
Perfusion	Permits antegrade blood flow to distal bed, except when filter is full	Blood flow distally is occluded, may cause ischemia if poor collateral circulation
Retrieval profile	May extrude embolic debris through pores during retrieval if filter is full	Low profile
Vessel visualization	Unhindered visualization of vessel allows accurate stent placement	Difficult to visualize vessel when balloon is inflated

Table 4
FDA-Approved Self-Expanding Carotid Stents

Stent	Manufacturer	Straight stents	Tapered stents	Clinical studies
ACCULINK™	Abbott Vascular	Diameter (mm): 5, 6, 7, 8, 9, 10 Length (mm): 20, 30, 40	Diameter (mm): 6–8, 7–10 taper Length (mm): 30, 40	ARCHeR CAPTURE CREATE II CREST
Xact®	Abbott Vascular	Diameter (mm): 7, 8, 9, 10 Length (mm): 20, 30	Diameter (mm): 6–8, 7–9, 8–10 taper Length (mm): 30, 40	ACT I SECURITY EXACT
Protégé®	eV3	Diameter (mm): 6, 7, 8, 9, 10 Length (mm): 20, 30, 40, 60	Diameter (mm): 6–8, 7–10 taper Length (mm): 30, 40	CREATE I
PRECISE™	Cordis	Diameter (mm): 5, 6, 7, 8, 9, 10 Length (mm): 20, 30, 40	Diameter (mm): 6–8, 7–9, 7–10 taper Length (mm): 30	SAPPHIRE
Nexstent®	Boston Scientific	Diameter (mm): 4–9 mm (one stent size for all) Length (mm): 30	N/A	CABERNET
Exponent®	Medtronic	Diameter (mm): 6, 7, 8, 9, 10 Length (mm): 20, 30, 40	N/A	MAVErIC I MAVErIC II

Table 5
FDA-Approved Embolic Protection Devices for CAS

EPD (Manufacturer)	Associated carotid stent	Filter size	Retrieval device profile	Filter pore size (μ)
ACCUNET™ (Abbott Vascular)	ACCULINK™	4.5, 5.5, 6.5, and 7.5 mm basket	4.9 Fr	115
Emboshield® (Abbott Vascular)	Xact®	3.0–6.0 mm basket	5.4 Fr	140
SPIDER™ (eV3)	Protégé®	3.0–7.0 mm basket	3.2 Fr	48–167
Angioguard® (Cordis)	PRECISE™	4.0–8.0 mm basket	5.1 Fr	100
Filterwire EZ™ (Boston Scientific)	Nexstent®	One size for 3.5–5.5 mm	6.0 Fr	110
Guardwire™ (Medtronic)	Exponent®	2.5–5.0 and 3.0–6.0 mm	N/A	N/A balloon occlusion

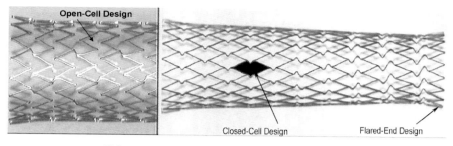

Fig. 4. Open-cell (Precise^{TM}) versus closed-cell (Xact$^{®}$) stents.

advantage either way. However, there have been some publications which have suggested a benefit to closed-cell design with regard to acute distal embolization. Nevertheless, it is likely the actual cell size and surface area coverage that are most important. The classification of open versus closed-cell designs depends on the number and arrangement of bridge connections. Closed-cell stents typically have adjacent rings that are connected at every junction, whereas open-cell stents usually have some (or all) of the connecting junctions absent between the rings.

In general, open-cell structure of carotid stents allows greater flexibility of the stent, which consequently allows the stent to be more deliverable in cases of difficult access or significant vessel tortuosity. Additionally, in vessels where there is a large discrepancy between the diameter of the CCA and ICA, open-cell design allows for improved stent conformability and wall apposition. Examples of open-cell design carotid stents include the Precise^{TM} (Cordis, Miami, FL, USA) stent, AccuLink^{TM} (Guidant Corporation, Santa Clara, CA, USA), Protégé^{TM} (ev3 Inc., Plymouth, MN, USA), and Exponent^{TM} (Medtronic, Minneapolis, MN, USA) stents.

Closed-cell stent designs tend to have more wall coverage due to the nature of the closed-cell design, which theoretically protects from distal embolization of plaque and atheroembolic debris. Closed-cell stents have increased radial force (expansive) as well as radial strength (resistive). These features make closed-cell designs the choice for lesions with a high plaque burden that has a predisposition to embolize, as well as heavily calcified lesions. Examples of nitinol closed-cell carotid stents include the Xact$^{®}$ (Abbott Vascular Devices, Redwood City, CA, USA) stent and Nexstent^{TM} (Boston Scientific, Natick, MA, USA), while the Wallstent$^{®}$ is a stainless steel closed-cell stent.

More recently, a new investigational carotid stent known as the Cristallo Ideale (Invatec, Roncadelle, BS, Italy) stent has been trialed in Europe. This stent combines a high scaffold central area which is closed cell with open-cell proximal and distal ends in a tapered stent. The stent is designed to maximize deliverability and conformability, with the safety of a closed-cell design in the high plaque burden section of the lesion. In addition, nitinol "mesh-like" stents with greater wall coverage are also being developed and investigated, which may potentially lower embolic events due to less plaque protrusion from greater scaffolding.

ACCULINK^{TM}, RX-ACCULINK^{TM} Stents and ACCUNET^{TM} EPD

The ACCULINK^{TM} and RX-ACCULINK^{TM} (Abbott Vascular, Santa Clara, CA, USA) carotid stent is a self-expanding nitinol stent, which has been used in several CAS trials, including the Acculink for Revascularization of Carotids in High-Risk Patients (ARCHeR) trial, the Carotid Acculink/Accunet Post Approval

Trial to Uncover Rare Events (CAPTURE) trial, the Carotid Stent Trial utilizing ev3's next generation SPIDER RX(TM) Embolic Protection Device with the Guidant AccuLinkRX(TM) Stent (CREATE II) trial, and the Carotid Revascularization Endarterectomy vs Stenting Trial (CREST). Being nitinol and an open-cell design, the stent is more conformable to the surrounding artery than a stainless steel stent and is crush resistant. Radial force is adequate but less than balloon-expandable stents, and hence lesions at the ostium of the CCA should be treated with balloon-expandable stents. It is 0.014″ guidewire compatible and compatible with 90 cm 6 Fr delivery sheaths or 100 cm 8 Fr guide catheters. Delivery of the stent and delivery of the EPD are both on monorail systems. The stent is also available in a tapered form to better conform to lesions which cross into the CCA, across the bifurcation of the internal carotid artery (ICA), and ECA. The stent design minimizes stent shortening on deployment, with manufacturer's figures from in-house testing suggesting only 1% shortening in a 7.0 × 40 mm stent. The stent ends are flared so as to facilitate passage of post-dilatation balloons. Additionally the deployment mechanism is designed to minimize stent migration on deployment, an issue that was common with initial self-expanding carotid stents.

Sizes for straight (cylindrical) stents range from 5.0 to 10 mm in diameter, increasing in 1.0 mm increments with lengths of 20, 30, and 40 mm. The tapered stents come in two sizes, with a 6.0–8.0 mm taper (suitable for ICA diameters of 4.3–5.4 mm and CCA diameters of 5.7–7.3 mm) and a 7.0–10.0 mm taper (suitable for ICA diameters of 5.0–6.4 mm and CCA diameters of 7.1–9.1 mm). They come in either 30 or 40 mm lengths.

The ACCUNET™ distal embolic protection system (Abbott Vascular, Santa Clara, CA, USA) has been used in conjunction with the ACCULINK™ and RX-ACCULINK™ carotid stents in the aforementioned trials (Fig. 5). It is a 0.014″ guidewire-based filter system with a flexible cage design to allow navigation through tortuosity and has good wall apposition. The filter is a nitinol basket-supported porous membrane with a maximum pore size of 115 μm. The sheath is "peel-away" after delivery. There are two lengths available, 190 and 300 cm with the 190 cm device having potential for "dock" wire attachment. Filter sizes are 4.5, 5.5, 6.5, and 7.5 mm basket diameters and are recommended for use in arteries from 3.25 to 7.0 mm. Filter sizing recommendation is 0.5 mm greater than the maximum reference vessel diameter (diameter of the pre-petrous carotid artery where the filter will be deployed). All sizes are 6 Fr sheath or 8 Fr guiding catheter compatible. Radiopaque markers are located on the guidewire tip, filter basket (four places), and delivery sheath. Recovery of the sheath is via either of two recovery catheters, which have shapeable tips for tortuous or difficult anatomy, and are 5.5 Fr in diameter profile. Newer versions have an improved retrieval sheath profile of 4.9 Fr.

XACT® Stent and Emboshield® EPD

The Xact® (Abbott Vascular, Santa Clara, CA, USA) carotid stent system is a rapid exchange nitinol stent which has been used in the Asymptomatic Carotid Trial (ACT 1), the Registry Study to Evaluate the Neuroshield Bare Wire Cerebral Protection System and X-Act Stent in Patients at High Risk for Carotid Endarterectomy (SECURITY), and the Emboshield and Xact Post Approval Carotid Stent Trial (EXACT). Vessel conformability due to its nitinol composition is high despite the closed-cell design. Again, the flared edges and lack of exposed cell struts have been

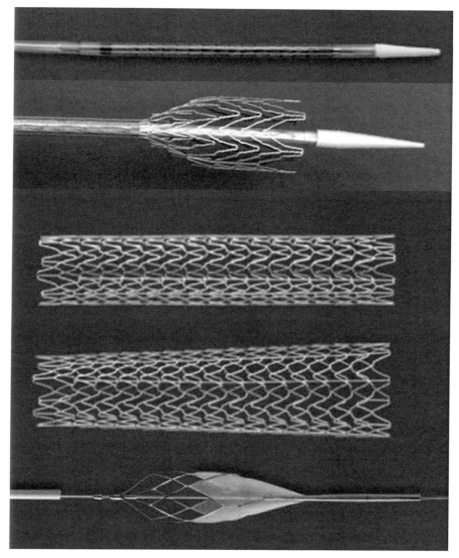

Fig. 5. ACCULINK™ and ACCUNET™ (Abbott Vascular, Santa Clara, CA, USA).

touted as facilitating passage of retrieval catheters and post-dilatation balloons. This stent is compatible with 0.014″ guidewires and 6 Fr delivery sheaths or 8 Fr guiding catheters.

Available stent sizes range from 7.0 to 10.0 mm in 1 mm size increments for the straight stent, and in 20 and 30 mm lengths. There are three tapered stents, 6–8, 7–9, and 8–10 mm, which come in 30 and 40 mm lengths.

The Emboshield® (Abbott Vascular, Santa Clara, CA, USA) distal embolic protection system was used in the aforementioned trials with the Xact® carotid stent (Fig. 6). The filter is 0.014″ guidewire based with a 0.018″ tip with independent 'BareWire' delivery to facilitate placement. The filter membrane itself is hydrophilic coated to minimize platelet, fibrin, or red blood cell adhesion. The design includes a

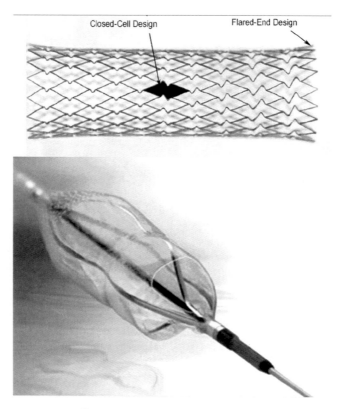

Fig. 6. Xact® and Emboshield® (Abbott Vascular, Santa Clara, CA, USA).

pore-free zone and helically staggered micropores (size 140 μm) to minimize plaque extrusion and optimize capture efficiency, respectively. The device is available in 190 and 315 cm lengths, with filter diameter sizes to cater for vessels between 2.8 and 6.2 mm (3.0, 4.0, 5.0, and 6.0 mm sizes). The devices have a crossing profile of 3.7–3.9 Fr and are 6 Fr sheath and 7 Fr guiding catheter compatible. The retrieval catheter profile is 5.4 Fr and has an expansile tip to maximize retrieval. The new Emboshield Pro® has an even smaller crossing profile and a slightly different basket design.

Protégé® GPS^{TM}, Protégé® RX Stents, and SPIDER^{TM} EPD

The Protégé® GPS and Protégé® RX stents (ev3 Inc., Plymouth, MN, USA) are open-cell, self-expanding nitinol carotid stents. This stent model has been investigated in and approved on the basis of the CREATE I (Carotid Revascularization with ev3, Inc. Arterial Technology Evolution) Trial. The nitinol composition is touted to allow excellent vessel conformability. The device is 0.014″ guidewire and 6 Fr sheath or 8 Fr guiding catheter compatible with a crossing profile of 0.78″. The stents are available in both straight and tapered forms. The straight stents come in 6, 7, 8, 9, and 10 mm diameter sizes, each available in 20, 30, 40, or 60 mm lengths. The tapered devices come in 30 and 40 mm lengths in 6–8 or 7–10 mm diameters. All the catheter lengths are 135 cm.

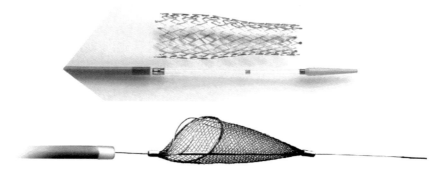

Fig. 7. Protégé® and SPIDER™ (ev3 Inc., Plymouth, MN, USA).

This stent has no significant foreshortening; furthermore, a new delivery system virtually eliminates stent "jumping" on deployment. Markers on each end of the stent aid in placement and the stent itself is radiopaque.

The SPIDER™ distal EPD (ev3 Inc., Plymouth, MN, USA) has been used in conjunction with the Protégé stent in the CREATE I trial (Fig. 7). The unique feature of this device is the fact that it uses a rapid exchange system of delivery of the filter over the operator's 0.014″ wire of choice. The filter is 3.2 Fr compatible, as is the retrieval catheter, and the pore size ranges from 48 to 167 μm. The only available length is 180 cm, and filter sizes are from 3 to 7 mm in diameter in 1 mm increments.

PRECISE™ Stent and Angioguard® XP EPD

The PRECISE™ over the wire (Cordis, Warren, NJ, USA) stent is a nitinol, open-cell design, self-expanding stent preloaded on either a 5.5 or 6 Fr sheathed delivery system. It has been evaluated in the Stenting and Angioplasty with Protection in Patients at High Risk for Endarterectomy (SAPPHIRE) study and approved on this basis. It is designed to accept up to a 0.018″ guidewire and the delivery system has a 135 cm working length. The stent comes in straight and tapered designs. The 5.5 Fr system has straight stent sizes with diameters of 5, 6, 7, and 8 mm with lengths of 20, 30, and 40 mm. There is one tapered 5.5 Fr device which measures 8 mm proximally, 6 mm distally, and 30 mm in length. In the 6 Fr-compatible stents, diameters are of 9 or 10 mm with lengths of 20, 30, or 40 mm. There are two tapered devices measuring either 9 or 10 mm proximally, 7 mm distally, and both are 30 mm in length. Foreshortening of the stent upon deployment ranges from 1.2% in the smallest devices to up to 8% in the larger straight stents. Stent selection should be based on oversizing the stent 1–2 mm to the reference vessel diameter, both proximally and distally, in order to ensure secure stent placement. There is a 1 mm flare at each end to minimize any difficulty in crossing the stent with post-dilatation balloons or the EPD retrieval catheter.

The Angioguard® XP (Cordis, Warren, NJ, USA) EPD has been used in conjunction with the PRECISE™ stent in the SAPPHIRE trial (Fig. 8). It is a 0.014″, 300 cm guidewire-based filter consisting of a polyurethane membrane umbrella with 100 μm pores. The distal tip is floppy and shapeable to allow steering and appropriate placement. The umbrella design is engineered to center the device in the middle of the vessel in order to ensure adequate vessel apposition to capture embolic

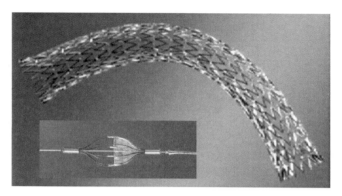

Fig. 8. PRECISE™ and AngioGuard™ (Cordis, Warren, NJ, USA).

debris. Radiopaque markers on four of the proximal ends of the eight nitinol umbrella struts facilitate visualization and show the operator that the device is fully deployed. The crossing profile of the device is 3.2 Fr, and it is 8 Fr guiding catheter or 6 Fr sheath compatible. Available filter basket diameter sizes range from 4 to 8 mm (in 1 mm increments) for vessels 3–7.5 mm in diameter. Recovery of the sheath is via a separate dedicated retrieval sheath which is 5.1 Fr compatible.

Nexstent® Stent and Filterwire EZ™ EPD

The Nexstent® (Boston Scientific, Natick, MA, USA) is a closed-cell design, self-expanding nitinol stent which has been approved on the basis of the Carotid Artery Revascularization Using the Boston Scientific FilterWire EX/EZ and the EndoTex NexStent (CABERNET) trial. There is one stent size to treat vessels 4–9 mm in diameter, and the stent length is 33 mm when mounted and 30 mm when deployed. The ends are flared to optimize retrieval of EPD. The system is 8 Fr guiding catheter and 6 Fr sheath compatible. The monorail and over-the-wire delivery sheaths are 135 cm in length, 0.014″, and 5 Fr compatible.

The Filterwire EZ™ (Boston Scientific, Natick, MA, USA) is a 0.014″ PTFE-coated wire-mounted distal protection device. It has been approved for carotid stenting based on the CABERNET trial where it was coupled to the Nexstent® (Fig. 9). The shapeable spring tip is 3.0 cm in length in the carotid device and is radiopaque. It is suitable for arteries 3.5–5.5 mm in diameter and has a minimum landing zone measuring 3.0 cm in length. The filter itself has 110 μm pores, and it is stabilized by a radiopaque nitinol loop which is designed to provide 360° vessel wall apposition. The crossing profile of the deployment catheter is 3.2 Fr with a smooth transition, which aims to simplify delivery. The new system has a preloaded, peel-away delivery sheath which is easy to prepare and provides rapid exchange-like convenience. The system comes in both 190 and 300 cm lengths, and there is also a bent tip retrieval catheter available for tortuous anatomy. The device is 6 Fr guiding catheter compatible.

Exponent® OTX, Exponent® RX, and Guardwire™ EPD

The Exponent® stent (Medtronic, Minneapolis, MN, USA) (Fig. 10) is an open-cell design, nitinol, self-expanding stent which has been approved on the basis of The Evaluation of the Medtronic AVE Self-Expanding Carotid Stent System in the Treatment of Carotid Stenosis (MAVErIC) I and II trials. There

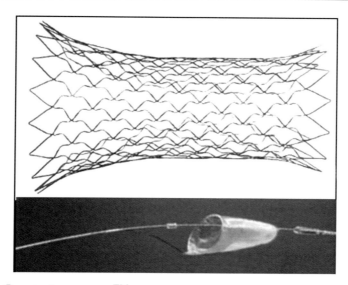

Fig. 9. Nexstent® and Filterwire EZ™ (Boston Scientific, Natick, MA, USA).

are two stent configurations, one for the 6.0 and 7.0 mm diameter size and one for the 8.0, 9.0, and 10.0 mm size. The smaller diameter stent has fewer crown segments with slightly thinner and wider struts than the larger diameter stent. Additionally, the larger stent has fewer longitudinal connections in its mid-segment in order to improve deliverability. Foreshortening is 0–4% and 0–6% in the smaller and larger diameter stents, respectively. The 6.0 and 7.0 mm stents are provided on a 5 Fr delivery platform, and the 8.0, 9.0, and 10.0 mm on a 6 Fr platform. Both have a 135 cm working length and are 0.014″ guidewire and EPD compatible. The Exponent® stents are available in 20, 30, or 40 mm lengths for all diameter sizes. The initial RX delivery system prompted complaints in Europe which resulted in a voluntary market withdrawal of the product in 2005. Following design changes which rectified the problem, the device was returned to the market in 2006.

The Guardwire® (Medtronic, Minneapolis, MN, USA) is a distal occlusion balloon and aspiration system for embolic protection. The guidewire is a 0.014″ specially constructed hollow kink-resistant nitinol hypotube, with an inflatable

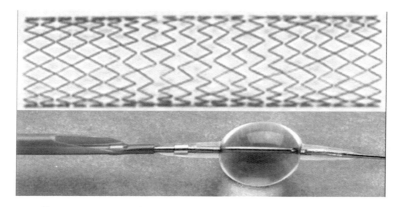

Fig. 10. Exponent® and Guardwire® (Medtronic, Minneapolis, MN, USA).

compliant balloon integrated near the distal end of the guidewire, and a 2.5 cm shapeable distal tip. The balloon occlusion system comes in two balloon sizes, 2.5–5.0 and 3.0–6.0 mm with the former having a 0.028″ crossing profile and the latter 0.036″. The shaft length comes in both 200 and 300 cm sizes with a minimum guide internal diameter requirement of 0.070″. The balloon itself is atraumatic and inflated to low pressure once the lesion is crossed to ensure an adequate cessation of flow, which is confirmed angiographically. The entire procedure may be performed under temporary balloon occlusion, or individual steps can be interrupted by aspiration and balloon deflation to allow antegrade flow.

Whether this system of vessel occlusion and subsequent aspiration is better than filter protection is debatable. One of the arguments in favor of an occlusion system is that in the evaluation of a balloon occlusion and aspiration system for protection from distal embolization during stenting in saphenous vein grafts (SAFE) study, 81% of particles were less than 96 μm in size which is the lower limit of filter pore size. Whether these small particles result in any clinically significant events in the carotid circulation remains to be determined. The retrieval catheter for the device is the Export® catheter which has a 1.0 mm aspiration lumen, is 0.014″ compatible, and is a monorail system with a length of 145 cm.

ASPIRATION CATHETERS

The aspiration of debris is mandatory during cases of slow antegrade flow due to basket filling and has been shown to reduce the incidence of neurological events with slow flow. The two most commonly used aspiration catheters in our institution are the Pronto™ V3 (Vascular Solutions, Minneapolis, MN, USA) and Export® (Medtronic, Minneapolis, MN, USA) systems. Both work on a similar principle, being monorail to advance into the vessel, and have a distal end-hole to aspirate thrombus by negative pressure via a syringe applied to the proximal end.

The Pronto™ V3 device comes in one size which is 6 Fr sheath compatible (requiring >0.070″ internal diameter). The catheter is rapid exchange (20 cm segment), has a 140 cm shaft length, has markers at 95 and 105 cm, and a marker band at 2 mm from the tip. It is a low profile device with a crossing profile of 0.053″ to enable passage into vessels as small as 1.5 mm in diameter. Deliverability is made easier by a hydrophilic coating. There is a separate 0.014″ wire port adjacent to the aspiration port which has a Silva tip (rather than a standard open tip) to maximize thrombus aspiration.

The Export® catheter (also used in conjunction with the Guardwire® distal occlusion embolic protection device) comes in 6 and 7 Fr guiding catheter-compatible sizes. The 6 Fr device is 5 Fr sheath compatible (minimum internal diameter 0.070″), and the 7 Fr device is compatible with a 6 Fr sheath (minimum internal diameter 0.080″). The devices are 140 and 145 cm in length, respectively. It is a monorail system and is 0.014″ guidewire compatible. The tip is open end and aspiration is performed using syringes placed at a negative pressure at the proximal end.

PROXIMAL BALLOON OCCLUSION EMBOLI PROTECTION DEVICES

The proximal balloon occlusion EPD design was intended to prevent emboli during all stages of CAS by interrupting or reversing blood flow in the ICA. Unlike the filter and distal balloon occlusion EPD where lesions have to be crossed with these devices prior to protection, the proximal balloon occlusion EPD allows cerebral protection prior to lesion crossing. This theoretically reduces distal embolization. Furthermore, operators can utilize 0.014″ guidewire of their choice, which would facilitate crossing critically tight lesions, as well as tortuous carotid arteries (especially those with 360° loops). There are two commercially available systems in Europe, the GORE Neuro Protection System (previously called Parodi Anti-Embolic System) (Gore, Flagstaff, AZ, USA) and the MO.MA system (Invatec, Roncadelle, Italy). The former is investigational only in the United States, and the latter is not yet available for sale in the United States.

Both these proximal devices have similar design, with a large compliant balloon integrated to the end of the guiding sheath for inflation in the CCA and a smaller compliant balloon delivered through the sheath to be inflated in the ECA (Fig. 11). Once the CCA and ECA balloons are inflated, the patient is protected from embolization and the operators then proceed with CAS using the guidewire, balloon, and stent of their choice (Fig. 11). With the balloons inflated in the CCA and ECA, retrograde blood flow through the ECA is prevented and forward flow through the ICA is prevented. In fact, reversal of flow is actually achieved with the GORE system by establishing a "fistula" with the lower pressure femoral venous system (via a 6 Fr venous sheath). The blood is directed through an external filter (with 180 μm pores) to collect aspirated debris, prior to re-entering the venous system. With the MO.MA device (Fig. 11), blood and debris are aspirated by the operator from the guiding sheath after post-dilatation and checked for debris, prior to deflating the CCA and ECA balloons.

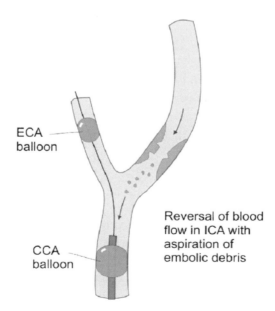

ECA balloon

CCA balloon

Reversal of blood flow in ICA with aspiration of embolic debris

Fig. 11. Schematic representation of a proximal balloon occlusion embolic protection device. A large compliant balloon is integrated to the end of the guiding sheath for inflation in the common carotid artery, and a smaller compliant balloon is delivered through the sheath and inflated in the external carotid artery. Negative suction is applied through the guiding sheath to enable retrograde flow in the internal carotid artery (ICA).

Preliminary data with these devices have been promising. In a nine patient experience with the Parodi device, no microembolic signals were detected with transcranial Doppler during CAS *(1)*. In the first 100 patient series reported by Parodi in 2001, there were again no embolic strokes; however, 8% of patients were intolerant of blood flow occlusion *(2)*. More recently in 2005, Parodi presented data on the first 200 patients with this device, reporting a technical success rate of 98.5%, 30-day death or stroke rate of 1.5%, and clamping intolerance rate of 3% *(3)*. For the MO.MA device, in the initial 42 patient experience, there were 2 transient ischemic attacks (TIA), 2 minor stroke events, and 12% were clamp intolerant. However, there was no major stroke or death at 3 months *(4)*. In the prospective PRIAMUS multicenter registry, 416 patients underwent CAS with the MO.MA device *(5)*. Technical success rate was 99%, with average of ~5 min clamp time. There were 24 (5.8%) patients who had transient intolerance to clamping, 12 of whom still completed the study with the MO.MA device, 7 required intermittent balloon deflation, and 5 required conversion to filter EPD. In-hospital stroke or death complication was 4.6% (0.7% TIA, 3.8% minor stroke, 0.2% major stroke, 0.5% death). Debris were retrieved in 59% of cases after filtration of the aspirated blood *(5)*. In a small 42 patient study comparing FilterWire EX^{TM} versus MO.MA, there were significantly lower number of microembolic signals on transcranial Doppler monitoring with the MO.MA device during the stages of guidewire lesion crossing, stent deployment, and post-dilatation *(6)*.

Although a great conceptual device with good preliminary data, up to 10% of patients do not tolerate this temporary occlusion of cerebral flow, especially those with contralateral stenosis or incomplete Circle of Willis. Furthermore, these devices are more cumbersome to use and the earlier generations required large ($\geq$10 Fr) femoral arterial access. The later devices are now lower profile, with the GORE device needing a 9 Fr access, and the newer model of the MO.MA device now compatible with an 8 Fr system (with a working inner diameter of 0.069″). They are unlikely to surpass the filter EPD as the protection device of choice, given their ease of use. However, they may have a niche market for patients with tortuous ICA where filter EPD is inaccessible and patients with critical lesions where filter EPD could not cross.

CONCLUSION

Many technical advances in the field of extracranial carotid artery stenting have allowed evolution of the technique to be safe and efficacious. Despite this, there remain further challenges such as improvement in stent design and emboli protection device to further reduce the occurrence of peri-procedural events. New stent design, incorporating positive features of both closed and open-stent design, will help achieve a balance between deliverability, scaffolding, embolization, and restenosis. Advancement in filter EPD designs with lower profile and better deliverability will further improve ease of use and technical success, especially for tight lesions and tortuous vessels. Proximal balloon occlusion EPD is not FDA approved yet; further evolution in design to reduce profile and improve ease of use will facilitate broader use and application.

REFERENCES

1. Whitlow PL, Lylyk P, Londero H, et al. Carotid artery stenting protected with an emboli containment system. Stroke 2002;33:1308–1314.
2. Parodi JC, Schonholz C, Ferreira M, Mendaro E, D'Agostino H. Parodi antiembolism system in carotid stenting: the first 100 patients. Presented at Society of Interventional Radiology 27th Annual Scientific Meeting, Baltimore, MD; 2002.
3. Parodi JC, Ferriera LM, Lamura R, Sicard G. Results of the first 200 cases of carotid stents using the ArteriA device. Presented at the International Congress of Endovascular Interventionx XVII, Scottsdale, AZ; 2005.
4. Diederich KW, Scheinert D, Schmidt A, et al. First clinical experiences with an endovascular clamping system for neuroprotection during carotid stenting. Eur J Vasc Endovasc Surg 2004;28:629–633.
5. Coppi G, Moratto R, Silingardi R, et al. PRIAMUS – Proximal flow blockage cerebral protection during carotid stenting: Results from a Multicenter Italian registry. J Cardiovasc Surg (Torino) 2005;46:219–227.
6. Schmidt A, Diederich KW, Scheinert S, et al. Effect of two different neuroprotection systems on microembolization during carotid artery stenting. J Am Coll Cardiol 2004;44:1966–1969.

13   The Endovascular Treatment of Acute Ischemic Stroke

Alex Abou-Chebl, MD *and Usman Khan,* MD

CONTENTS

ABSTRACT

The treatment of acute ischemic stroke has advanced greatly in the last decade. Currently, intravenous tissue plasminogen activator, intra-arterial recombinant pro-urokinase, and mechanical embolectomy have all been shown to be effective in treating acute ischemic stroke patients. This endovascular treatment remains very complex, and operators need to continuously balance between the drive to achieve rapid recanalization and the risk of intracranial bleeding.

Keywords Ischemic stroke; Embolization; Thrombolysis; Mechanical clot disruption; Aspiration; Thrombectomy; Angioplasty

INTRODUCTION

The treatment of acute ischemic stroke (IS) has advanced greatly in the last decade. Prior to 1995 there were no proven or approved treatments for IS. Since then intravenous (IV) tissue plasminogen activator (tPA), intra-arterial (IA) recombinant pro-urokinase, and mechanical embolectomy have all been shown to be effective in treating stroke patients or have received Food and Drug Administration (FDA) approval for use in the United States. Currently, newer approaches and novel treatments are under development or clinical study and are rapidly growing.

With this expanding armamentarium, more and more of the 750,000 annual cases of stroke in the United States are being treated *(1)*. However, the choice of

From: *Contemporary Cardiology: Carotid Artery Stenting: The Basics*
Edited by: J. Saw, DOI 10.1007/978-1-60327-314-5_13,
© Humana Press, a part of Springer Science+Business Media, LLC 2009

treatment must be individualized because of the heterogeneous nature of IS. Unlike the more homogenous acute coronary syndrome, which in the vast majority of patients is the result of an atherosclerotic plaque rupture, ischemic stroke can be caused by a plethora of mechanisms such as cardiac embolism, extracranial atherosclerosis/thrombosis, intracranial atherosclerosis or penetrating artery disease (i.e., lipohyalinosis), among others. This, coupled with the multiple variables that affect clinical response to treatment, makes the approach to the patient with acute IS complex, requiring not only exceptional endovascular technical skills but also a thorough knowledge of cerebral anatomy and physiology, stroke pathophysiology and clinical manifestations, and medical management *(2)*.

THE UNIQUENESS OF THE CEREBROVASCULAR CIRCULATION

The cerebral vessels most commonly involved in the pathogenesis of clinically severe IS include the intracranial internal carotid artery (ICA), the middle cerebral artery (MCA), the anterior cerebral artery (ACA), the intracranial vertebral artery (VA), the basilar artery (BA), and the posterior cerebral artery (PCA). These vessels are interconnected via three anastomotic channels at the base of the brain: the paired posterior communicating arteries (PCom) and the single anterior communicating artery (ACom). Together with the ICA, ACA, and PCA these anastomotic channels form the Circle of Willis, the major source of potential collateral blood supply.

The cerebral arteries lose the adventitia and external elastic lamina within 1 cm of entering the skull base and the tunica muscularis thins; most muscular arteries elsewhere in the body have dual elastic lamina and substantial adventitia. The cerebral arteries course on the surface of the brain within the subarachnoid space. As a result, perforation or rupture of an artery often results in intracranial hemorrhage (ICH), most commonly subarachnoid hemorrhage (SAH) or less commonly, intraparenchymal hemorrhage. Intracranial hemorrhage can lead to a rapid and marked elevation of intracranial pressure (ICP), which in turn can lead to the cessation of cerebral blood flow when the ICP approaches mean arterial pressure (MAP) or to herniation and brainstem compression, both of which often lead to immediate tissue injury and death *(3, 4)*. Another important and unique characteristic of the brain and cerebral circulation is that the brain is extremely sensitive to embolization. In the peripheral tissues, except for massive embolization in a patient with poor collaterals, embolization is not often of clinical consequence. In the brain, on the other hand, even microscopic emboli may lead to disabling neurological deficits if exquisite and eloquent areas of the brain are involved.

Another salient characteristic of the cerebral circulation is that reperfusion following ischemia or revascularization of a chronically stenosed artery may trigger reperfusion neuronal injury and cerebral hyperperfusion. The former results in neuronal apoptosis and neurological deterioration and the latter may cause ICH. Thus even a technically flawless and successful endovascular procedure may paradoxically result in brain injury or death.

With the above in mind it becomes clear that the endovascular treatment of acute IS is much more demanding and risky, but no less rewarding than endovascular treatment of other vascular beds. Careful attention to meticulous technique in every aspect of the procedure must be used to minimize the risk of embolization, and finesse and gentle technique rather than brute force should be used.

ACUTE ISCHEMIC STROKE TREATMENT

Most of the data on the endovascular approaches to acute stroke treatment are from small case series or non-randomized safety studies, all of which have differed greatly in their methodologies and patient populations studied. As a consequence, there are no standardized or widely accepted endovascular techniques for the treatment of acute IS. These difficulties are all attributable not only to the risk of ICH but also to the heterogeneous nature of ischemic stroke. In contrast with the most common cause of the acute coronary artery syndrome – atherosclerotic plaque rupture and thrombosis – acute strokes have a number of potential causes. Eighty-five percent of strokes are ischemic and the remainders are hemorrhagic. Ischemic stroke is caused by cardiogenic embolism in 20%, atherosclerosis/thrombosis (i.e., artery to artery embolism from cervical atherosclerosis or intracranial stenosis leading to occlusion or embolism) in 20%, and penetrating artery disease, aka small vessel disease, in 25% *(5)*. Thirty percent of strokes have no identifiable cause and the remainders are caused by a multitude of conditions such as migraine, arterial dissection, hypercoagulable states, etc. Therefore, no single approach or pharmacological agent will be effective in all cases, and treatment must be individualized based on the needs of each patient and on the probable mechanism of ischemia. To date, there has been only one FDA-approved pharmacological treatment for acute IS – intravenous (IV) administration of recombinant tissue plasminogen activator (rt-PA) – and only one randomized trial of endovascular treatment for acute IS – PROACT II (Prolyse in Acute Cerebral Thromboembolism II) *(6)*. In addition, there have been several safety/feasibility studies of mechanical embolectomy devices which have been FDA approved for clot and foreign body retrieval (Merci, Multimerci, and Penumbra).

PROACT II is the only placebo-controlled, randomized trial that evaluated the safety and efficacy of IA thrombolysis. PROACT II studied the effects of recombinant pro-urokinase (r-pro-UK) in 180 patients with MCA occlusion. In this study IA thrombolysis had superior recanalization efficacy with approximately 66% TIMI grade 2 or 3, compared to 33% with IV thrombolysis, and much superior compared to placebo *(7)*. With the high recanalization rate there was a 15% absolute benefit (58% relative benefit) for the treatment group over the placebo group with a symptomatic hemorrhage rate that was only 10% (for comparison the ICH rate in the definitive IV rt-PA study that led to FDA approval was 6%) *(8)*. Although the PROACT II trial was positive, intra-arterial thrombolysis with r-pro-UK is not yet FDA approved *(9)*. There have been no randomized or direct studies of the clinical efficacy of IA compared with IV thrombolysis; it is generally accepted, however, that larger vessels and greater clot burdens (e.g., occlusions of the ICA, MCA, or BA) are more resistant to thrombolysis, particularly IV thrombolysis, and that intra-arterial thrombolysis is the best option for those patients *(10, 11)*. Most clinicians accept the PROACT II results as a proof of the safety and efficacy of IA thrombolysis for strokes of less than 6 h duration and many have adopted the "PROACT protocol" for IA thrombolysis (other thrombolytic agents are used in place of r-pro-UK).

The PROACT protocol was remarkable for its stringent inclusion criteria and standardized protocol. All patients received the same dose of peri-procedural heparin, which consisted of a 2,000 U bolus at the start of the procedure, and was then followed by a 500 U/h infusion for 4 h only. The r-pro-UK dose was 9 mg infused over 2 h in all patients irrespective of the clot burden, and mechanical disruption of the thrombus was not permitted. As a result, although there was nearly 70% recanalization at 2 h, the complete, TIMI 3 recanalization rate was only 19% *(6)*.

In addition to the longer time window for treatment (6 h for IA and 3 h for IV) and the higher recanalization rates, intra-arterial thrombolysis is useful in circumstances where IV thrombolysis is contraindicated such as for patients with recent non-cerebral hemorrhage, major organ surgery or arterial puncture in a non-compressible site, and patients on systemic anticoagulation. Although the risk of hemorrhage exists with IA thrombolysis in these circumstances, in general, smaller doses of thrombolytics are needed so the risks are minimized *(12)*.

A major concern regarding the use of intra-arterial thrombolysis is the amount of time required for the interventional team to be available as well as the time it takes to obtain arterial access and to perform cerebral angiography. In contrast, IV tPA may be given with minimal delay once a head CT and blood work are obtained. However, not all patients qualify for IV therapy and many patients (approximately 2/3) treated with IV tPA do not improve neurologically. In addition, many patients treated with intravenous tPA have residual occlusion of the involved vessel. To overcome the limitations of both approaches, an innovative treatment approach in which an attempt was made to combine a rapid infusion of IV tPA with local intra-arterial thrombolysis was studied in the Emergency Management of Stroke Bridging Trial *(13)*. This was a double-blind, randomized, placebo-controlled, multicenter feasibility study with 35 enrolled patients, in which intravenous plus intra-arterial tPA (IV/IA) treatment was compared with placebo plus intra-arterial tPA (placebo/IA). The rate of symptomatic ICH at 72 h ranged from 5.5% (IV/IA group) to 11.8% (placebo/IA group). Primary outcome measures were not different between treatment groups at 90 days of follow-up; because the number of patients was so small in this study, no definitive conclusions could be drawn except that combination intravenous/intra-arterial therapy is feasible and appears safe and deserves further investigation. This study also showed a direct correlation between the National Institutes of Health Stroke Scale (NIHSS) score and the presence of thrombus in a "major cerebral artery". This finding could be explored in future studies as a marker to identify patients who may benefit from intra-arterial thrombolysis.

Since r-pro-UK is not commercially available and no randomized trials have compared intra-arterial therapy with best medical treatment for acute ischemic stroke clinicians must rely on whatever data are available. A recent meta-analysis of 27 reports with a total of 1,117 patients compared treatment results against prognostic models of natural history adjusted for NIHSS scores and age. The combined data showed that there was no net benefit for thrombolysis with percent differences from predicted outcomes varying from −51 to + 24.6% for mortality and −30.3 to + 28.7% for good functional outcome. There was, however, an indication that the use of lower doses of thrombolytics (urokinase in particular) was associated with better outcomes. Such analyses are inherently flawed but are nevertheless helpful and emphasize the need for prospective trials of IA thrombolysis.

Patient Selection

All patients should be evaluated clinically as well as with laboratory tests and cerebral imaging before an intervention is contemplated. Clinical assessments of stroke severity are typically performed using the NIHSS *(14)*, which has been validated as a reliable tool for this task. This scale, which ranges from 0 (normal) to 42 (no neurological function), is based on a 12-item focused neurological examination. In general, strokes in the 0–3 range are considered minor, those between 4 and 7 are considered mild, those between 8 and 15 are moderate, and strokes with scores of more than 15 are severe. The NIHSS value can also suggest the size of the vessel involved and is of prognostic value. Deficits with a score of <4 are more likely to resolve completely; these patients should not be considered for IA thrombolysis because in these patients the prognosis for recovery is usually good and the probability of finding a large artery occlusion which would be amenable to IA thrombolysis is small. In contrast, patients with a score >20 are less likely to derive benefit from any treatment, including IV or IA thrombolysis (6). Patients with a score of 8–20 are the most likely to benefit from intervention and are also less likely than those with more severe strokes to have hemorrhagic transformation, so they are the ideal group of patients to select for IA thrombolysis.

The time of stroke onset must be known with certainty before an intervention can be performed, because the duration of ischemia is a predictor of prognosis and the risk of ICH *(15, 16)*. In most circumstances, 6 h appears to be the upper limit for safe intervention; however, emerging clinical experience suggests that longer durations of ischemia may still be treatable in appropriately selected patients or that delayed recanalization may be beneficial (Abou-Chebl et al. unpublished data) *(17)*. Despite these data the earlier the treatment can be started the better the prognosis *(18)*.

It is of great value to try to determine the likely etiology of the stroke before beginning the intervention so that as much planning is done beforehand as possible since, for example, the approach to the patient with a fresh cardioembolic stroke may be different than that for a patient with a long atherosclerotic ICA occlusion. Although there are no completely reliable means of determining etiology, particularly without angiography, there may be historical or clinical facts that may be of value. For example, the presence of atrial fibrillation or a history of it in someone who is not anticoagulated greatly increases the likelihood that it is the cause. Similarly a history of atherosclerosis (e.g., known coronary artery disease, peripheral vascular disease) especially if there is known carotid artery disease should raise the possibility of atherothrombosis as the mechanism of stroke. In African-Americans and those of Asian descent who have no cardiac history and who have vascular risk factors, particularly diabetes and renal failure, there is a high likelihood that intracranial atherosclerosis and thrombosis will be the mechanism of stroke *(19, 20)*. Therefore, without delay, as much clinical history as possible should be obtained before the intervention.

A computerized tomographic (CT) scan of the brain is mandatory in all patients presenting with acute IS. Computerized tomography is currently the standard means of evaluating the brain in the setting of acute IS primarily because of its high sensitivity and specificity for ICH. Magnetic resonance imaging (MRI) is a more sensitive and specific tool for the assessment of cerebral ischemia and can also provide data on the viability of brain tissue as well as the area of brain at risk. The major limitation of MRI is the prolonged imaging and processing time (up to 15–30 min or longer) compared with CT, which can be performed within seconds on the latest generation of multi-detector spiral scanners. A full discussion of the merits of one imaging modality over another is beyond the scope of this chapter.

The interventionist should therefore work in concert with a colleague in neurology who is familiar with the evaluation of stroke patients to determine the best imaging study and to determine which patients are candidates for intervention.

A history of ICH at any time in the recent or remote past should be considered an absolute contraindication in most cases. Similarly, patients with Alzheimer's disease who are predisposed to ICH due to amyloid angiopathy should be considered as very high risk for IA lysis *(21)*. Other factors such as patient age over 80 years old, elevated serum glucose level, active treatment with heparin or a heparinoid, therapy with high-dose aspirin, clopidogrel, or platelet GP IIb/IIIa receptor antagonists should be considered as potential contraindications as they all are associated with an increased risk of ICH *(15, 22)*. The clinician deciding on whether to treat an individual patient should weigh all of these factors together. For example, an octogenarian with no other risk factors and stroke duration of 3 h with no evidence of ischemia on initial CT scan may be a better candidate than a 55-year-old receiving dual antiplatelet therapy with aspirin and clopidogrel, who also has profound hyperglycemia and elevated blood pressure, presenting at 5.5 h after stroke onset with some evidence of ischemia on CT scan.

In addition to a non-contrast-enhanced CT scan of the brain an assessment of the size of the ischemic core and ischemic penumbra may be an effective means of determining whether a patient is appropriate for interventional treatment. Animal studies and preliminary human clinical data suggest that the more the brain tissue at risk of complete infarction, but which is not yet irreversibly damaged (i.e., the penumbra), and the smaller the volume of the irreversibly injured brain tissue (i.e., the ischemic core), the greater the benefit and the lower the risk of reperfusion therapy *(20, 23–25)*. The best means of determining ischemic core from penumbra is not yet clear, but MRI and CT technologies are both clinically available and are currently being tested. These tests may be most helpful in cases of clinical uncertainty (e.g., early CT scan changes) or in cases where the time of onset is unknown or is quite prolonged to determine if it is appropriate to intervene or not. Again a full discussion of these imaging modalities and their merits are beyond the scope of this chapter.

In summary the indications for IA thrombolysis are the following:

○ Acute, ischemic stroke <6 h in duration
○ Stroke is significant, i.e., disabling or life threatening
○ Suspected occlusion of a large artery, i.e., non-lacunar stroke syndrome
○ No hemorrhage on screening computed tomography (CT) scan

The contraindications to IA thrombolysis are all based on the need to decrease the risk of ICH *(16)* and include the following:

○ Intracerebral hemorrhage is suspected or evident on CT
○ Initial CT scan shows evidence of acute ischemia in a large portion of the affected territory (i.e., more than 1/3 of the middle cerebral artery territory)
○ History of ICH or SAH
○ The presence of an arteriovenous malformation or large thrombosed aneurysm (non-thrombosed, unruptured aneurysms are not an absolute contraindication to thrombolysis if the clinical deficit is severe enough)
○ Uncontrolled hypertension >185/110 mmHg
○ Profound hyperglycemia

○ History of dementia of Alzheimer's type
○ Stroke duration is unknown or is >6 h (unless some radiological assessment of ischemic core:penumbra volumes indicates a favorable ratio)
○ Recent stroke within 3 months
○ Bleeding diathesis, elevated INR>1.7, or thrombocytopenia <100,000 cells/mm^3

INTERVENTIONAL APPROACH

Diagnostic Angiography

Access should be obtained rapidly via the femoral artery and a 5 Fr diagnostic catheter is used for diagnostic angiography. If time permits and the patient is very old or known to have severe untreated hypertension, an arch angiogram should be performed to assess the tortuosity of the vessels and therefore the complexity of engaging the symptomatic vessel. In most cases, however, arch aortography is not needed. This step will determine the equipment used for access. If the ICA or MCA are the symptomatic vessels, ipsilateral common carotid artery (CCA) angiography should be performed, as well as angiography of the carotid bifurcation and ICA origin. The intracranial ICA and MCA are best visualized with both an antero-posterior (AP) image (with slight, 10–15° of cranial angulation) and a true lateral image. For suspected ischemia in the vertebrobasilar (VB) circulation, the subclavian artery should be cannulated first and the ostium of the VA visualized. The left subclavian and VA are usually more easily cannulated than the right VA. If the left VA cannot be found arising from the subclavian artery, the right subclavian artery should be cannulated and angiography of the right VA then performed. Of note, the left VA rarely can arise from the aorta, usually in between the left common carotid and left subclavian artery origins. In addition many individuals have a dominant VA on one side with the other, smaller VA ending in the posterior inferior cerebellar artery (PICA), which does not contribute significant flow to the BA and the brainstem. Lastly the VA supplies small arterial feeders to the anterior spinal artery, which arise medially from its cervical portion; therefore, the wire tip should be pointed laterally when possible to avoid precipitation of a spinal cord infarct.

When performing digital subtraction angiography, image capture should be continued until the end of the venous phase. Branch occlusions are sometimes only indicated angiographically by delayed arterial filling and emptying, which sometimes can be subtle. Following angiography of the symptomatic vessel and if time allows, cannulation of the contralateral carotid artery and at least one vertebral artery, whichever is appropriate, should be performed to search for evidence of collateral blood flow from either the ACom, the PCom, or pial collaterals from the PCA to the MCA or ACA or vice versa. The presence of collaterals is a positive prognostic sign and their presence suggests a high probability of recanalization success with a lower risk of ICH. Conversely their absence suggests a high likelihood of infarction of the affected territory even if rapid recanalization is achieved *(26)*. In addition, angiography is performed to exclude the presence of large, thrombosed aneurysms or arteriovenous malformations or vascular brain tumors, all of which should be considered to be contraindications to thrombolysis because of the risk of ICH. In most cases brought to the interventional suite, a non-invasive assessment (magnetic resonance angiography or CT angiography) of the vasculature and collaterals should have already been completed while the interventional team and lab are being prepared. Therefore, catheter angiography of collaterals is not as essential in those cases.

Spontaneous dissections of the extracranial or intracranial vessels do not represent contraindications to thrombolysis; however, these are conditions that do increase the risk of subarachnoid hemorrhage (even without the use of thrombolytics and anticoagulants) and can make access to the intracranial vessels difficult and risky and should be handled with extreme caution.

Access

Due to the tortuosity and sharp angles of the cervico-cranial vessels, the most critical technical factor that determines procedural failure or success is stable access to the site of occlusion or stenosis. In those patients who have straight vessels both proximally and distally, a 6 Fr guide catheter in the distal cervical ICA or distal cervical VA provides sufficient support to allow equipment access to the most distal intracranial vessels. Road mapping or trace subtraction should be considered, as they greatly increase the margin of safety. In patients with tortuous vessels the approach may be different. Proximal tortuosity prevents the effective transmission of kinetic energy to the tips of wires and catheters, which when combined with distal tortuosity makes delivery very difficult, particularly for stiff equipment such as balloon-mounted stents. In addition to the tortuosity, the vessels in the elderly are stiff and noncompliant which makes equipment navigation that much more difficult. For this reason, the use of a more supportive guide catheter or a long sheath should be considered. If there is extreme iliac tortuosity or abdominal aorta dilation (but with straight cerebral vessels) a 6 Fr 55 cm long sheath may be sufficient. If there is a great deal of proximal aortic arch or great vessel tortuosity and redundant loops then 7 or 8 Fr 70–80 cm length sheaths should be used; of note, 90 cm sheaths are too long and will not permit sufficiently high guide catheter placement since most guide catheters are only 100 cm in length.

For ICA and MCA interventions, the sheath should be placed in the distal CCA. Sheath placement that high within the CCA carries a risk of vessel injury and the approach we have found to be most effective and safest is to use the telescoping technique frequently used in obtaining access for carotid artery stenting. Using road mapping and the 5 Fr diagnostic catheter, place a stiff-angled 0.035″ hydrophilic wire in the external carotid artery (ECA). After the wire is placed in the ECA the diagnostic catheter is advanced into the ECA and the hydrophilic wire is exchanged for a super-stiff 0.035″ wire; this wire will straighten out most tortuous segments and will give sufficient support even for cannulation of a right CCA that is arising from a very low-lying innominate artery. The diagnostic catheter is then removed. The sheath exchange is carried out over the super-stiff wire keeping it securely within the ECA. The sheath should be inserted with its introducer securely in place rather than over the diagnostic or guide catheters to avoid dissection of the CCA. The introducers are quite stiff and caution should be used not to dissect the ICA as the tip approaches the CCA bifurcation. The stiff wire and introducer are carefully removed after the sheath is placed just below the carotid bifurcation while back traction is maintained on the sheath to prevent it from "jumping" into the ICA.

For VB interventions a variation of the procedure described above can be used but since the sheath is only needed within the proximal subclavian, if there is not severe innominate or subclavian tortuosity, there is no need for exchange of the hydrophilic wire for a super-stiff wire. This wire is placed in the axillary artery and unless a super-stiff wire is needed the sheath can be inserted over it; if a super-stiff wire will be needed then as was described for CCA placement, a 5 Fr diagnostic catheter is placed distally in the axillary or distal subclavian artery and the wires exchanged. VB access can be quite difficult if there is severe tortuosity as even a rigid sheath may have a tendency to fall out of the subclavian, particularly the right subclavian. In those cases there are two options. The first is to place a 0.018″ stiff wire or 0.035″ non-hydrophilic wire distally within the axillary or brachial arteries for sheath support. If that is not adequate and stable access cannot be obtained via a femoral approach, then the second option is to obtain brachial access with insertion of a 6 Fr sheath into the subclavian just distal to the VA origin.

Following the sheath exchange a 2,000 U bolus of heparin is given and is followed by a 500 U/h infusion for 4 h. This was the heparin regimen that was validated in the PROACT II trial *(6)*. This regimen is the most commonly used with pure pharmacological thrombolysis, but in our experience higher doses of heparin with an activated clotting time (ACT) of 1 ½–2 times baseline or a value of 250–300 s is often needed if angioplasty and stenting are to be performed but not if the patient was treated with GP IIb/IIIa inhibitors or high doses of thrombolytics, or if the patient has had recalcitrant hypertension or if a large infarct is suspected. Under those circumstances the PROACT regimen discussed above may be more appropriate and in addition the heparin may be reversed with protamine sulfate at the end of the procedure if an excellent recanalization result was achieved. Prolonged or post-procedural heparinization is of no value in the authors' opinion and may greatly increase the risk of ICH.

When stable access to the appropriate vessel has been obtained, a 6 Fr soft-tipped and curved guide catheter is then placed within the distal cervical ICA or VA. This is typically performed over a soft, hydrophilic 0.035″ wire or over a small coronary balloon which has been advanced over a 0.014″ wire. If resistance is felt force should not be used to advance the guide, rather a very gentle injection of contrast can be performed to look for spasm or dissection. These vessels have a high propensity for spasm, particularly in younger patients. If spasm is found then nitroglycerin 200–400 μg should be given directly into the vessel or the guide catheter can be withdrawn slightly to alleviate the spasm. With the availability of embolectomy devices designed specifically for the neurovascular tree, placement of a balloon occlusion guide catheter rather than a conventional neuro-guide may be more prudent in cases with a high likelihood of cardioembolism. Doing so will facilitate embolectomy and obviate the need to exchange guide catheters in the middle of the case.

A 0.014″ hydrophilic, soft-tipped wire should then be passed through the stenotic or occluded segment and placed distally. Crossing an occluded segment should be performed very carefully remembering that the intracranial vessels have no adventitia and are easily perforated. The wire tip should always be free and mobile: any buckling or loss of ability to torque the wire tip should raise the possibility of subintimal migration. In advancing the wire through an occluded segment the operator must also be aware of the normal branches arising from the occluded segment and their usual course so that the wire does not perforate the artery and is not directed inadvertently into one of the small branches which can easily be perforated. The essential branches to be aware of are the ophthalmic artery arising anteriorly from the distal cavernous ICA, the PCom arising posteriorly from the carotid siphon, and the smaller anterior choroidal also arising posteriorly just above the PCom. The MCA has multiple perforators (the lenticulostriate arteries) which arise superiorly (dorsally) along the length of the main trunk; the wire tip should be kept pointing downward in the AP view when it is being passed through this segment of the MCA. The MCA bifurcation can be variable in its location and branching pattern: it can bifurcate normally with a long trunk and two main branches arising just as the MCA enters the Sylvian fissure and takes an upward (dorsal) course or the bifurcation can be very proximal to the ICA terminus. Also instead of a bifurcation there can be a trifurcation or quadrifurcation. Another common variant is for the anterior temporal artery to arise antero-inferiorly (ventrally) from the mid to distal MCA trunk.

The VA has several muscular branches in its distal cervical segments and the posterior inferior cerebellar artery (PICA) can often arise extracranially at the C1 level and should not be cannulated inadvertently. Intracranially the VA gives off the PICA dorsally, and just before the VB junction each VA gives off a very small vessel, the anterior spinal artery to the spinal cord, dorsomedially. The BA has multiple nearly microscopic perforating branches posteriorly (dorsal) that supply the pons and midbrain as well as the large paired anterior inferior cerebellar arteries (AICA) arising laterally at the juncture of the proximal and middle thirds and the paired superior cerebellar arteries (SCA) arising laterally at the BA terminus just before the BA bifurcation into the PCA. The wire tip should be carefully maneuvered into the third order MCA and PCA branches for adequate support. If road mapping is available and sufficient flow, either antegrade or retrograde, is present, the wire should be placed into the largest possible branch. Careful shaping of the wire tip is essential; not enough of a tip can lead to perforation and the inability to navigate very tortuous vessels and too much of a curve on the tip can make manipulation of the wire difficult in the smaller distal branches. A two-component curve on the wire tip, a very small and short (1–2 mm) distal curve with a slightly longer secondary curve 1–2 mm more proximally, is highly effective.

Wire placement can be greatly facilitated by loading the wire through a microcatheter or small balloon angioplasty catheter, which is then advanced with the wire leading. If there is a low likelihood of underlying atherosclerotic plaque as the cause of the vessel occlusion and thrombolysis is the first planned treatment then a microcatheter may be more appropriate so that thrombolysis can be immediately begun. However, if there is a high likelihood of underlying stenosis then loading the wire through a small 1.5–2.5 mm diameter, flexible over-the-wire balloon catheter will allow for more rapid angioplasty. An over-the-wire balloon catheter is preferred to a rapid-exchange or monorail system because it permits wire exchanges and is generally more deliverable to tortuous segments. Also, if needed angiography can be performed through the central lumen of the balloon catheter just as with a microcatheter. Regardless of whether a microcatheter or balloon is used, the device should be advanced into the occluded segment and thrombus.

Recanalization Technique

Several approaches to achieve recanalization have been described. Most of the published series have reported on the use of thrombolytics alone similar to the PROACT II protocol but without the use of r-pro-UK *(27)*. More recently some have reported on the use of a combination of pharmacological agents, while a few series have described a purely mechanical approach *(28)*. A multimodal approach combining multiple pharmacological agents and mechanical disruption may be superior to a single modality approach because IS is heterogeneous *(29, 30)*. Not all thrombi are composed of the same platelet and fibrin components and not all emboli are thrombi; therefore, the treatment approach should be adjusted to the needs of each patient. For example, in cases with a high likelihood of cardioembolism as the cause of the stroke, higher doses of thrombolytics may be preferred, whereas in patients with an atherothrombotic lesion GP IIb/IIIa inhibitors may be combined with thrombolytics and angioplasty or even stenting alone. However, in standard clinical practice, the first line treatment remains the infusion of a single thrombolytic agent. This approach has been performed with significant differences in the technique. Some interventionists do advance the microcatheter distally to the occluded segment with the goal of defining the distal-most extent of the occlusion or to permit infusion of thrombolytic agent distally. This approach carries a risk of distal embolization and some recent data suggest that microcatheter dye injections distal to the occlusion may increase the risk of ICH *(31)* so another approach is to place the microcatheter within the thrombus and to infuse the pharmacologic agents directly into the thrombus. Other aspects of IA thrombolysis that vary from one center to another include the choice of pharmacological agent as well as the dose, the rate of infusion, and the duration of the infusion.

The most widely used thrombolytic agent is rt-PA *(32, 33)*, but other agents have also been used including streptokinase, urokinase, reteplase, and TNKase *(28, 34, 35)*. The only agent whose efficacy and safety were validated in a controlled trial, r-pro-UK, is not commercially available. One agent in particular, streptokinase, is no longer used and should be avoided because in early studies it was associated with excessive risks of ICH *(36)*. Although rt-PA is the most commonly used, there are data suggesting that it may not be ideal because it has some neurotoxic effects and it may be associated with higher risks of ICH *(37)*. The optimal dose of each agent is unknown because of the significant variation in the doses used in the various reported series, which have ranged from 5–50 mg of rt-PA, 250,000–1,000,000 U of urokinase, and 1–8 U of reteplase, for example. In general lower doses are preferred and excessive dosing may not only increase the risk of ICH, but it may also lead to a paradoxical increase in thrombosis. The doses of each agent should be adjusted to the needs of each patient based on the presence or absence of several patient characteristics that are associated with higher risks of ICH or poor prognosis, namely increasing patient age (especially >80 years), hypertension (especially if >185/110 mmHg and if difficult to control), elevated serum glucose, duration of ischemia >4 h, the absence of collateral blood flow, underlying large brain infarct >1/3 of the MCA territory, large clot burden (e.g., complete ICA occlusion from bulb to MCA), other extenuating circumstances (e.g., anticoagulant use or coagulopathy, thrombocytopenia), or the intended use of other agents or aggressive mechanical manipulation during the intervention *(38)*. The presence of several of these factors may best be handled by avoiding thrombolytics alltogether or by using a purely mechanical approach whereas the absence of all of the factors would favor an aggressive approach particularly if the clinical deficit is severe. No systematic prospective study of IA thrombolysis has yet been done other than PROACT II and no approach has been proven to be superior to another.

In regard to the dosing frequency and infusion rate the authors follow the rule that "the more rapid the recanalization the better the chance of a good neurological outcome". Therefore, two to three boluses of thrombolytic given over 30 min may be superior than the 2-h infusion used in the PROACT II trial. Yet again, as with practically all aspects of this procedure, clinical data are lacking on the best approach.

Adjunctive Pharmacotherapy

In a few small reported series, platelet GP IIb/IIIa receptor antagonists have been used successfully in combination with thrombolytics in order to treat patients with acute IS without significantly increasing the risk of ICH *(28, 29)*. These agents may have a facilitatory effect on thrombolysis when combined with a thrombolytic agent because thrombi are often composed of a combination of aggregated platelets bound with fibrin strands *(39)*. Moreover if a balloon angioplasty is planned, a GP IIb/IIIa receptor antagonist is typically administered since there is a risk of endothelial injury and may be essential if a stent is to be placed *(16)*. The two most commonly used agents are abciximab and eptifibatide. The typical doses are similar to those used to treat patients with an acute coronary syndrome, although it is the authors' preference to start slowly and give more as needed, e.g., abciximab in 1/4 bolus increments. The GP IIb/IIIa inhibitor doses are then alternated with boluses of thrombolytic agent. The GP IIb/IIIa antagonists are typically infused IV, but IA administration directly into the thrombus through the microcatheter may facilitate thrombolysis by saturating the platelets within the thrombus *(29)*. A continuous (12-h) infusion should rarely be considered following successful thrombolysis and only in the event that a stent is placed, or if there is an underlying atherosclerotic plaque and small doses of thrombolytics were used. The risk of ICH appears to be low with this approach, but this has not been studied in a randomized fashion; it should, therefore, not be considered in all patients and should be used by centers with some experience using these agents in patients undergoing cerebrovascular interventions.

Clot Disruption

Manipulation of the thrombus with the wire is of possible benefit for fresh thrombi, that is to say those complicating endovascular procedures, e.g., coronary catheterization or cerebral angiography, or for small clot burdens, e.g., an MCA branch occlusion. Mechanical clot disruption can be performed with repeated passes of the microwire or microcatheter through the thrombus, although the efficacy of this approach is unclear. In some instances, the clot may migrate distally due to wire manipulation, which may be of benefit if the clot passes beyond a critical vessel (e.g., the rolandic artery supplying blood flow to the motor cortex or out of the M1 into the M2 segments in patients who have good pial collateral flow); however, it may also block off collateral channels (e.g., occluding the origin of the ipsilateral ACA which may have been supplying collateral flow to the MCA). Mechanical manipulation increases the risks of the intervention, so great care should be taken not to injure the vasculature. Wire passes and manipulation should be performed with close attention to the wire tip.

Both larger occlusions and those due to an atherosclerotic plaque are unlikely to be disrupted sufficiently with wire manipulation. In these cases a more elaborate approach, such as angioplasty, is warranted, especially in the latter group; these patients often have typical risk factors (especially poorly controlled diabetes mellitus) and are more likely to be of African or Asian descent *(40)*.

Adjunct balloon angioplasty for acute stroke has been reported both in combination with other techniques and as the sole treatment *(29, 41–43)*. We often perform gentle balloon angioplasty with undersized coronary balloons in patients who do not respond quickly to thrombolysis. Balloon inflations should be somewhat prolonged, up to 2 min in duration, and multiple inflations may be required. Adjunctive GP IIb/IIIa antagonists can be considered in patients treated with angioplasty because of the likelihood of either iatrogenic or pre-existing endothelial injury. This approach is similar to that used to treat patients with ACS. In some circumstances, angioplasty is inadequate and stenting of the occluded vessel may be needed. We, and others, have reported on the use of stenting without thrombolysis for the treatment of acute IS. Most of these patients have had severe underlying stenoses, either of the intracranial or extracranial vessel *(44)*. Such lesions may have a high propensity for re-occlusion, both early and delayed, with purely pharmacological treatments. Stenting may, therefore, allow for both early recanalization and definitive treatment of the causative lesion, thus reducing the risk of re-occlusion. Adequate platelet inhibition is important in these cases, and GP IIb/IIIa antagonists should be considered as discussed above. Following stent placement, patients also receive clopidogrel and aspirin to prevent early stent thrombosis. This approach should not be considered as a standard of care, but in selected patients it can be performed probably with a low risk of ICH.

Clot Extraction

Mechanical embolectomy, or clot removal, is an emerging alternative to thrombolysis. In some circumstances, pharmacological thrombolysis, even IA thrombolysis, may be contraindicated (e.g., active systemic bleeding) or be associated with a high risk of ICH (e.g., moderate early infarct signs or recent neurosurgery). Another major limitation of thrombolysis is the speed of recanalization. In PROACT II thrombolysis was carried out over 2 h. When combined with the time it takes to activate the interventional team and obtain access, etc., several hours may pass and a previously salvageable penumbra may become ischemic core. Mechanical embolectomy may greatly increase the speed of recanalization and potentially lead to better outcomes than those reported using thrombolysis. Moreover, mechanically removing the clot may greatly reduce or alleviate the necessity for administration of thrombolytics and anticoagulants and their associated complications.

Driven by these needs, several devices for mechanical embolectomy have been developed. However, it was not until August of 2005 that the FDA approved the first device for clot removal. The MERCI^{TM} (Mechanical Embolus Removal in Cerebral Ischemia) clot retriever, manufactured by Concentric Medical Inc., was FDA approved based on the data from the single-arm MERCI trial. A total of 151 patients with various large vessel occlusions were enrolled, but the device could be deployed in only 141 patients. The recanalization rate of the target vessels with the MERCI device only was 45% as compared to 56.3% with adjunctive thrombolysis. Serious device-related events occurred in only 3.5% of patients, and symptomatic ICH occurred in 8%. The overall mortality at 90 days was 39%, but among patients in whom embolectomy was unsuccessful, the mortality was nearly 61%. Good outcome, defined as a modified Rankin Score ≤2 at 90 days, was achieved in 28% of patients in the MERCI trial, a figure similar to the percentage of patients with a good outcome in the placebo arm of PROACT II. Based on these findings and the fact that there was no concomitant control arm to the study, the FDA approved the device for the "removal of clots" and not for stroke therapy.

The MERCI retriever system consists of a helically shaped nitinol wire, a micro-catheter, and a balloon occlusion guide catheter. The device is passed through the microcatheter distal to the thrombus, and the catheter is removed; the clot is then trapped in the wire helix and withdrawn from the vessel under negative pressure applied through the balloon occlusion guide catheter. The device is available in two models, the stiffer X6 and the softer X5. Both require Concentric Medical's proprietary microcatheters for delivery.

With the goal of improved recanalization, enhancements were made to the original "X-series" MERCI retriever to yield the "L-series" of retrievers, which have a 90° bend at the junction of the wire and the helix and several filaments attaching the distal end of the helix with the proximal end (Fig. 1). Like the "X-series" these devices are available in different sizes and degrees of

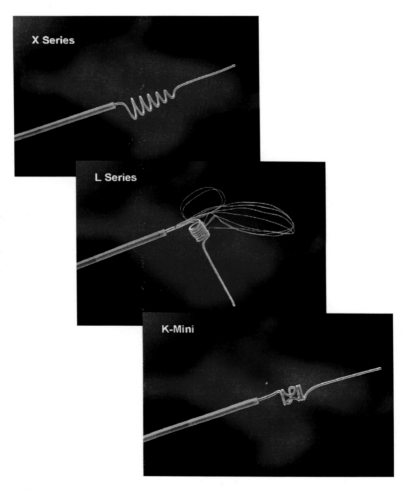

Fig. 1. Mercy Retriever system.

stiffness. The first of these, the L5 series, was tested in the Multi-MERCI trial, which was an international, multicenter, prospective, single-arm trial of thrombectomy in patients with large vessel stroke treated within 8 h of symptom onset. In this trial, 164 patients received thrombectomy, of which 131 were initially treated with the L5 Retriever. Mean age ± SD was 68 ±16 years, and baseline median NIHSS was 19 (15–23). Patients with persistent large vessel occlusion after IV tissue plasminogen activator treatment were included. The primary outcome of the trial was recanalization of the target vessel. Treatment with the L5 Retriever resulted in successful recanalization in 57.3% in treatable vessels and in 69.5% after adjunctive therapy (intra-arterial tPA). Overall, favorable clinical outcomes (mRS 0–2) occurred in 36% and mortality was 34%; both outcomes were significantly related to vascular recanalization. Symptomatic ICH occurred in 9.8% of patients. Clinically significant procedural complications occurred in 5.5% of patients. Although higher rates of recanalization were associated with the newer generation thrombectomy device compared with first-generation devices, these differences did not achieve statistical significance. However, mortality trended lower and the proportion of good clinical outcomes trended higher than historical controls.

Both the MERCI and Multi-MERCI trials showed a higher proportion of favorable outcomes in patients with recanalization than in those without it. In MERCI, revascularization was an independent predictor of favorable outcome (odds ratio [OR]: 12.82; 95% confidence interval [CI]: 2.95–55.75) and lower mortality (OR: 0.33; 95% CI: 0.14–0.77), identified by multivariate modeling. In the Multi-MERCI, 49% (95% CI: 40–59) of recanalized patients had a favorable outcome compared with 9.6% (95% CI: 1.6–18) of those that were not recanalized ($p<0.001$), and mortality was halved in the recanalized group (25 vs. 52%; 95% CI: 17–33, $p<0.001$). A post hoc analysis of the 27 patients from both trials with vertebrobasilar strokes (26 with basilar artery occlusions) – a group known for its dismal natural history – revealed favorable outcomes in 43% of revascularized patients compared to 0% of non-revascularized patients; mortality was 43 and 50% in the two groups, respectively.

More recently, another mechanical embolectomy device, the Penumbra™ system (Fig. 2), has been FDA approved to reduce clot burden within 8 h of acute ischemic stroke. This system consists of a series of three variously sized microcatheters, a "separator wire", and a continuous suction device that applies one atmosphere of suction through the microcatheter. The separator wire is then moved in and out of the tip of the microcatheter to break up the thrombus as it enters the microcatheter so that it can be aspirated out of the artery. The major difference between this system and the MERCI system is that access to the thrombus and vessel is not lost with every pass of the device. The multicenter, international, prospective, single-arm study that led to approval of the Penumbra™ system involved 125 patients with baseline NIHSS of eight points or higher. Patients had to have either no perfusion or faint antegrade flow beyond the occlusion, as indicated by scores of 0–1 on the TIMI scale. Use of the device led to successful revascularization in nearly 82% of treated vessels. Additionally, 41.6% of patients had a favorable outcome, defined as improvement of four points or more on the NIHSS at discharge, or a 30 day mRS of two points or less. Outcomes from the MERCI trial were used as the historical controls and the comparison showed that the Penumbra system was associated with a significantly better revascularization

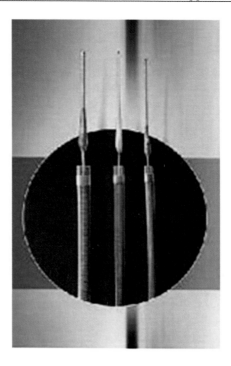

Fig. 2. Penumbra system.

rate – 82 versus 48% for MERCI. Such comparisons are of dubious merit since the patient populations are not comparable and the definitions of recanalization are often different. Nevertheless, the newer generation devices do appear to be more efficacious at recanalizing occluded cerebral vessels.

Other devices are commercially available and can also be used for embolectomy; all, however, are snares designed for the removal of foreign bodies. Nonetheless we, and others, have used these devices in the pre-MERCI era to successfully remove thrombi in patients with acute ischemic stroke *(45, 46)*. One such device is the GooseNeck (MicroVena Corp.) snare, which acts essentially as a lasso (Fig. 3). Snaring should be considered in patients who have cardioembolism because such emboli are less likely to be affixed to an underlying plaque (unpublished data). The technique of snaring involves the passage of a microwire and microcatheter through the occlusion. The wire is then exchanged for the GooseNeck snare, which (we have found) should be slightly oversized for the occluded artery. The lasso of the snare is deployed just distal to the occluded segment by unsheathing of the microcatheter; then the snare and microcatheter are withdrawn together into the thrombus. The snare is engaged into the thrombus and the microcatheter is advanced slightly in order to tighten the snare, but not so tightly as to tear through the thrombus. Finally, the microcatheter and snare are withdrawn as a unit into the guide catheter while negative pressure is applied within the guide catheter to facilitate the removal of the thrombus and decrease the likelihood of distal embolization. Retrograde flow is induced by applying negative pressure within the guide catheter just as with the MERCI Retriever. The creation of a negative pressure differential can be greatly facilitated by the use of a balloon occlusion guide catheter that can be inflated gently

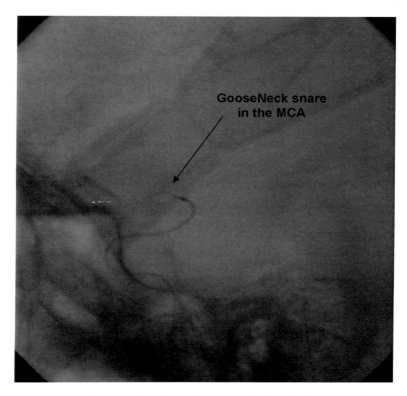

Fig. 3. Fluoroscopy image showing the GooseNeck snare in the middle cerebral artery (MCA) for embolus retrieval.

within the ICA to occlude all antegrade flow. A similar procedure can be performed with a balloon guide in the subclavian artery or, if large enough, the VA in cases of VB occlusion. When successful, this technique can lead to very rapid recanalization and excellent clinical outcomes with a very low risk of complications (Fig. 4).

The disadvantage of the technique is the loss of access to the lesion with every snaring attempt. Additionally the guide catheter often has to be completely removed if the retrieved thrombus becomes lodged within the guide lumen. It is because of the latter that the placement of a sheath in the common carotid or subclavian artery can be very helpful, permitting rapid recanalization of the target vessel. In addition these devices have the potential to cause arterial perforation, dissection, or distal embolization.

Peri-procedural Medical Management

A complete discussion of medical vascular neurology and neurological critical care is beyond the scope of this chapter and so only a cursory discussion of the most pressing matters will be discussed. The reader is referred to several excellent text-books on these subjects for further reading.

Maintaining a patient's airway, breathing, and circulation is mandatory in the rush to recanalize the occluded vessel. Although most patients are able to breathe spontaneously (patients with diffuse lower brainstem ischemia notwithstanding), those with a depressed level of consciousness may run the risk of hypoventilation or

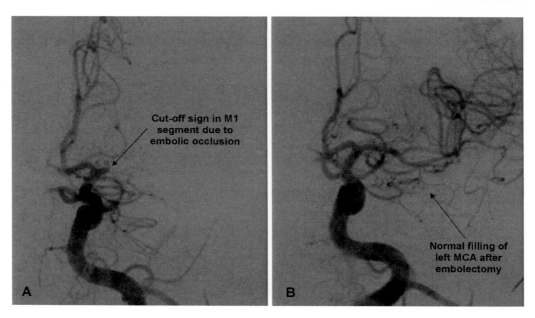

Fig. 4. Intracranial angiograms showing embolic occlusion of the left middle cerebral artery in the M1 segment (**A**) in a patient with unanticoagulated atrial fibrillation, followed by normal intracranial filling of the MCA after successful embolectomy (**B**).

aspiration. If there is a high likelihood that the patient will need artificial ventilation or airway protection then the patient should be intubated and mechanically ventilated prior to beginning the intervention but without delaying the initiation of recanalization therapy. Intubating and sedating all patients is unnecessary despite the widespread misconception that it is important for patient safety. In the authors' experience the loss of the neurological examination and the ability to communicate with the patient are tremendous drawbacks which make endovascular therapy riskier. By not sedating our patients, we are able to monitor the response to treatment and if a patient begins to markedly improve we may terminate a procedure even if the angiographic appearance is not perfect; after all, the goal of therapy is neurological recovery, not purely vessel recanalization. More importantly, awake patients are able to express signs of pain and discomfort, which may permit the early detection of complications. Headache, for example, is a potentially important indication of vascular irritation and intracerebral bleeding. The occurrence of such headache during an intervention always requires a clinical re-evaluation of the patient as well as a reassessment of the operative technique and equipment positioning (particularly that of the wire) *(47)*. If there is no vessel perforation on angiography and the headache resolves without clinical deterioration, then the intervention can be continued. If a patient's headache (or severe agitation in the case of non-verbal patients) persists, then strong consideration should be given to termination of the procedure in order to obtain a CT scan or at least a thorough angiographic and clinical re-evaluation.

Blood pressure (BP) control is the most important peri-procedural clinical factor. Under ischemic conditions the cerebral arteries maximally vasodilate to maintain cerebral blood flow (CBF) in the optimal range (i.e., *cerebral autoregulation*). As a direct result of this vasodilatation, CBF becomes linearly proportional to the mean arterial pressure (MAP). Cerebral ischemia can, therefore, be potentiated by iatrogenic or spontaneous declines of MAP, resulting in decreased CBF below the critical levels for tissue survival *(7)*. Similarly, excessive elevations of MAP may lead to marked elevations of CBF and an increased risk of reperfusion injury and hemorrhage – particularly in cases where recanalization is successful. The optimal range for BP varies for each patient, but in general MAP should be maintained between 110 (150/90 mmHg) and 135 mmHg (185/110 mmHg) for patients receiving thrombolytics *(5)*. Beta-blockers are safe and very useful in controlling BP, but nicardipine can also be considered for persistently and severely elevated blood pressures. Although nitroglycerin is effective, it can cause headache, which can mimic or mask the headache of ICH. Nitroprusside should generally be avoided because of its deleterious effects on increased intracranial pressure.

In general, it is preferable not to lower arterial blood pressures before recanalization is achieved unless the blood pressures are significantly elevated (i.e., >220/130 mmHg) *(48)*. If complete recanalization is achieved, then pressures can be lowered into the normal to high-normal ranges. In certain circumstances where the risk of ICH may be high (e.g., long duration of ischemia, large doses of thrombolytics, or GP IIb/IIIa antagonists were administered, a long-standing arteriosclerotic lesion is treated) blood pressures should be lowered into the low normal or occasionally into hypotensive ranges *(49)*. It is critical to keep in mind that the prevention of ICH is the single most important task following any cerebral intervention. Intracerebral hemorrhage has no effective treatment and is fatal in up to 80% of cases.

Furthermore, if needed, we recommend giving all patients oxygen via a nasal cannula or non-rebreather face mask during the procedure. Supplemental oxygen increases brain tissue oxygenation and is generally safe. Although there is some concern that high oxygen levels may worsen reperfusion injury, we feel that preserving the ischemic penumbra is paramount.

The management of post-stroke and ICH patients can be complex and is best performed with the assistance of an experienced neurointensivist and stroke neurologist. For this purpose, after the procedure all patients should be sent to a neurological intensive care unit for monitoring. Frequent neurological checks should be performed, at least every 15 min. Particular attention should be paid to the occurrence of headache, the worsening of deficits, or the development of a decreased level of consciousness, all of which could be the signs of ICH. If any of the above develops, a quick neurological assessment followed by an urgent CT scan of the brain should be obtained. The management of ICH following thrombolysis is quite difficult, and the prognosis is greatly worsened if ICH develops. If symptomatic ICH is present or a hematoma with mass effect develops, any residual doses or effects of anticoagulants, thrombolytics, or antiplatelets should be immediately reversed if possible. Neurosurgical consultation should be obtained immediately, but it is unclear if there is in fact a role for neurosurgical intervention in this setting *(10, 26)*. It is unclear what should be done if a patient develops asymptomatic petechial hemorrhagic conversion which is very common. Although a frank hematoma with mass effect may develop following petechial conversion, it is not guaranteed, and the overall clinical status of the patient should be considered along with the risk of precipitating acute thrombosis and vessel occlusion (e.g., following stent placement) before antithrombotics and antiplatelet agents are reversed or withheld. Also the interventionist should be aware that often immediate post-procedural CT scans show marked contrast enhancement of the ischemic tissue. This finding likely represents breakdown of the blood–brain barrier and likely is a marker for increased risk of ICH but is not always so. Therefore, it should be differentiated from ICH particularly if the patient is doing well. Repeat scanning often shows resolution within 24–48 h.

CONCLUSION

Endovascular treatment of acute IS remains very complex with the continuous need to balance between the drive to achieve rapid recanalization and the risk of intracranial bleeding. Management of these patients requires a thorough understanding of the intracranial cerebral vasculature and the pathophysiology of stroke. Nonetheless, a variety of tools and pharmacological agents are available, and excellent clinical results can be achieved with a thoughtful approach to the patients with IS and individualization of the treatment to the needs of each patient. Although more randomized controlled trials are needed to help find the most efficacious treatment strategy, pharmacologic intra-arterial lysis with or without thrombectomy appear to be effective recanalization strategies with the potential for greatly improving neurological outcomes.

REFERENCES

1. Rosamond W, Flegal K, Furie K et al. Heart disease and stroke statistics–2008 update: a report from the American Heart Association Statistics Committee and Stroke Statistics Subcommittee. Circulation 2008; 117(4):e25–e146.
2. Caplan LR. TIAs: we need to return to the question, 'What is wrong with Mr. Jones?'. Neurology 1988; 38(5):791–793.
3. Juvela S, Heiskanen O, Poranen A et al. The treatment of spontaneous intracerebral hemorrhage. A prospective randomized trial of surgical and conservative treatment. J Neurosurg 1989; 70(5):755–758.
4. Batjer HH, Reisch JS, Allen BC, Plaizier LJ, Su CJ. Failure of surgery to improve outcome in hypertensive putaminal hemorrhage. A prospective randomized trial. Arch Neurol 1990; 47(10):1103–1106.
5. Foulkes MA, Wolf PA, Price TR, Mohr JP, Hier DB. The Stroke Data Bank: design, methods, and baseline characteristics. Stroke 1988; 19(5):547–554.
6. Furlan A, Higashida R, Wechsler L et al. Intra-arterial prourokinase for acute ischemic stroke. The PROACT II study: a randomized controlled trial. Prolyse in Acute Cerebral Thromboembolism. JAMA 1999; 282(21):2003–2011.
7. Haley EC, Jr., Brott TG, Sheppard GL et al. Pilot randomized trial of tissue plasminogen activator in acute ischemic stroke. The TPA Bridging Study Group. Stroke 1993; 24(7):1000–1004.
8. Tissue plasminogen activator for acute ischemic stroke. The National Institute of Neurological Disorders and Stroke rt-PA Stroke Study Group. N Engl J Med 1995; 333(24):1581–1587.
9. Moskowitz M, Caplan LR, editors. Thrombolytic treatment in acute stroke: review and update of selective topics. Cerebrovascular Diseases. 19th Princeton Stroke Conference. Boston: Butterworth-Heinemann, 1995.
10. del Zoppo GJ, Ferbert A, Otis S et al. Local intra-arterial fibrinolytic therapy in acute carotid territory stroke. A pilot study. Stroke 1988;19(3):307–313.
11. del Zoppo GJ, Poeck K, Pessin MS et al. Recombinant tissue plasminogen activator in acute thrombotic and embolic stroke. Ann Neurol 1992; 32(1):78–86.
12. Katzan IL, Masaryk TJ, Furlan AJ et al. Intra-arterial thrombolysis for perioperative stroke after open heart surgery. Neurology 1999; 52(5):1081–1084.

13. Lewandowski CA, Frankel M, Tomsick TA et al. Combined intravenous and intra-arterial r-TPA versus intra-arterial therapy of acute ischemic stroke: Emergency Management of Stroke (EMS) Bridging Trial. Stroke 1999;30(12):2598–2605.

14. Brott T, Adams HP, Jr., Olinger CP et al. Measurements of acute cerebral infarction: a clinical examination scale. Stroke 1989;20(7):864–870.

15. Adams HP, Jr., Brott TG, Furlan AJ et al. Guidelines for thrombolytic therapy for acute stroke: a supplement to the guidelines for the management of patients with acute ischemic stroke. A statement for healthcare professionals from a Special Writing Group of the Stroke Council, American Heart Association. Circulation 1996;94(5):1167–1174.

16. Hacke W, Ringleb P, Stingele R. How did the results of ECASS II influence clinical practice of treatment of acute stroke. Rev Neurol 1999;29(7):638–641.

17. Wunderlich MT, Goertler M, Postert T et al. Recanalization after intravenous thrombolysis: does a recanalization time window exist? Neurology 2007;68(17):1364–1368.

18. Hacke W, Donnan G, Fieschi C et al. Association of outcome with early stroke treatment: pooled analysis of ATLANTIS, ECASS, and NINDS rt-PA stroke trials. Lancet 2004;363(9411): 768–774.

19. Sacco RL, Kargman DE, Gu Q, Zamanillo MC. Race-ethnicity and determinants of intracranial atherosclerotic cerebral infarction. The Northern Manhattan Stroke Study. Stroke 1995;26(1): 14–20.

20. Jovin TG, Yonas H, Gebel JM et al. The cortical ischemic core and not the consistently present penumbra is a determinant of clinical outcome in acute middle cerebral artery occlusion. Stroke 2003;34(10):2426–2433.

21. McCarron MO, Nicoll JA. Cerebral amyloid angiopathy and thrombolysis-related intracerebral haemorrhage. Lancet Neurol 2004;3(8):484–492.

22. Suarez JI, Sunshine JL, Tarr R et al. Predictors of clinical improvement, angiographic recanalization, and intracranial hemorrhage after intra-arterial thrombolysis for acute ischemic stroke. Stroke 1999;30(10):2094–2100.

23. Sunshine JL, Bambakidis N, Tarr RW et al. Benefits of perfusion MR imaging relative to diffusion MR imaging in the diagnosis and treatment of hyperacute stroke. AJNR Am J Neuroradiol 2001;22(5):915–921.

24. Kidwell CS, Alger JR, Saver JL. Beyond mismatch: evolving paradigms in imaging the ischemic penumbra with multimodal magnetic resonance imaging. Stroke 2003;34(11):2729–2735.

25. Thomalla GJ, Kucinski T, Schoder V et al. Prediction of malignant middle cerebral artery infarction by early perfusion- and diffusion-weighted magnetic resonance imaging. Stroke 2003;34(8):1892–1899.

26. Barr J. Cerebral angiography in the assessment of acute cerebral ischemia: guidelines and recommendations. J Vasc Interven Radiol 2004;15(1): S57–S66.

27. Furlan AJ. Acute stroke therapy: beyond i.v. tPA. Cleve Clin J Med 2002;69(9):730–734.

28. Lee DH, Jo KD, Kim HG, et al. Local intraarterial urokinase thrombolysis of acute ischemic stroke with or without intravenous abciximab: a pilot study. J Vasc Interv Radiol 2002;13(8): 769–774.

29. Abou-Chebl A, Krieger D, Bajzer C, Yadav J. Multimodal therapy for the treatment of severe ischemic stroke combining GPIIb/IIIa antagonists and angioplasty after failure of thrombolysis. Stroke 2003;34(1).

30. Gupta R, Vora NA, Horowitz MB, et al. Multimodal reperfusion therapy for acute ischemic stroke: factors predicting vessel recanalization. Stroke 2006;37(4):986–990.

31. Khatri R, Khatri P, Khoury J, Broderick JP, Carrozzella J, Tomsick T. Microcatheter contrast injections during intraarterial thrombolysis increase parenchymal hematoma risk: registry experience. Stroke 2008;38(2):454–455.

32. Hacke W, Kaste M, Fieschi C, et al. Intravenous thrombolysis with recombinant tissue plasminogen activator for acute hemispheric stroke. The European Cooperative Acute Stroke Study (ECASS). JAMA 1995;274(13):1017–1025.

33. del Zoppo GJ, Sasahara AA. Interventional use of plasminogen activators in central nervous system diseases. Med Clin North Am 1998;82(3):545–568.

34. Qureshi AI, Ali Z, Suri MF, et al. Intra-arterial third-generation recombinant tissue plasminogen activator (reteplase) for acute ischemic stroke. Neurosurgery 2001;49(1):41–48.

35. Arnold M, Schroth G, Nedeltchev K, et al. Intra-arterial thrombolysis in 100 patients with acute stroke due to middle cerebral artery occlusion. Stroke 2002;33(7):1828–1833.

36. Thrombolytic therapy with streptokinase in acute ischemic stroke. The Multicenter Acute Stroke Trial – Europe Study Group. N Engl J Med 1996;335(3):145–150.
37. Figueroa BE, Keep RF, Betz AL, Hoff JT. Plasminogen activators potentiate thrombin-induced brain injury. Stroke 1998;29(6):1202–1207.
38. Yokogami K, Nakano S, Ohta H, Goya T, Wakisaka S. Prediction of hemorrhagic complications after thrombolytic therapy for middle cerebral artery occlusion: value of pre- and post-therapeutic computed tomographic findings and angiographic occlusive site. Neurosurgery 1996;39(6): 1102–1107.
39. Collet J, Montalescot G, Lesty C, et al. Disaggregation of in vitro preformed platelet-rich clots by abciximab increases fibrin exposure and promotes fibrinolysis. Arterioscler Thromb Vasc Biol 2001;21:142–148.
40. Sacco RL, Kargman DE, Gu Q, Zamanillo MC. Race-ethnicity and determinants of intracranial atherosclerotic cerebral infarction. The Northern Manhattan Stroke Study. Stroke 1995; 26(1):14–20.
41. Ringer AJ, Qureshi AI, Fessler RD, Guterman LR, Hopkins LN. Angioplasty of intracranial occlusion resistant to thrombolysis in acute ischemic stroke. Neurosurgery 2001;48(6):1282–1288.
42. Nakano S, Iseda T, Yoneyama T, Kawano H, Wakisaka S. Direct percutaneous transluminal angioplasty for acute middle cerebral artery trunk occlusion: an alternative option to intra-arterial thrombolysis. Stroke 2002;33(12):2872–2876.
43. Qureshi AI, Siddiqui AM, Suri MF et al. Aggressive mechanical clot disruption and low-dose intra-arterial third-generation thrombolytic agent for ischemic stroke: a prospective study. Neurosurgery 2002; 51(5):1319–1327.
44. Li SM, Miao ZR, Zhu FS, et al. Combined intraarterial thrombolysis and intra-cerebral stent for acute ischemic stroke institute of brain vascular diseases. Zhonghua Yi Xue Za Zhi 2003; 83(1):9–12.
45. Wikholm G. Mechanical intracranial embolectomy: a report of two cases. Interventional Neuroradiology 1998;4:159–164.
46. Chopko BW, Kerber C, Wong W, Grorgy B. Transcatheter snare removal of acute middle cerebral artery thromboembolism: technical case report. Neurosurgery 2000; 46(6):1529–1531.
47. Abou-Chebl A, Krieger DW, Bajzer CT, Yadav JS. Intracranial angioplasty and stenting in the awake patient. J Neuroimaging 2006;16(3):216–223.
48. Adams HP, Jr., Brott TG, Crowell RM, et al. Guidelines for the management of patients with acute ischemic stroke. A statement for healthcare professionals from a special writing group of the Stroke Council, American Heart Association. Circulation 1994;90(3):1588–1601.
49. Abou-Chebl A, Reginelli J, Bajzer CT, Yadav JS. Intensive treatment of hypertension decreases the risk of hyperperfusion and intracerebral hemorrhage following carotid artery stenting. Catheter Cardiovasc Interv 2007; 69(5):690–696.

V

COMPLICATIONS AND POST-PROCEDURAL MONITORING

14 Complications Related to Carotid Stenting

Peter Ruchin, MD
and Jacqueline Saw, MD, FRCPC

CONTENTS

ABSTRACT

Complications associated with angioplasty and stenting of the carotid arteries have dramatically decreased over the past two decades. Experienced operators in high-volume centers can now safely perform carotid stenting with an acceptably low rate of complications, both neurological and cardiovascular. There remain high-risk patient subsets where further efforts to lower the rate of adverse events is required.

Keywords: Complications; Ischemia; Embolization; No reflow; Stroke; Transient ischemic attack; Hyperperfusion; Restenosis

INTRODUCTION

Carotid artery angioplasty and carotid artery stenting (CAS) were first performed in 1981 and 1989, respectively. From the early balloon angioplasty studies to the modern day use of stents, embolic protection devices (EPD), and antiplatelet regimens, the rate of complications has progressively decreased. Since its inception, the theoretical benefits of CAS have been in limiting complications over the

From: *Contemporary Cardiology: Carotid Artery Stenting: The Basics*
Edited by: J. Saw, DOI 10.1007/978-1-60327-314-5_14,
© Humana Press, a part of Springer Science+Business Media, LLC 2009

traditional, more invasive surgical revascularization. Thus, not only should CAS be successful in preventing the occurrence of future neurological events, it should do so with fewer peri-procedural complications than carotid endarterectomy (CEA). Yet, despite significant advances, there continue to be adverse events due to the unforgiving nature of the neurological vasculature. Hence, it is safe to say that the minimization of complications is the most important aspect of mechanical treatment of carotid disease and is essential before operators can offer this percutaneous method for routine management of carotid artery stenosis.

FACTORS AFFECTING COMPLICATION RATES OF CAROTID REVASCULARIZATION

The natural history of carotid artery stenosis varies depending on the symptomatic status of the individual and, to a lesser extent, on the degree of stenosis in the vessel. Therefore, when looking at the overall incidence of complications, it is important that we divide patients into symptomatic and asymptomatic groups. In the two largest trials looking at the surgical treatment of asymptomatic patients with a carotid stenosis of $\geq 60\%$, the event rate in the medical management arm at 5 years was an aggregate risk of ipsilateral stroke and any stroke or death of 11% in the Asymptomatic Carotid Artery Endarterectomy trial (ACAS) and 11.8% in the Asymptomatic Carotid Surgery Trial (ACST) *(1, 2)*. It is important to note that in these trials, events such as myocardial infarction (MI) were not included in the cumulative end point. In the symptomatic population from the North American Symptomatic Carotid Endarterectomy Trial (NASCET), the 5-year risk increased significantly with an ipsilateral stroke rate in the medically managed arm of 22.2% in those with a 50–69% carotid stenosis, and 26% in those with a 70–99% carotid stenosis. What is not reflected in these figures is that although there was significant benefit in the prevention of stroke from carotid surgery, there was an increased risk of surgical complications such as MI, especially in patients with a history of angina, MI, or hypertension. Furthermore, complications such as cranial nerve palsy (7.6%), wound hematoma (5.5%), and wound infection (3.4%) were not infrequent *(3)*. From this surgical data it was deduced that the benefits of carotid revascularization were lost if the 30-day rate of stroke or death exceeded 6% for symptomatic patients and 3% for those who were asymptomatic. These figures have formed the basis for the American Heart Association/Society of Vascular Surgery guidelines *(4)*.

These trials have shown that the greater the stenosis and, more importantly, the presence of symptoms, the greater the increase in future neurological events by over 200%. Similarly when looking at the meta-analysis of CAS by Wholey et al., we see that this relationship extends to the rate of complications post-CAS in these different populations *(5)*. In this review of 11,243 patients who underwent 12,392 CAS procedures, the 30-day risk of stroke or death was 4.94% in the symptomatic population and 2.95% in the asymptomatic population, translating to 1.7-fold higher risk in the symptomatic group. Similarly, in a more recent comparison of symptomatic versus asymptomatic patients undergoing CAS by Kastrup et al., the rate of 30-day death or stroke was over three times greater in the symptomatic patients (9.4 versus 3.1%) *(6)*.

In a recent review by Roubin et al., increased peri-procedural CAS risk was determined by several medical, anatomic, and procedural characteristics. Age over 80 years was judged to significantly increase the risk of peri-procedural events, possibly due to the lack of cerebrovascular reserve required to protect against microscopic distal embolization. Decreased cerebral reserve was considered more likely to be present in patients with prior stroke or multiple lacunar infarcts, intracranial microangiopathy, or dementia (presumably due to prior vascular events). Angiographically, lesions with excessive tortuosity, defined as two or more 90° bends within 5 cm of the lesion, or heavy concentric calcification (≥3 cm in width) were also thought to increase the risk of CAS *(7)*.

OVERALL COMPLICATION RATES

The complications of carotid artery catheterization and stenting range from minor bruising at the vascular access site to major stroke and death. Their prevalence varies depending on technical aspects of the procedure and patient-specific risk factors. Table 1 summarizes the potential complications and approximate prevalence associated with CAS in the modern era.

Prevalence of Major Complications (Death, Stroke, and MI)

Major studies of CEA and CAS have emphasized the prevalence of the most disabling adverse sequelae, namely death and stroke. The prevalence of peri-procedural MI is also reported in the majority of CAS trials, since this is a major adverse event and is associated with higher-risk populations and prognosticates worse cardiovascular outcomes *(8)*.

In the early developmental stages of CAS, the complication rate of strokes was high, attributable to the learning curve of mastering the percutaneous technique and the lack of EPD use. In the angioplasty-alone era, rates of peri-procedural stroke were found to be as high as 12% *(9)*. Not surprisingly, this was highest in patients who were symptomatic. The early Carotid and Vertebral Artery Transluminal Angioplasty Study (CAVATAS), which randomized symptomatic and asymptomatic patients to carotid angioplasty (only 26% had stent use, and embolic

Table 1
Estimated Complication Rates of Carotid Stenting in the Modern Era
in Experienced Centers

Complications	*Estimated prevalence (%)*
Death (30 day)	0.5–2
Major stroke (30 day)	0.5–2
Minor stroke (30 day)	1–3
Transient ischemic attack	1–3
Death or stroke (30 day)	2–5
Myocardial infarction (30 day)	0–2
Retinal embolization	1–2
Slow flow	10
Prolonged bradycardia and/or hypotension	20–30
Hyperperfusion syndrome	1
Intracranial hemorrhage	<1
Acute stent thrombosis	<1
In-stent restenosis	<5
Vascular access complications	1–3.1

protection was not utilized) versus CEA, showed comparable 30-day rate of disabling stroke or death of 6%, and a 30-day any stroke or death rate of 10% in both groups *(10)*. These figures were much higher than the ideal rate of $\leq 6\%$ for symptomatic patients and $\leq 3\%$ for asymptomatic patients.

Along with the development of self-expanding carotid stents came the use of EPD. Early trials and registries showed that the rates of stroke with CAS were higher when EPD were not utilized, especially in high-risk patient subsets such as the elderly *(11)*. In a meta-analysis by Kastrup et al., they compared 40 single-center studies of CAS without EPD and 14 studies of CAS with EPD. They found a much higher 30-day death or stroke rate of 5.5% in those undergoing CAS without EPD, compared to 1.8% in those who underwent CAS with EPD *(12)*. These two groups were well matched for risk factors, although it could be argued that most studies where EPD were not used were older studies that employed no stents or balloon-expandable stents and utilized less contemporary anticoagulation and antiplatelet regimens. However, similar conclusions were drawn from a more contemporary study, the Endarterectomy versus Angioplasty in Patients with Symptomatic Severe Carotid Stenosis (EVA-3S) trial, where the 30-day stroke rate was 26.7% without EPD versus 8.6% with EPD. This led to early termination of the non-EPD arm of CAS by the study's safety committee *(13)*. Overall, these studies supported the use of EPD as an essential component of CAS to prevent peri-procedural strokes.

In the Stenting and Angioplasty with Protection in Patients at High Risk for Endarterectomy (SAPPHIRE) trial of CAS with EPD versus CEA in high-risk patients, the 30-day death, stroke, or MI rate was 4.4% with CAS and 9.9% with CEA. This advantage held out to 1 year with rates of 12.0 versus 20.1%, respectively. Importantly, when divided into individual events, the rates in the actual treatment arm at 30 days and 1 year were stroke 3.1% CAS and 5.8% CEA, death 0.6% CAS and 7% CEA, and MI 1.9% CAS and 2.5% CEA *(8)*. These figures highlight the high-risk nature of this population, from both a neurologic and cardiac perspective.

More recent registry data using contemporary techniques have also added to the morbidity and mortality figures associated with CAS. In the Carotid Revascularization Endarterectomy Versus Stenting Trial (CREST) lead-in study, which included 749 patients (symptomatic with $\geq 50\%$ stenosis or asymptomatic with $\geq 70\%$ stenosis), the stroke and death rate at 30 days was 4.4% for symptomatic patients and 0.8% for asymptomatic patients *(14)*. The Acculink for Revascularization of Carotids in High-Risk Patients (ARCHeR) study assessed 581 patients at high risk for CEA (80% with high-risk surgical or medical comorbidities and 15% octogenarians) and found higher rates of major peri-procedural events. The 30-day stroke or death rate was 6.9%, with a composite stroke, death, or MI rate at 1 year of 8.3% *(15)*. The high-risk nature of subjects was highlighted by the 30-day death rate of 2.1% compared to the usual range of 0.5–0.8% in most other CAS trials *(8, 14, 16–18)*. A similar 30-day mortality rate of 1.9% was seen in the Carotid Revascularization with ev3 Arterial Technology Evolution (CREATE) registry, which also recruited a high-risk patient cohort *(19)*. The European Pro-CAS registry for CAS enrolled 3,267 patients and found a 30-day combined rate of death and permanent neurologic deficit of 2.8% and a 30-day death and any stroke rate of 4.2% *(17)*.

The recently published Carotid ACCULINK/ACCUNET Post-Approval Trial to Uncover Unanticipated or Rare Events (CAPTURE) registry is a prospective, multicenter registry of 3,500 patients, which was designed to assess outcomes of CAS in the "real-world" practice using the RX Acculink™ self-expanding nitinol stent and the RX Accunet™ (Abbott Vascular, IL) EPD system. It represents the largest, neurologically audited, independently adjudicated database of high surgical risk CAS in the United States to date. The 30-day rate of major stroke or death was 2.9% with a 30-day rate of death, stroke, and MI of 6.3%. The patient population included 14% symptomatic patients who had suffered a stroke, transient ischemic attack (TIA), or amaurosis fugax within the preceding 180 days. Again it was found that there were comparatively more events in the symptomatic patients and in octogenarians *(20)*.

Octogenarians constitute a high-risk group with regard to major complications following carotid revascularization. In a subset analysis of the CREST lead-in phase, being 80 years of age or older was associated with a statistically significant higher rate of peri-procedural stroke and death. In fact, there was a trend to increased mortality, but the main difference was a 12.1% rate of stroke at 30 days compared to 4.0% for non-octogenarians ($p<0.0001$) *(14)*. In another albeit retrospective analysis of 75 patients $\geq$80 years of age (56% symptomatic, 44% asymptomatic), the rate of stroke was 10.7%, again higher than would be expected in a general cohort of patients undergoing CAS *(12)*. This trend of increasing risk with age is not unique to CAS; in fact, a similar pattern of increasing mortality was seen in patients undergoing CEA, alluding to confounding comorbidities that accompany age *(21)*.

In summary, the rates of peri-procedural stroke, death, and MI with modern day pharmacotherapy and EPD use is acceptably low with rates of 30-day death between 0.6 and 2.1%, major stroke 0.6–4.01% and MI 0–2.4% depending on the underlying risk of the patient subset (Table 2). There are patients in which the risks are elevated and early identification can aid both accurate informed consent and management. Just as important is the operator's experience and technical knowledge, in order to reduce peri-procedural event rates and expedite appropriate management of any complications.

PROCEDURAL COMPLICATIONS

Complications following CAS can be grouped into procedural and post-procedural events (Table 3). Procedural events include the categories of complications related to vascular access, distal embolization of atherosclerotic debris on cannulation of the common carotid artery, and complications arising from the crossing and stenting of the culprit lesion.

Vascular Access Complications

Vascular access complications include bleeding, infection, retroperitoneal bleeding, femoral artery pseudoaneurysm, and dissection at the access point (usually a femoral arterial approach). While an in-depth description of access techniques is beyond the scope of this chapter, the risk of such complications lies to a great extent in the expertise of both the operator and staff involved in the management and removal of the arterial sheath. Appropriate femoral access at the level of the femoral head to allow adequate artery compression will significantly reduce any risks of

Table 2
Overview of Major Complications with Carotid Angioplasty and Stent in Major Trials and Registries

Study	EPD use	Symptom status	End points	Stroke major (%)	Stroke minor (%)	MI (%)	Death (%)	Combined end points (%)
CAVATAS (10) (2001), n=251 angioplasty	No EPD Only 26% had stents	96% Symp	30-day death or stroke	4	4	0	3	10
SAPPHIRE (8) (2004), n=159 stent	96% EPD	70% Asymp 30% Symp	30-day death, stroke, or MI	0.6	3.1	1.9	0.6	4.4
CREST (14) (2004), n=749 stent registry	88% EPD	69% Asymp 31% Symp	30-day death or stroke	Stroke-major and minor 4.01		NA	0.8	4.41
Pro-CAS (17) (2004), n=3,270 stent registry	72% EPD	44% Asymp 56% Symp	30-day death or stroke	1.2	1.3	NA	0.6	2.8
CABERNET (76) (2005), n=454 stent registry	96% EPD	76% Asymp 24% Symp	30-day death, stroke, or MI	1.3	2.1	0.2	0.5	3.9
ARCHeR (15) (2006), n=581 stent registry	95.5% EPD	76% Asymp 24% Symp	30-day death, stroke, or MI	1.5	4.0	2.4	2.1	8.3
EVA-3S (13) (2006), n=261 stent	92% EPD	100% Symp	30-day death or stroke	2.7	6.1	0.4	1.2	9.6
SPACE (16) (2006), n=599 stent arm	27% EPD	100% Symp	30-day death or ipsilateral stroke	4.01	3.5	NA	0.67	6.84
CREATE (19) (2006), n=419 stent registry	97.4% EPD	83% Asymp 17% Symp	30-day death, stroke, or MI	3.5	1.0	1.0	1.9	6.2
CAPTURE (20) (2007), n=3,500 stent registry	100% EPD (attempted)	86% Asymp 14% Symp	30-day death, stroke, or MI	2.0	2.9	0.9	1.8	6.3

Asymp = asymptomatic; Symp = symptomatic; MI = myocardial infarction.

Table 3
Complications Related to Carotid Artery Stenting

(A). Procedural complications
    (1) Vascular access complications
    (2) Ischemic embolization
        (a) Carotid artery access complications during guide or sheath placement
        (b) Complications with emboli protection devices
        (c) Embolization during pre-dilatation, stent placement, and post-dilatation
    (3) Slow flow, no reflow, and abrupt closure
    (4) Retinal embolization
    (5) Reflex bradycardia and hypotension
(B) Early post-procedural complications
    (1) Delirium
    (2) Cerebral hyperperfusion syndrome
    (3) Stent thrombosis
    (4) Distal embolization
    (5) Contrast-induced nephropathy
(C) Late post-procedural complications
    (1) Late distal embolization
    (2) Stent deformation
    (3) In-stent restenosis

both retroperitoneal bleed (and subsequent complications) or pseudoaneurysm. Vascular access complications in the main CAS trials have been recorded at between 1 and 3.1% *(8, 10, 15)*. There is, of course, a risk of retroperitoneal bleeding merely due to the anticoagulation used; however, this is low (<1%). Access site dissection requiring surgery and infection are quite rare with rates of <1% for each complication *(22)*. Careful monitoring of the ACT if heparin is the anticoagulant of choice, ensuring it remains between 250 and 299 s, can also help reduce the incidence of access site bleeding and bleeding complications overall when compared to levels of 300–350 s *(23)*.

Ischemic Embolization

Cannulation of the carotid system carries a risk of morbidity due to possible arterial dissection or, more commonly, distal embolization of atherosclerotic or thrombotic debris. Contralateral or posterior circulation stroke may occur due to catheter manipulation in the aortic arch, innominate and subclavian arteries. Fortunately the rates of such complications are low; however, they are more likely to occur in cases where there is significant tortuosity of the vasculature, a difficult aortic arch anatomy such as a type III arch or a bovine arch, and in cases with associated ostial common carotid disease. The presence of significant aortic arch atheroma (echocardiographic grades III and IV) predisposes to a higher risk of embolization of debris on catheter manipulation. For this reason, time of catheter manipulation in the arch should be minimized, and this can be achieved by careful selection of equipment after the aortic arch anatomy has been assessed. Choice of a reverse-curved catheter such as a Vitek (Cook Inc., Bloomington, IN) or Simmons (Terumo, Somerset, NJ) catheter can enable easier cannulation of vessels in a type

III aortic arch; however, the greater complexity and need of manipulation of these catheters in the aortic arch may increase the likelihood of cerebral emboli. Telescoping of a 5 Fr catheter through a larger guide or use of a sheath with its tapered dilator can both serve to reduce plaque dislodgement at the ostium or the proximal portion of the common carotid artery, allowing a smoother passage of equipment to the desired position *(24)*.

The combination of crossing of the lesion, pre-dilatation, stent deployment, and post-dilatation comprises the highest risk component of the CAS procedure. Since the advent of diagnostic carotid angiography it has been known that even injection of saline or contrast media produces microscopic air emboli *(25)*. More recently the use of both transcranial Doppler during CAS and diffusion-weighted magnetic resonance imaging (MRI) pre- and post-CAS has revealed the extent of micro- and macroscopic emboli during the procedure itself and its neurological imaging sequelae. A study by Ackerstaff et al. found that multiple microemboli (greater than five showers) were associated with neurological deficits post-procedure *(26)*. The different stages of CAS, sheath insertion, wire crossing, pre-dilatation, stent deployment, and post-dilatation, carry different risks of distal embolization. This was confirmed in a study comparing microembolic signals (MES) seen on transcranial Doppler (TCD) during CAS with and without EPD. In this study the highest risk stage by far was stent deployment which resulted in over two times the MES of pre-dilatation and nearly three times the MES as post-dilatation (Fig. 1). With the use of EPDs there was a statistically significant drop in MES in all three stages, to a degree comparable to the wiring stage *(27)*. This again highlights that the use of EPD should not be considered optional and that the risk of major complications in cases where one is not used is undoubtedly higher.

MRI has also given many insights into the occurrence of distal embolization and the subsequent neurological ramifications. In a study of over 200 patients, MRI diffusion-weighted images (DWI) were used to compare patients undergoing CAS

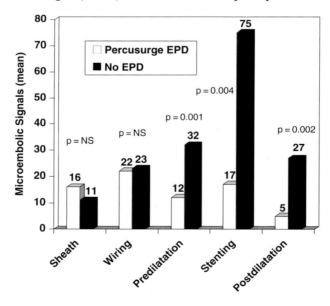

Fig. 1. Microembolic signals on transcranial Doppler at various stages of carotid stenting and the effect of embolic protection. Adapted from Al-Mubarak N. et al. *(27)*.

with and without EPD. There were significantly less DWI lesions on MRI when EPD were used. Although the majority of emboli were asymptomatic, the number of new MRI DWI lesions was significantly higher in patients who developed a peri-procedural stroke *(12)*. This and other indirect evidence has led to the general belief that the use of EPD is imperative in order to minimize the risk of peri-procedural stoke. Incredibly, distal embolization, enough to cause a detectable lesion on DWI, occurred in 67% of patients without an EPD and 49% of those patients where one was deployed. Clinically the occurrence of any stroke or death was 7.5% at 30 days in the group without protection and 4.3% in those with protection, highlighting the largely asymptomatic nature of small particle distal embolization. This corresponds to previous CEA trials that show distal particulate embolization to be nearly ubiquitous *(28)*. It is hoped that the new proximal embolic protection devices such as the Parodi (ArteriA, San Francisco, CA) and Mo.Ma (Invatec, Roncadelle, Italy) systems where a stagnant column of blood is formed and then aspirated along with debris will further reduce microscopic distal embolization *(29, 30)*. Furthermore, in a prospective look at 24 patients undergoing CEA and 20 undergoing CAS with pre- and post-MRI DWI, the investigators found a significantly lower rate of new lesions, albeit asymptomatic, after CEA. However, EPD were not used in this study and the carotid lesion was mostly crossed with a 0.038″ or 0.035″ wire and not a 0.014″ coronary wire which is the current standard. This would have placed patients at increased risk of plaque dislodgement and distal propagation of debris *(31)*. In a larger review of CAS in 105 patients with 6 month follow-up, there were new DWI lesions in 21% of patients, with 3.1% also visible on T2-weighted images. These were neurologically silent and at 6 months, only 3.1% were still visible on MRI scanning. Only one patient (0.95%) was neurologically symptomatic at 6 month follow-up, leading the authors to conclude that the vast majority of MRI-detectable lesions post-procedure are not clinically significant, especially if only seen on DWI and not on T2-weighted images *(32)*. Almost identical results were found by Schluter et al., with 22.7% of patients found to have MRI DWI lesions post-procedure, but only one patient (2.3%) suffering a neurological deficit. Importantly, this was the only patient whose MRI changes did not resolve at follow-up *(33)*.

The concept of reducing peri-procedural events by direct stenting of the stenosis after deployment of the embolic protection device has also been investigated recently. In as yet unpublished data which was presented in abstract form, Montorsi et al. randomized 205 consecutive, unselected carotid stent cases to either pre-dilatation or direct stenting. There was no significant difference in terms of peri-procedural neurological events between the two groups and there were no crossovers from the direct stenting group. There was no difference in outcome between the two groups at 30 days, with no major strokes or death in either arm. Macroscopic debris was discovered significantly more frequently in the filters of the pre-dilatation versus the direct stenting arm (50 versus 36%). Not surprisingly, procedural time was significantly shorter in the direct stenting group. Although the sample size is relatively small, this may represent another technique to simplify the stenting process and maybe limit the occurrence of distal embolic propagation *(34)*.

Slow Flow/No Reflow/Abrupt Vessel Closure

Like in the coronary vasculature, CAS carries with it the risk of post-stenting slow flow, no reflow, and abrupt vessel closure. Possible causes of these problems include large amounts of plaque and/or thrombus embolizing distally, dissection of the distal vessel with luminal obstruction, filling of the EPD with debris occluding flow, and spasm of the distal vessel. The occurrence of these events has diminished by the near-universal use of carotid stents, as well as the avoidance of lesions with large thrombus burden. In addition, the preparation of patients from a pharmaco-logical standpoint with pretreatment of dual antiplatelet therapy, meticulous peri-procedural anticoagulation, and possibly the use of HMG Co-A reductase inhibitors (statins) may also minimize this risk. In a study looking at the routine use of EPD, spasm occurred in 4.2% and was reversed immediately by giving intra-arterial nitroglycerin. The same group noted a 7.9% slow flow rate due to filter obstruction, which resolved after filter retrieval. In this study of 753 patients there were 7 cases (0.9%) of non-occlusive distal dissection, all of which were treated successfully without neurological sequelae *(35)*.

A single center study by Casserly et al. prospectively identified a group of 42 patients who suffered the slow-flow phenomenon with the use of filter-type embolic protection devices and compared them to patients who did not. Slow flow was more common after post-dilatation (71.4%) and stent deployment (26.2%). Only 2.4% of patients developed slow flow after the initial balloon angioplasty. Those who developed this phenomenon were significantly older, more often had symptomatic carotid lesions, and were more likely to have suffered an anterior circulation TIA or stroke within the previous 6 months. With regard to the angiographic appearance of lesions, slow flow was more frequent with ulcerated lesions, larger diameter stents, and smaller post-dilatation balloons. Importantly, 9.5% of patients with slow flow suffered a stroke compared to 1.7% in the group who had normal flow, and 2.4% suffered an MI compared to 1.2%. This resulted in significantly decreased event-free survival on a Kaplan–Meier estimate despite restoration of flow with retrieval of the EPD. In an attempt to minimize the rates of neurological injury, the authors recommended aspiration of the stagnant flow with a catheter prior to retrieval of the EPD *(36)*.

With specific regard to abrupt vessel closure, this complication is now exceed-ingly rare and predominantly limited to the balloon angioplasty-only period. Its occurrence was most often associated with dissections at the site of dilatation and less commonly due to thrombosis or significant hypotension. With the near-universal use of dedicated carotid stents, modern day antiplatelet and antic-oagulation regimens, and close hemodynamic monitoring, the rates are now less than 1%.

In the modern era, the combined overall risk of such events is below 10%, and significant neurologic sequelae are infrequent. Appropriate and timely response to these events is required to help further lower the risk of complications. For instance, in the setting of no reflow or slow flow after carotid stent placement or post-dilatation, it is recommended that operators promptly aspirate the stagnant column of blood that is proximal to the deployed filter EPD. This can be achieved by using commercially available thrombectomy devices such as the Export® (Medtronic, Santa Rosa, CA) or Pronto™ (Vascular Solutions Inc., Minneapolis, MN) extrac-tion catheters or simply using a 5 Fr 125 cm multipurpose catheter. Figure 2 shows an example of aspirated debris from a full filter. Following aspiration, the filter EPD should be promptly retrieved and final intracranial angiography taken to assess for any distal cerebral embolization.

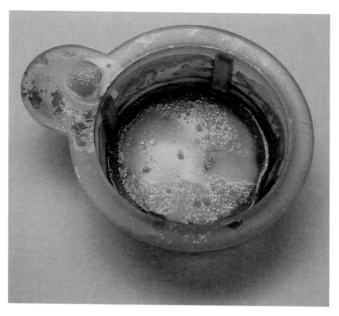

Fig. 2. Debris obtained from aspirating the stagnant column of blood during a slow flow case after carotid stent deployment and post-dilatation.

Retinal Artery Embolization

The arterial supply of the retina is via the central retinal artery or its branches which originate from the ophthalmic artery, off the internal carotid artery. There is often a collateral arterial supply, both intra- and extracerebrally, via the vertebral arteries or external carotid artery branches in the orbit. Carotid artery disease, especially disease of the internal carotid artery, may lead to episodes of transient monocular blindness known as amaurosis fugax *(37)*. Retinal embolization during CAS can thus be caused by showering of emboli or atherosclerotic debris via the internal carotid and ophthalmic arteries or via the external carotid artery and its collateral network. The latter event has been highlighted with the use of the Theron embolic protection system where routine flushing toward the external carotid artery with balloon occlusion of the distal internal carotid artery is performed. In one series, 13.2% of patients suffered a retinal event compared to 1.3% of the patients with the Percusurge® (Medtronic, Minneapolis, MN) system where there was no flushing of debris to the external carotid system *(38)*. Newer proximal protection devices such as the Mo.Ma system may predispose to this risk if debris is not well aspirated. This is because the occlusion balloon in the external carotid is routinely deflated first, allowing flushing of any residual debris to the lower risk territory. However, with regular aspiration of the column of blood and debris, such a risk should theoretically be much lower than the Theron and possibly the Percusurge® systems.

The occurrence of retinal emboli with filter EPD is largely unknown, but appears to be relatively infrequent. In cases of slow flow due to basket filling with debris or thrombus, it is conceivable that larger particles may pass and thus increase the risk of embolization to the retina via the internal carotid and ophthalmic arteries. As suggested previously, thorough aspiration of material prior to basket retrieval is recommended in this scenario in an endeavor to reduce the risk of distal propagation of embolic debris *(36)*.

Fortunately, less than half of the retinal embolic events are symptomatic and amongst these, many are only transient. When a significant retinal embolus is suspected, urgent ophthalmological review is mandatory in an attempt to dislodge or dissolve (in the case of thrombus) the embolus. Methods include ocular massage, decreasing intra-ocular pressure pharmacologically with acetazolamide or mechanically with an anterior chamber paracentesis, hyperbaric oxygen or the use of intravenous heparin or thrombolytics to lyse thrombus *(39)*. Of course, the use of anticoagulants and thrombolysis must be weighed against the risks of bleeding, especially considering that patients are already on dual antiplatelet therapy.

Reflex Bradycardia and Hypotension

One of the most important hemodynamic consequences of CAS involves significant bradycardia and hypotension which often accompanies balloon dilatation of the carotid bulb. Carotid angioplasty almost always stimulates the carotid baroreceptors, which via vagal stimulus results in bradycardia and reduced cardiac inotropy (Fig. 3). This cascade of events is mediated via stimulation of the nerve

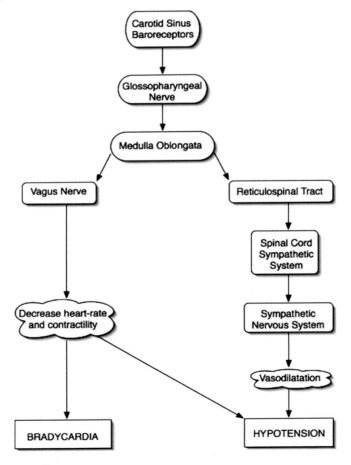

Fig. 3. Baroreceptor reflex.

of Herring, a branch of the glossopharyngeal nerve which serves as the afferent arc of the reflex to the nucleus tractus solitarius in the caudal medulla oblongata. The efferent arc comprises vagally induced decreased inotropy and chronotropy as well as inhibition of the reticulo-spinal tract, which via a cascade of negative inhibition of the sympathetic nervous system leads to vasodilatation and hypotension *(37)*. Significant bradycardia is very common with carotid balloon dilatation and occurred in 71% of patients in a study of 107 patients undergoing CAS *(40)*. These episodes were short-lived and there was only one case where a permanent pacemaker was required several days later. Due to this high prevalence, some interventionalists advocate routinely administering prophylactic atropine (0.6–1 mg) prior to carotid bulb dilatation.

Of more clinical importance is the development of sustained hypotension, which can last up to 48 h post-procedure. Qureshi et al. found that prolonged hypotension occurred in 22.4% of patients and lasted a mean of 25.7 h (range 18–43). They also found prolonged bradycardia in 27.5% of patients. Prolonged post-procedural hypotension was more common in patients who developed intra-procedural hypotension and bradycardia *(41)*. Usually, as with bradycardia, hypotension is short-lived and resolves spontaneously or with small bolus of intravenous saline or small doses of intravenous peripherally acting vasoconstrictors such as phenylephrine, metaraminol, norepinephrine, or dopamine. It is important to note that although infusion of intravenous fluid may help initially, sustained hypotension may be resistant to fluid resuscitation, and aggressive intravenous therapy may precipitate pulmonary edema in patients with a history of congestive heart failure or significant diastolic dysfunction. Patients with sustained hypotension can usually be treated with regular oral pseudoephedrine 30–60 mg q4 hourly prn or low-dose peripheral vasoconstrictor infusions. The aim should be to keep the systolic blood pressure between 90 and 140 mmHg, depending on the patient's pre-procedural blood pressure, to ensure adequate cerebral perfusion pressure and minimize the risk of stent thrombosis.

POST-PROCEDURAL COMPLICATIONS

Delirium

Delirium in the elderly patient is a common event, especially in the setting of hospitalization *(42)*. Post-CAS, there are numerous potential mechanisms including cerebral hypoperfusion (due to carotid baroreceptor-induced systemic hypotension), the cerebral hyperperfusion syndrome, and drug-induced confusion. Some operators routinely give sedatives prior to CAS, whereas others abstain entirely from sedation peri-procedurally to allow prompt monitoring for acute neurologic changes. Atropine is routinely administered in many centers prior to carotid bulb angioplasty and/or post-dilatation or may be given if there is significant bradycardia with pre- or post-dilatation *(43)*. Atropine is an anticholinergic agent which can lead to anxiety, agitation, confusion, hallucination, dysarthria, delirium, paranoia, and psychosis and even coma or seizures. Signs of an anticholinergic reaction include cutaneous vasodilatation, anhidrosis, and subsequent hyperthermia and a non-reactive mydriasis due to inhibition of pupillary constriction and accommodation resulting in blurred vision. Usually treatment is conservative and supportive. Sedation with benzodiazepines is only used as a last resort, so as not to mask an underlying neurological event. Sedatives such as phenothiazines and butyrophenones should never be used to treat atropine-induced confusion or psychosis as they are themselves anticholinergic. The pharmacological antidote for anticholinergic overdose is the acetylcholinesterase inhibitor physostigmine; however, its use should be only for extreme cases and in conjunction with a toxicologist and neurologist *(44)*.

The Hyperperfusion Syndrome

Successful carotid revascularization may be complicated by the hyperperfusion syndrome, which can manifest as ipsilateral headaches, vomiting, confusion, ipsilateral focal seizures, and hemorrhage. Fortunately this is an infrequent complication, occurring in 1.1% of 450 consecutive cases of CAS in one retrospective database *(45)*. In this particular group, the event occurred at a median time of 10 h post-stenting with a range of 6 h–4 days. In the limited data available on this event, specific risk factors for the syndrome appear to be a high-severity lesion (mean stenosis >95%), a significant contralateral lesion (>80%) or occlusion of the contralateral artery, and the presence of hypertension pre-procedure. Also of note was the fact that patients who went on to develop an intracerebral bleed were found to have a hypertensive (>180 mmHg systolic) period which preceded the bleed. The rate of intracerebral hemorrhage (ICH) in this group was 0.67% with two of the three cases of bleeding proving fatal. In this retrospective review, the presence of hypertension, a contralateral stenotic lesion of >80%, and an ipsilateral stenotic lesion >90% gave a 16% risk of post-CAS hyperperfusion syndrome. It is interesting to note that the incidence of hyperperfusion syndrome is not limited to CAS. CEA trials have shown rates between 0.75 and 3% with a hyperperfusion-related ICH rate of 0.3–1.2% *(46–50)*.

Mortality following hyperperfusion-related ICH is 37–80% in CEA trials and is likely similar after CAS due to the similarity in the underlying physiological process *(47, 49)*. Possible preventative strategies include the use of antihypertensive agents in patients with elevated BP post-procedure, using TCD to monitor middle cerebral artery velocities, and withholding antiplatelet agents until BP control is satisfactory *(45)*. These methods have not been proven in randomized trials; however, their implementation is based on biologic plausibility.

Stent Thrombosis

As is the case with coronary artery stenting, the abrupt thrombosis of a carotid stent is disastrous and usually results in severe morbidity or mortality. Its occurrence has not been widely studied, but several smaller studies quoted risks between 0.5 and 2% depending on the criteria used *(51, 52)*. What is apparent with the limited data available is that there appears to be a common thread, namely cessation of one or both antiplatelet agents as a precipitating event. Buhk et al. reported on three cases occurring after 1 week, but before 3 months post-procedure, where aspirin and clopidogrel were ceased because of a concomitant medical problem (two cases of cancer and a case of deep venous thrombosis requiring warfarin). These cases highlight the need for dual antiplatelet therapy as well as the importance of good communication between treating physicians. In none of these cases was the neurointerventionalist consulted before the cessation of the antiplatelet agents *(53)*. Another case report of two patients who had not received any antiplatelet therapy before or after stenting and who died following carotid stent thrombosis further highlights this point *(54)*. This emphasizes a clear failure of appropriate peri-procedural pharmacotherapy and once again suggests that much of the risk of carotid artery stent thrombosis is preventable. Dual antiplatelet therapy with aspirin and clopidogrel for at least 30 days and then aspirin indefinitely as per the 2007 ACCF/SCAI/SVMB/SIR/ASITN Clinical Expert Consensus on Carotid Stenting is mandatory and patients must be informed as to the critical nature of this therapy *(55)*. Family physicians and other medical specialists closely involved with the patient's acute care should also be informed as to the importance and the duration of dual antiplatelet therapy.

Late Distal Embolization

The CAPTURE registry reviewed the timing of post-procedural strokes, both major and minor, after CAS. Interestingly it was found that only 22% of strokes occurred during the procedure itself. More importantly, 38% occurred beyond 24 h after the stent procedure *(56)*. The cause of these events is debatable; however, the most likely culprit is distal embolization of atherosclerotic material protruding through the stent struts, the so-called cheesegrater effect. As in the CAPTURE registry these late events usually manifest as a TIA or minor stroke with a major stroke being much less common. It is also important to note that rarely is any specific therapy required other than continuing the patient's current dual antiplate-let therapy and usual cardiovascular medications *(20)*. The sudden onset of a severe neurological deficit, however, should prompt urgent investigation including a CT scan to exclude a hemorrhagic event and possibly angiographic investigation with a view to mechanical intervention. Other, rarer causes of late distal embolization include disruption of aortic atheromatous plaque or thrombus with late dehiscence secondary to pulsatile aortic flow.

Restenosis

In-stent restenosis (ISR) in the carotid arteries has been defined as stenosis of ≥50% inside or within 5 mm of a previously implanted carotid stent. Fortuitously, this event is less common in the carotid arteries than in the coronary or the peripheral circulation. The rates of carotid stent ISR vary between 2.7 and 6% *(40, 57–60)*. A review of 34 trials showed an ISR rate of 6% at 1 year, which is lower than that expected with CEA. CEA restenosis has been shown to be >10%; for example, it was 14% in the CAVATAS trial (against 4% in the CAS arm) when routine carotid Doppler ultrasound (US) was performed *(8, 10, 61)*. Similarly, the SAPPHIRE trial showed an increased restenosis rate of 4.6% in the CEA group versus 0.7% in the CAS group when symptomatic target vessel revascularization (TVR) was the end point at 1 year in the actual treatment analysis. Even in the early CAS period with use of balloon-expandable stents, the rates of restenosis at 6 months follow-up was <5% *(62)*. Other early CAS experience showed only 1 case of flow-limiting ISR in a sample size of 110 patients at 7 month follow-up when patients were routinely screened with carotid US *(52)*. In an Austrian study of 279 patients followed over 45 months, ISR was defined using a cutoff of ≥70% by carotid US and confirmed by carotid angiography. Over a median 12 month follow-up period there were nine cases (3%) of ISR, six occurring late (>30 days) of which three were located at the distal edge of the stent at the kinking of the ICA, and were diagnosed within 30 days. These restenosis events were all treated successfully by repeat stenting *(63)*.

In a recent publication looking at predictors of restenosis in a single center study of 399 procedures with a mean follow-up of 24 months, there were 15 cases of ISR (3.8%). Restenosis was most often asymptomatic and was diagnosed with carotid US. The treatment was restenting, angioplasty alone, or medical management (four patients). The only two predictors of ISR were previous CEA and a prior history of neck radiotherapy *(64)*. The treatment of CAS ISR is generally lower risk than treatment of de novo carotid stenosis, due to the lower embolic risk from the fibrotic restenotic lesions.

The diagnosis of ISR non-invasively after CAS is potentially a challenge with pitfalls when using carotid US. The most plausible mechanism for this difficulty is a change in vessel compliance by the stent, which either changes the blood flow velocity or the Doppler signal. From initial experience, Robbin et al. found that standard US velocity criteria would significantly overestimate the degree of ISR in carotid arteries *(65)*. Another group reviewed patients post-CAS and determined that a more accurate method of assessing significant ISR was an increase in peak systolic velocity (PSV) of at least 100% over baseline. This required a baseline procedure to be performed soon after stenting. However, the results varied and even using a $\geq$80% increase in internal carotid artery to common carotid artery velocity ratio (ICA:CCA) did not produce a reliable method of diagnosing ISR in previously stented carotid arteries. These parameters could, however, guide one into a more judicious use of invasive investigations and thereby avoid a proportion of unnecessary repeat carotid angiography *(66)*.

More recently a study by Stanziale et al. looked at 118 patients who had paired carotid US and angiography. The group set out new parameters to determine restenosis which included a PSV of $\geq$225 cm/s rather than the cutoff of 125 cm/s (for non-stented carotid arteries) to diagnose stenosis of $\geq$50%. To improve the sensitivity and specificity of this test, it is best combined with the ICA:CCA velocity ratio of $\geq$2.5 which gives a sensitivity of 95%, a specificity of 99%, a positive predictive value (PPV) of 95%, and, more importantly, a negative predictive value (NPV) of 99%. With restenotic lesions $\geq$70% in stenosis, a PSV $\geq$350 cm/s (rather than a PSV of $\geq$250 cm/s in non-stented carotid arteries) gives 100% sensitivity, 96% specificity, a 55% PPV, and a 100% NPV *(67)* (see Table 4).

Contrast-Induced Nephropathy

Contrast-induced nephropathy (CIN) represents a potentially preventable iatrogenic complication which accounts for 12% of hospital-acquired acute renal failure *(68)*. There are numerous factors which predispose patients to this complication, including underling renal dysfunction, diabetes, concomitant use of nephrotoxic agents, hydration state of the patient, amount of contrast agent administered, and the type of agent used. CIN correlates with increased morbidity and mortality of patients and increases length of hospitalization. Its occurrence is also relatively common with rates up to 50% in patients with underlying severe renal dysfunction and diabetes who undergo coronary angiography *(68–72)*.

In order to prevent the occurrence of CIN, patients at increased risk should be pre-hydrated with intravenous normal saline (1 L over 12 h) or sodium bicarbonate

Table 4
Carotid US Criteria for Non-invasive Diagnosis of Carotid In-Stent Restenosis

	Sensitivity for stenosis ≥50% (%)	Specificity for stenosis ≥ 50% (%)	Positive predictive value (%)	Negative predictive value (%)
PSV ≥225 cm/s	90	97	86	98
PSV ≥225 cm/s and ICA/CCA ≥2.5	95	99	95	99
PSV ≥225 cm/s and ICA/CCA ≥4.75	100	95	50	100

	Sensitivity for stenosis ≥ 70% (%)	Specificity for stenosis ≥ 70% (%)	Positive predictive value (%)	Negative predictive value (%)
PSV ≥350 cm/s	100	96	55	100
ICA/CCA ≥4.75	100	92	50	100

Adapted from Stanziale SF et al. (67).
PSV = Peak systolic velocity; ICA/CCA = Internal carotid artery to common carotid artery velocity ratio.

(150 mEq in 850 mL of 5% Dextrose at 3 mL/kg/h to a maximum of 330 mL/h for 1 h pre-procedure and 6 h post) *(66, 68–70)*. Antihypertensive medications, especially angiotensin-converting enzyme inhibitors (ACEIs) or angiotensin receptor blockers (ARBs), should be withheld at least the day of the procedure (preferably 24 h for ACEIs and ARBs) if the blood pressure allows this. Other nephrotoxic agents such as non-steroidal anti-inflammatory drugs (NSAIDs) should be withheld for 24 h pre- and at least 48 h post-procedure if possible. Although contentious, the use of *N*-acetyl cysteine (NAC) 600 mg bid two doses pre- and post-procedure carries little risk to the patient and should be considered.

The type of contrast agent used is also important in the prevention of CIN. The use of high-osmolar agents has been universally accepted to increase the risk of CIN. However, there is ongoing debate regarding whether iso-osmolar contrast agents are superior to low osmolar agents. The most important single factor by far with regard to contrast use is the amount administered. Minimizing the use of contrast by limiting to essential cineangiographic views, diluting contrast with heparinized saline, and the use of road map techniques can all be helpful. In cases of severe renal impairment, staging of diagnostic and interventional procedures with an interval of at least 72 h may also aid in the reduction of renal function deterioration *(72)*.

Hypotension in the peri-procedural period may add to the risk of CIN and is a particular problem with CAS. Due to the increased frequency of hypotension with carotid bulb dilatation, prophylactic atropine should be given to minimize this hemodynamic change. Close blood pressure monitoring and management of hypotension is thus essential in the peri-procedural period.

Finally, it is important that the occurrence of CIN in the at-risk population is properly assessed. The peak serum creatinine level with CIN is seen at 48–72 h post-procedure. In fact, creatinine is often artificially decreased the day after the procedure, mainly due to volume hydration. All too often is this mistaken as a sign that CIN has not occurred, only to then miss the true creatinine peak in a further 24–48 h. Although this should not delay patient discharge from hospital, creatinine levels should be repeated at an outpatient laboratory at 72 h post-procedure.

Stent Deformity

The risk of late stent deformation now appears only to be historical. In the early period of CAS, there were concerns regarding the use of the balloon-expandable Palmaz® stent and its predisposition to late deformation and compression. An early review of 70 patients who underwent CAS with a Palmaz® stent and who returned for repeat angiography showed that 11 of 70 (16%) had suffered stent collapse or deformity *(73)*. Importantly, only a small proportion of these could be detected on ultrasound. In a prospective review of patients undergoing CAS, of the 71 (66%) who returned for repeat angiography there were 8 cases of Palmaz® stent deformity, 2 were considered severe *(40)*. In a group of early studies, the rates of stent deformation ranged from 0 to 16% *(73–75)*. Due to these results, the use of balloon-expandable stents in the carotid arteries has been abandoned in favor of self-expanding stents.

CONCLUSION

In conclusion, the complications associated with angioplasty and stenting of the carotid arteries have been greatly reduced over the past two decades *(76, 77)*. Experienced operators in high-volume centers can now safely perform carotid stenting with an acceptably low rate of complications, both neurological and cardiovascular. There remain high-risk patient subsets where further efforts to lower the rate of adverse events is required. With continued advances in equipment, neurovascular protection, and pharmacotherapy, one can anticipate carotid artery stenting complications to further decrease in the future.

REFERENCES

1. Executive committee for Asymptomatic Carotid Atherosclerosis Study. Endarterectomy for asymptomatic carotid artery stenosis. JAMA 1995;273:1421–1428.
2. Halliday A, Mansfield A, Marro J, Peto C, Peto R, Potter J, Thomas D. MRC Asymptomatic Carotid Surgery Trial (ACST) Collaborative Group. Prevention of disabling and fatal strokes by successful carotid endarterectomy in patients without recent neurological symptoms: randomised controlled trial. Lancet 2004;363(9420):1491–1502.
3. NASCET Collaborators. Beneficial effect of carotid endarterectomy in symptomatic patients with high-grade carotid stenosis. N Engl J Med 1991;325:445–453.
4. Biller J, Feinberg WM, Castaldo JE, Whittemore AD, Harbaugh RE, Dempsey RJ, Caplan LR, Kresowik TF, Matchar DB, Toole JF, Easton JD, Adams HP Jr, Brass LM, Hobson RW 2nd, Brott TG, Sternau L. Guidelines for carotid endarterectomy: a statement for healthcare professionals from a Special Writing Group of the Stroke Council, American Heart Association. Circulation 1998 Feb 10;97(5):501–509.
5. Wholey MH, Al-Mubarek N, Wholey MH. Updated review of the global carotid artery stent registry. Catheter Cardiovasc Interven 2003;60(2):259–266.
6. Kastrup A, Groschel K, Schulz JB, Nagele T, Ernemann U. Clinical predictors of transient ischemic attack, stroke, or death within 30 days of carotid angioplasty and stenting. Stroke 2005;36(4):787–791.
7. Roubin GS, Iyer S, Halkin A, Vitek J, Brennan C. Realizing the potential of carotid artery stenting: proposed paradigms for patient selection and procedural technique. Circulation 2006;113(16):2021–2030.
8. Yadav JS, Wholey MH, Kuntz RE, Fayad P, Katzen BT, Mishkel GJ, Bajwa TK, Whitlow P, Strickman NE, Jaff MR, Popma JJ, Snead DB, Cutlip DE, Firth BG, Ouriel K. Stenting and angioplasty with protection in patients at high risk for endarterectomy investigators. Protected carotid-artery stenting versus endarterectomy in high-risk patients. New Engl J Med 2004 Oct ;51(15):1493–1501.
9. Bagley L. Carotid Angioplasty. Interventional Radiology and Vascular Imaging, 5th Annual Course, Philadelphia, 1997.
10. CAVATAS Investigators. Endovascular versus surgical treatment in patients with carotid stenosis in the Carotid and Vertebral Artery Transluminal Angioplasty Study (CAVATAS): a randomised trial. Lancet 2001;357(9270):1729–1737
11. Alberts, MJ. Results of a multicenter prospective randomized trial of carotid artery stenting vs carotid endarterectomy. (abstract). Stroke 2001;32:325.
12. Kastrup A, Nagele T, Groschel K, Schmidt F, Vogler E, Schulz J, Ernemann U. Incidence of new brain lesions after carotid stenting with and without cerebral protection. Stroke 2006;37(9): 2312–2316.
13. Mas JL, Chatellier G, Beyssen B, Branchereau A, Moulin T, Becquemin JP, Larrue V, Lievre M, Leys D, Bonneville JF, Watelet J, Pruvo JP, Albucher JF, Viguier A, Piquet P, Garnier P, Viader F, Touze E, Giroud M, Hosseini H, Pillet JC, Favrole P, Neau JP, Ducrocq X, EVA-3S Investigators. Endarterectomy versus stenting in patients with symptomatic severe carotid stenosis. New Engl J Med 2006;355(16):1660–1671.
14. Hobson RW 2nd, Howard VJ, Roubin GS, Brott TG, Ferguson RD, Popma JJ, Graham DL, Howard G, CREST Investigators. Carotid artery stenting is associated with increased complications in octogenarians: 30-day stroke and death rates in the CREST lead-in phase. J Vasc Surg 2004;40(6):1106–1111.
15. Gray WA, Hopkins LN, Yadav S, Davis T, Wholey M, Atkinson R, Cremonesi A, Fairman R, Walker G, Verta P, Popma J, Virmani R, Cohen DJ, ARCHeR Trial Collaborators. Protected carotid stenting in high-surgical-risk patients: the ARCHeR results. J Vasc Surg 2006;44(2): 258–268.
16. SPACE Collaborative Group, Ringleb PA, Allenberg J, Bruckmann H, Eckstein HH, Fraedrich G, Hartmann M, Hennerici M, Jansen O, Klein G, Kunze A, Marx P, Niederkorn K, Schmiedt W,

Solymosi L, Stingele R, Zeumer H, Hacke W. 30 day results from the SPACE trial of stent-protected angioplasty versus carotid endarterectomy in symptomatic patients: a randomised non-inferiority trial. Lancet 2006;368(9543):1239–1247.

17. Theiss W, Hermanek P, Mathias K, Ahmadi R, Heuser L, Hoffmann FJ, Kerner R, Leisch F, Sievert H, von Sommoggy S, German Societies of Angiology and Radiology. Pro-CAS: a prospective registry of carotid angioplasty and stenting. Stroke 2004;35(9):2134–2139.

18. Hopkins LN. The Carotid Artery Revascularization Using the Boston Scientific EPI Filterwire EX/EZ and the EndoTex NexStent trial results. (Presentation). Transcatheter Therapeutics. Washington DC, 2005.

19. Safian RD, Bresnahan JF, Jaff MR, Foster M, Bacharach JM, Maini B, Turco M, Myla S, Eles G, Ansel GM, CREATE Pivotal Trial Investigators. Protected carotid stenting in high-risk patients with severe carotid artery stenosis. J Am Coll Cardiol 2006;47(12):2384–2389.

20. Gray WA, Yadav JS, Verta P, Scicli A, Fairman R, Wholey M, Hopkins LN, Atkinson R, Raabe R, Barnwell S, Green R. The CAPTURE registry: results of carotid stenting with embolic protection in the post approval setting. Catheter Cardiovasc Interven 2007;69(3):341–348.

21. Fisher ES, Malenka DJ, Solomon NA, Bubolz TA, Whaley FS, Wennberg JE. Risk of carotid endarterectomy in the elderly. Am J Public Health. 1989;79(12):1617–1620.

22. Applegate RJ, Grabarczyk MA, Little WC, Craven T, Walkup M, Kahl FR, Braden GA, Rankin KM, Kutcher MA. Vascular closure devices in patients treated with anticoagulation and IIb/IIIa receptor inhibitors during percutaneous revascularization. J Am Coll Cardiol 2002;40(1):78–83.

23. Saw J, Bajzer C, Casserly IP, Exaire E, Haery C, Sachar R, Lee D, Abou-Chebl A, Yadav JS. Evaluating the optimal activated clotting time during carotid artery stenting. Am J Cardiol 2006 Jun;97(11):1657–1660.

24. Saw J, Exaire JE, Lee DS, Yadav JS. Handbook of Complex Percutaneous Carotid Intervention. Humana Press, New York, 2007.

25. Markus H, Loh A, Israel D, Buckenham T, Clifton A, Brown MM. Microscopic air embolism during cerebral angiography and strategies for its avoidance. Lancet 1993;341(8848):784–787.

26. Ackerstaff RG, Suttorp MJ, van den Berg JC, Overtoom TT, Vos JA, Bal ET, Zanen P, Antonius Carotid Endarterectomy, Angioplasty, and Stenting Study Group. Prediction of early cerebral outcome by transcranial Doppler monitoring in carotid bifurcation angioplasty and stenting. J Vasc Surg 2005;41(4):618–624.

27. Al-Mubarak N, Roubin GS, Vitek JJ, Iyer SS, New G, Leon MB. Effect of the distal-balloon protection system on microembolization during carotid stenting. Circulation 2001;104(17):1999–2002.

28. Ackerstaff RG, Jansen C, Moll FL, Vermeulen FE, Hamerlijnck RP, Mauser HW. The significance of microemboli detection by means of transcranial Doppler ultrasonography monitoring in carotid endarterectomy. J Vasc Surg 1995;21(6):963–969.

29. Coppi G, Moratto R, Silingardi R, Rubino P, Sarropago G, Salemme L, Cremonesi A, Castriota F, Manetti R, Sacca S, Reimers B. PRIAMUS – proximal flow blockage cerebral protection during carotid stenting: results from a multicenter Italian registry. J Cardiovasc Surg 2005;46(3):219–227.

30. Parodi JC, Schonholz C, Parodi FE, Sicard G, Ferreira LM. Initial 200 cases of carotid artery stenting using a reversal-of-flow cerebral protection device. J Cardiovasc Surg 2007;48(2): 117–124.

31. Roh HG, Byun HS, Ryoo JW, Na DG, Moon WJ, Lee BB, Kim DI. Prospective analysis of cerebral infarction after carotid endarterectomy and carotid artery stent placement by using diffusion-weighted imaging. Am J Neuroradiol 2005;26(2):376–384.

32. Hauth EA, Jansen C, Drescher R, Schwartz M, Forsting M, Jaeger HJ, Mathias KD. MR and clinical follow-up of diffusion-weighted cerebral lesions after carotid artery stenting. Am J Neuroradiol 2005;26(9):2336–2341.

33. Schluter M, Tubler T, Steffens JC, Mathey DG, Schofer J. Focal ischemia of the brain after neuroprotected carotid artery stenting. J Am Coll Cardiol 2003 Sep;42(6):1007–1013.

34. Montorsi P, Galli S, Ravagnani P, Fabbiocchi F, Lualdi A, Trabattoni D, Calligaris G, Grancini L, Bartorelli AL. Direct vs predilation carotid artery stenting: acute and long-term results. 16th Annual Symposium Transcatheter Cardiovascular Therapeutics, Washington 30/9/2004. Am J Cardiol 2004;94(Supplement):161E.

35. Reimers B, Schluter M, Castriota F, Tubler T, Corvaja N, Cernetti C, Manetti R, Picciolo A, Liistro F, Di Mario C, Cremonesi A, Schofer J, Colombo A. Routine use of cerebral protection during carotid artery stenting: results of a multicenter registry of 753 patients. Am J Med 2004; 116(4):217–222.

36. Casserly IP, Abou-Chebl A, Fathi RB, Lee DS, Saw J, Exaire JE, Kapadia SR, Bajzer CT, Yadav JS. Slow-flow phenomenon during carotid artery intervention with embolic protection devices: predictors and clinical outcome. J Am Coll Cardiol 2005;46(8):1466–1472.
37. Ropper AH, Brown RH. Adams and Victor's Principles of Neurology. 8th Edition. McGraw-Hill Companies Inc., New York, 2005.
38. Wilentz JR, Chati Z, Krafft V, Amor M. Retinal embolization during carotid angioplasty and stenting: mechanisms and role of cerebral protection systems. Catheter Cardiovasc Interven 2002;56(3):320–327.
39. Yanoff M, Duker JS (eds): *Ophthalmology*. London: Mosby, 1999.
40. Yadav JS, Roubin GS, Iyer S, Vitek J, King P, Jordan WD, Fisher WS. Elective stenting of the extracranial carotid arteries. Circulation 1997;95(2):376–381.
41. Qureshi AI, Luft AR, Sharma M, Janardhan V, Lopes DK, Khan J, Guterman LR, Hopkins LN. Frequency and determinants of postprocedural hemodynamic instability after carotid angioplasty and stenting. Stroke 1999;30(10):2086–2093.
42. Iseli RK, Brand C, Telford M, LoGiudice D. Delirium in elderly general medical inpatients: a prospective study. Internal Medicine Journal 2007;37(12); 806–811.
43. Hanson MR, Galvez-Jimenez N. Management of dementia and acute confusional states in the perioperative period. Neurol Clin 2004;22(2):vii–viii, 413–422.
44. Burns MJ, Linden CH, Graudins A, Brown RM, Fletcher KE. A comparison of physostigmine and benzodiazepines for the treatment of anticholinergic poisoning. Ann Emerg Med 2000;35(4):374–381.
45. Abou-Chebl A, Yadav JS, Reginelli JP, Bajzer C, Bhatt D, Krieger DW. Intracranial hemorrhage and hyperperfusion syndrome following carotid artery stenting: risk factors, prevention, and treatment. J Am Coll Cardiol 2004;43(9):1596–1601.
46. Penn AA, Schomer DF, Steinberg GK. Imaging studies of cerebral hyperperfusion after carotid endarterectomy. Case report. J Neurosurg 1995;83(1):133–137.
47. Connolly ES. Hyperperfusion syndrome following carotid endarterectomy. In: Loftus CM, editor. Carotid Artery Surgery. Thieme Medical Publishers, New York, 2000, pp. 493–500.
48. Jansen C, Sprengers AM, Moll FL, Vermeulen FE, Hamerlijnck RP, van Gijn J, Ackerstaff RG. Prediction of intracerebral haemorrhage after carotid endarterectomy by clinical criteria and intraoperative transcranial Doppler monitoring. Eur J Vasc Surg 1994;8(3):303–308.
49. Piepgras DG, Morgan MK, Sundt TM Jr, Yanagihara T, Mussman LM. Intracerebral hemorrhage after carotid endarterectomy. [Comparative Study] J Neurosurg 1988;68(4):532–536.
50. Ouriel K, Shortell CK, Illig KA, Greenberg RK, Green RM. Intracerebral hemorrhage after carotid endarterectomy: incidence, contribution to neurologic morbidity, and predictive factors. J Vasc Surg 1999;29(1):82–87; discussion 87–89.
51. Roubin GS, Yadav S, Iyer SS, Vitek J. Carotid stent-supported angioplasty: a neurovascular intervention to prevent stroke. Am J Cardiol 1996;78(3A):8–12.
52. Diethrich EB, Ndiaye M, Reid DB. Stenting in the carotid artery: initial experience in 110 patients. J Endovasc Surg 1996;3(1):42–62.
53. Buhk JH, Wellmer A, Knauth M. Late in-stent thrombosis following carotid angioplasty and stenting. Neurology 2006 May;66(10):1594–1596.
54. Chaturvedi S, Sohrab S, Tselis A. Carotid stent thrombosis: report of 2 fatal cases. Stroke 2001;32(11):2700–2702.
55. Carotid Stenting: ACCF/SCAI/SVMB/SIR/ASITN 2007 Clinical Expert Consensus Document on: J Am Coll Cardiol 2007;49:126–170.
56. Fairman R, Gray WA, Scicli AP, Wilburn O, Verta P, Atkinson R, Yadav JS, Wholey M, Hopkins LN, Raabe R, Barnwell S, Green R, for the CAPTURE Trial Collaborators. The CAPTURE registry: analysis of strokes resulting from carotid artery stenting in the post approval setting: timing, location, severity, and type. Ann Surg 2007;246(4):551–556; discussion 556–558.
57. Wholey MH, Al-Mubarek N, Wholey MH. Updated review of the global carotid artery stent registry. Catheter Cardiovasc Interven 2003;60(2):259–266.
58. Setacci C, de Donato G, Setacci F, Pieraccini M, Cappelli A, Trovato RA, Benevento D. In-stent restenosis after carotid angioplasty and stenting: a challenge for the vascular surgeon. Eur J Vasc Endovasc Surg 2005;29(6):601–607.
59. Shawl FA. Carotid artery stenting: acute and long-term results. Curr Opin Cardiol 2002;17(6):671–676.

60. Levy EI, Hanel RA, Lau T, Koebbe CJ, Levy N, Padalino DJ, Malicki KM, Guterman LR, Hopkins LN. Frequency and management of recurrent stenosis after carotid artery stent implantation. J Neurosurg 2005;102(1):29–37.

61. Groschel K, Riecker A, Schulz JB, Ernemann U, Kastrup A. Systematic review of early recurrent stenosis after carotid angioplasty and stenting. Stroke 2005;36(2):367–373.

62. Roubin GS, Yadav S, Iyer SS, Vitek J. Carotid stent-supported angioplasty: a neurovascular intervention to prevent stroke. Am J Cardiol 1996;78(3A):8–12.

63. Willfort-Ehringer A, Ahmadi R, Gschwandtner ME, Haumer M, Lang W, Minar E. Single-center experience with carotid stent restenosis. J Endovasc Ther 2002;9(3):299–307.

64. Younis GA, Gupta K, Mortazavi A, Strickman NE, Krajcer Z, Perin E, Achari A. Predictors of carotid stent restenosis. Catheter Cardiovasc Interven 2007;69(5):673–682.

65. Robbin ML, Lockhart ME, Weber TM, Vitek JJ, Smith JK, Yadav J, Mathur A, Iyer SS, Roubin GS. Carotid artery stents: early and intermediate follow-up with Doppler US. Radiology 1997;205(3):749–756.

66. Ringer AJ, German JW, Guterman LR, Hopkins LN. Follow-up of stented carotid arteries by Doppler ultrasound. Neurosurgery 2002;51(3):639–643; discussion 643.

67. Stanziale SF, Wholey MH, Boules TN, Selzer F, Makaroun MS. Determining in-stent stenosis of carotid arteries by duplex ultrasound criteria. J Endovasc 2005;12(3):346–353.

68. Pannu N, Wiebe N, Tonelli M, Alberta Kidney Disease Network. Prophylaxis strategies for contrast-induced nephropathy. JAMA 2006;295(23):2765–2779.

69. Hoste EA, Kellum JA. Acute kidney dysfunction and the critically ill. Minerva Anestesiologica 2006;72(3):133–143.

70. Zagler A, Azadpour M, Mercado C, Hennekens CH. N-acetylcysteine and contrast-induced nephropathy: a meta-analysis of 13 randomized trials. Am Heart J 2006;151(1):140–145.

71. Barrett BJ, Parfrey PS. Clinical practice. Preventing nephropathy induced by contrast medium. New Engl J Med 2006;354(4):379–386.

72. Bartorelli AL, Marenzi G. Contrast Induced Nephropathy in Interventional Cardiovascular Medicine. Taylor & Francis Publishers, London; 2005.

73. Mathur A, Dorros G, Iyer SS, Vitek JJ, Yadav SS, Roubin GS. Palmaz stent compression in patients following carotid artery stenting. Catheter Cardiovasc Diagn 1997;41(2):137–140.

74. Bergeron P, Becquemin JP, Jausseran JM, Biasi G, Cardon JM, Castellani L, Martinez R, Fiorani P, Kniemeyer P. Percutaneous stenting of the internal carotid artery: the European CAST I Study. Carotid Artery Stent Trial. J Endovasc Surg 1999;6(2):155–159.

75. Wholey MH, Wholey M, Mathias K, Roubin GS, Diethrich EB, Henry M, Bailey S, Bergeron P, Dorros G, Eles G, Gaines P, Gomez CR, Gray B, Guimaraens J, Higashida R, Ho DS, Katzen B, Kambara A, Kumar V, Laborde JC, Leon M, Lim M, Londero H, Mesa J, Musacchio A, Myla S, Ramee S, Rodriquez A, Rosenfield K, Sakai N, Shawl F, Sievert H, Teitelbaum G, Theron JG, Vaclav P, Vozzi C, Yadav JS, Yoshimura SI. Global experience in cervical carotid artery stent placement. Catheter Cardiovasc Interven 2000;50(2):160–167.

76. Hopkins LN, for the CABERNET Investigators. Results of Carotid Artery Revascularization Using the Boston Scientific FilterWire EX/EX and the Endo Tex NexStent. Results from the CABERNET Clinical Trial. Paper presented at: EuroPCR Conference; May 24–27, 2005; Paris, France.

77. Villalobos HJ, Harrigan MR, Lau T, Wehman JC, Hanel RA, Levy EI, Guterman LR, Hopkins LN. Advancements in carotid stenting leading to reductions in perioperative morbidity among patients 80 years and older. Neurosurgery 2006;58(2):233–240; discussion 233–240.

15

Post-Procedural Monitoring and Follow-Up

Simon Walsh, MD

and Jacqueline Saw, MD, FRCPC

CONTENTS

ABSTRACT

Complications associated with carotid artery stenting can occur during or following the procedure, which can be divided into early post-procedural and late post-procedural complications. After the completion of a successful CAS procedure, management and monitoring is targeted toward the cardiovascular hemodynamic status and neurological status of the patients, to promptly identify early complications.

Keywords: Post-procedural monitoring; Complications; Follow-up

INTRODUCTION

Complications associated with carotid artery stenting (CAS) can occur during or following the procedure (see Chapter 14). The latter can be divided into early post-procedural complications and late post-procedural complications (see Table 3 in Chapter 14). Several early post-procedural complications are important to assess for, including persistent reflex bradycardia and hypotension, delirium, hyperperfusion syndrome, distal embolization, and stent thrombosis. Late post-procedural

From: *Contemporary Cardiology: Carotid Artery Stenting: The Basics*
Edited by: J. Saw, DOI 10.1007/978-1-60327-314-5_15,
© Humana Press, a part of Springer Science+Business Media, LLC 2009

complications may occur soon after hospital discharge to months after the CAS procedure and include late distal embolization, stent deformation, and in-stent restenosis.

PROCEDURAL AND EARLY POST-PROCEDURAL MONITORING

After the completion of a successful CAS procedure, management and monitoring is targeted toward the cardiovascular hemodynamic status and neurological status of the patients, to promptly identify early complications. To facilitate frequent monitoring of these patients, we routinely admit our CAS patients into our Cardiac Care Unit post-procedure, where cardiac telemetry and intensive nursing support is available. At our institution, we utilize pre-printed standardized carotid stent post-procedural orders (Figs. 1 and 2) to familiarize nursing staffs, residents, and fellows to the management of these patients. These orders help emphasize the frequency of hemodynamic and neurological monitoring (which differs from other interventional procedures) and alert support staffs to contact the interventionalists promptly with any complications.

A key element in the post-procedural care of these patients involves education of the critical care nursing staffs. Although the vast majority of patients (~90%) are likely to be hemodynamically stable without neurological symptoms after the

---

POST CAROTID STENT ORDERS (page 1 of 2)

Date: _____   Time: _____

1. Admit to   ☐ CCU2   ☐ Other: _____

2. Cardiovascular Service: Dr. _____

3. Neuro checks: Q15 min x 4 hours;   begin @ _____
                    Then, Q30 min x 4 hours;
                    Then, Q1 hour x 4 hours;
                    Then, Q4 hours

4. Notify Carotid Physician, Dr. _____ with any changes

5. Report stat to Carotid Physician or Interventional Fellow Dr. _____

     SPB < _____ or SBP > _____ , arrhythmias or angina pain.

6. Report any headache or neurological findings to Carotid Physician.

7. Stop all oral medications.

8. No sedation to be given without consulting the Physician.

<u>**Post-Procedure Standard Orders:**</u>

1. Bed rest overnight: (Head of bed may be elevated to 30°)

2. Check Vital Signs, groin sheaths, pedal pulses Q15min x 4hrs then, Q30min x 4hrs, then Q1h while sheath are in place.

3. Push PO fluids to 1L over 4 hours if tolerated.

4. Diet-clear fluids and crackers until 1h after groin sheaths out, then DAT.

5. ECG on return to ward if no VGH ECG on chart + STAT ECG for angina or nausea PRN

6. Foley catheter or In and Out catheterization PRN.

7. If closure device used: Bed rest until _____
                                  If subcutaneous ooze develops, light clamp x _____ min.
                                  if ooze continues or hematoma forms, call MD

8. If no closure device used follow standard insertion site orders.

Fig. 1. Routine post-procedure monitoring of carotid stent patients at Vancouver General Hospital (page 1).

POST CAROTID STENT ORDERS (page 2 of 2)

Date: _____   Time: _____

Antiplatelet therapy

☐ Plain ASA 325 po daily   ☐ _____ mg po daily.

☐ Enteric-coated ASA 325 po daily   ☐ _____ mg po daily.

☐ Clopidogrel 75mg od po daily.

IV Fluids

☐ Normal LV _____ @ 150ml/hr. x 1 liter, then 75ml/hr to KVO in a.m.

☐ Moderate LV _____ @ 100ml/hr. x 1 liter, then 75ml/hr to KVO in a.m.

☐ Severe LV _____ @ 75ml/hr. x 1 liter, then KVO in a.m.

Routine Laboratory and ECG orders

1. ECG in a.m.

2. Creatinine, CBC, CK and Troponin in a.m.

3. Hgb PRN – if suspected bleeding.

4. Ultra-sensitive CRP in a.m.

5. Carotid Doppler in a.m. before discharge.

6. Neuro consult post-procedure.

Other Medication

1. ☐ Ace-inhibitor: _____

2. ☐ Beta-blocker: _____

3. ☐ Statin therapy: _____

Fig. 2. Routine post-procedure monitoring of carotid stent patients at Vancouver General Hospital (page 2).

procedure *(1)*, a small proportion could develop complications that require prompt recognition and management. Thus, operators should educate their nursing colleagues about potential complications post-CAS and their management strategies. In our institution, a videotape on carotid stenting and complications by our carotid interventionalist was recorded and is shown to new nursing staffs looking after our CAS patients. Table 1 lists the major components that need to be monitored during and following the CAS procedure.

Cardiovascular Hemodynamic Monitoring

The most commonly encountered post-procedural complications are transient hemodynamic changes (hypotension or hypertension) or bradycardia. Typically these features are present during and immediately following stent deployment and will be apparent before the patient is transferred to the recovery unit. As indicated in Figs. 1 and 2, all our CAS patients are aggressively monitored post-procedure. Both cardiovascular vital signs and neurovitals are checked by nursing staffs every 15 min for the first 4 h, followed by every 30 min for the next 4 h, followed by hourly for another 4 h, followed by every 4 h thereafter. We educate our nursing staffs to alert

Table 1
Cardiovascular and Neurological Monitoring with CAS

Stages of CAS procedure	*Assess for*
(1) Throughout procedure	Blood pressure and heart rate
	Ask patient for symptoms: headache, vision, speech, sensory and motor
(2) During balloon inflation	Level of consciousness
	Bradycardia and hypotension
	Throat fullness or pain
(3) Immediately after CAS	Blood pressure and heart rate
	Ask patient for symptoms: headache, vision, speech, sensory and motor
	Mentation and orientation
	Check: speech, motor, pupils
(4) Monitoring in recovery unit	Blood pressure and heart rate
	Ask patient for symptoms: headache, vision, speech, sensory and motor
	Mentation and orientation
	Check: speech, motor, pupils

the carotid interventionalist if the systolic blood pressure falls below 90 mmHg or rises above 140 mmHg. Likewise, the interventionalist will be alerted to any symptomatic bradycardia.

REFLEX HYPOTENSION

In general, reflex hypotension is usually transient, mild, and asymptomatic. If the patient is asymptomatic and the systolic blood pressure is >80 mmHg, observation may be all that is required. Volume replacement with a crystalloid solution can be instituted with good effects in most cases. If the patient is symptomatic (e.g., feeling lightheaded, diaphoretic) or their systolic blood pressure is <80 mmHg, they should be administered crystalloid solution (e.g., normal saline) and oral pseudoephedrine (typical doses at 30–60 mg q4h prn). With persistent hypotension, intravenous infusion of inotropic vasoconstricting agents (e.g., dopamine or norepinephrine) may be required.

REFLEX BRADYCARDIA

Reflex bradycardia rarely develops after the patient has been transferred to the recovering unit. Typically this occurs during the CAS procedure with balloon inflation or stent deployment. However, it is possible for the bradycardia to deteriorate after the procedure. Symptomatic sinus bradycardia will usually respond to the administration of intravenous atropine (0.6 mg repeated as necessary to a maximum of 3 mg). In more severe cases, an infusion with dopamine or even temporary pacemaker may be required, although this is extremely rare.

HYPERPERFUSION SYNDROME

The development of hypertension is particularly worrisome after a carotid intervention, as this can be a result of or lead to cerebral hyperperfusion syndrome.

Again, it is imperative that the nursing staffs are educated regarding this rare but potentially catastrophic complication. In general, hypertension is usually noted before or during the procedure. Most frequently this is a pre-existing diagnosis, worsened by withholding their antihypertensive medications prior to the CAS procedure. The use of intravenous nitroglycerin is sometimes necessary to control the blood pressure during and post-procedure. Most patients' blood pressure will drop as a consequence of the carotid sinus reflex during carotid intervention. Stimulation of the carotid bulb leads to baroreceptor stimulation, and an efferent reflex to the sympathetic nervous system results in vasodilatation. Patients with persistent hypertension post-CAS should have their antihypertensive medications reinstituted soon after the procedure, with intravenous nitroglycerin overlapping until the oral medications take effect. It is extremely important to keep their systolic blood pressure less than 140 mmHg to avoid precipitating hyperperfusion syndrome.

Patients with hyperperfusion syndrome often complain of headache (classically unilateral symptoms on the side that underwent CAS), which may be accompanied by nausea and vomiting, confusion, reduced level of consciousness, seizures, focal neurological deficits, and intracranial hemorrhage. Thus, nursing staffs are warned to alert the interventionalists of any neurological changes, even if the headaches are mild. Prompt recognition is the key to successful management of hyperperfusion syndrome, followed by careful blood pressure (beta-blockers and diuretics) and seizure control. Antiplatelet therapy may need to be withheld until the blood pressure is adequately controlled.

Neurological Monitoring

Close neurological monitoring post-procedure is vital to diagnose distal embolization, cerebral hyperperfusion, encephalopathic delirium, stent thrombosis, and intracranial hemorrhage after CAS. Although the majority of these neurologic complications are rare, it is important that nursing staffs and operators are familiar with these complications (discussed in Chapter 14).

Immediately after the completion of CAS, the patient should be examined while still on the catheterization table (see Table 1). This is followed by frequent routine neurovital checks as alluded to earlier (see Figs. 1 and 2). These brief neurologic examinations should include assessment of headaches, orientation, speech, motor strength, vision (and pupils), and sensory changes (see Table 2). Nursing staffs should be instructed to evaluate these findings regularly. Current guidelines also recommend a formal neurological assessment within 24 h of the procedure, including scoring with the NIH Stroke Scale (see Chapter 6) *(1)*.

Table 2
Summary of Routine Neurological Assessment

Headache
Orientation (mental status)
Talk (assess speech: dysarthria, dysphasia, aphasia)
Motor (upper and lower extremities strength)
Eyes (assess vision and pupils)
Numb (upper and lower extremities sensory changes)

NEUROLOGICAL COMPLICATIONS

If the patient develops any neurologic symptoms, they should be fully assessed by the interventionalist and a neurologist without delay. Delirium post-CAS should prompt evaluation to rule out cerebral hyperperfusion or cerebral embolization. Focal neurologic deficits most often indicate ischemic distal embolization (e.g., extrusion of atheromatous plaque through stent struts). Sudden catastrophic neurologic event should raise concerns of acute stent thrombosis or intracranial hemorrhage, fortunately both are extremely rare. A prompt CT or MRI head scan is frequently warranted to assess for ischemic or hemorrhagic events and consideration for emergent cerebral angiography if distal embolization or stent thrombosis is suspected.

RETINAL EMBOLIZATION

Retinal cholesterol embolization is a unique complication that warrants further discussion (see Chapter 14). Fortunately, most events are asymptomatic or transiently symptomatic. Patients may complain of blurred vision or visual field loss. An opthalmology consultation should be obtained promptly, and potential treatments to dislodge the emboli include ocular massage, decreasing intra-ocular pressure pharmacologically with acetazolamide or mechanically with an anterior chamber paracentesis, or the use of hyperbaric oxygen. In the case of thrombotic emboli, attempts to lyse the thrombus may be achieved by intravenous heparin or thrombolytic agents.

PRE-DISCHARGE INVESTIGATIONS, MEDICATIONS, AND FOLLOW-UP

Prior to hospital discharge, the access site should be examined for the presence of vascular complications (e.g., hematoma, pseudoanuerysm, arterio-venous fistula). Repeat neurologic and cardiovascular vital signs should be evaluated prior to discharge.

Carotid Doppler

A baseline post-CAS carotid Doppler should be performed the day following the stenting procedure. This provides a baseline set of values for comparison during long-term follow-up, which is relevant since carotid velocities tend to be higher in the presence of stents despite lack of significant stenosis. This is supposedly due to increased stiffness in the stented segment of the carotid artery. A higher threshold of peak systolic velocity and internal carotid artery/common carotid artery ratio should be used to correctly identify the presence of restenosis *(2)*. It is also important to assess the change in contralateral internal carotid artery velocities following CAS among patients with bilateral carotid artery stenosis. Data from the Cleveland Clinic have shown a significant drop in contralateral peak systolic velocity (by 60.3 cm/s, $p = 0.005$) and end-diastolic velocity (by 15.1 cm/s, $p = 0.03$) after ipsilateral CAS among patients with bilateral stenosis *(3)*.

During follow-up, subsequent carotid duplex surveillance is recommended at 1 month, 6 months, and annually to assess for restenosis *(1)*.

Medications

Evidence-based medical therapy for patients with carotid disease has been discussed in Chapter 1. In the absence of contraindications, patients should be discharged home on aspirin (to continue lifelong) and clopidogrel (recommended for a minimum of 4 weeks after a carotid stent) *(1)*. There is no direct evidence for the use of dual antiplatelet therapy with aspirin and clopidogrel after carotid stenting. These recommendations were made on the basis of previous experience with bare-metal stents in the coronary circulation *(4, 5)* and extrapolated to the carotid population. Some centers arbitrarily recommend 6- or 12-week courses of aspirin and clopidogrel post-procedure on the basis of operator preference. It should be noted that dual antiplatelet therapy is indicated to allow the stent to endothelialize and negate the risk of stent thrombosis. However, there is no evidence of improved efficacy for long-term dual antiplatelet therapy in preventing cerebrovascular events *(6, 7)*.

Optimal medical therapy and aggressive risk factor modification are important adjuncts to carotid revascularization to lower cerebrovascular events in patients with carotid disease. Accordingly, patients should be advised to quit smoking and have their hypertension, hyperlipidemia, and diabetes mellitus aggressively managed. In a Cleveland Clinic prospective carotid registry ($n = 616$), patients discharged on a statin had a lower 30-day death or stroke event rate (3.4% statin vs. 9.0% no statin, $p = 0.005$) *(8)*. In the absence of contraindications, patients are discharged on appropriate doses of angiotensin-converting enzyme inhibitors and statins. Those with ischemic heart disease should also be considered for beta-blockers.

CONCLUSION

Self-limited and benign cardiovascular events of reflex bradycardia and hypotension occur frequently post-carotid stent procedures. On the contrary, hypertension post-CAS need to be closely monitored and treated to prevent hyperperfusion syndrome. Neurological complications are uncommon post-procedure, but need to be promptly diagnosed for acute management, which may prevent permanent neurologic deficits. Therefore, post-CAS monitoring should be carried out in a closely monitored setting where cardiac telemetry and intensive nursing support are available. Operators and nursing staffs should be familiar with the potential hemodynamic and neurologic complications and educated about the management strategies.

REFERENCES

1. Bates ER, Babb JD, Casey DE, Jr, et al. ACCF/SCAI/SVMB/SIR/ASITN 2007 clinical expert consensus document on carotid stenting: a report of the American College of Cardiology Foundation Task Force on Clinical Expert Consensus Documents (ACCF/SCAI/SVMB/SIR/ASITN Clinical Expert Consensus Document Committee on Carotid Stenting). J Am Coll Cardiol 2007;49:126–170.
2. Lal BK, Hobson RW, 2nd, Goldstein J, Chakhtoura EY, Duran WN. Carotid artery stenting: is there a need to revise ultrasound velocity criteria? J Vasc Surg 2004;39:58–66.
3. Sachar R, Yadav JS, Roffi M, et al. Severe bilateral carotid stenosis: the impact of ipsilateral stenting on Doppler-defined contralateral stenosis. J Am Coll Cardiol 2004;43:1358–1362.

4. Bertrand ME, Rupprecht HJ, Urban P, Gershlick AH. Double-blind study of the safety of clopidogrel with and without a loading dose in combination with aspirin compared with ticlopidine in combination with aspirin after coronary stenting: the clopidogrel aspirin stent international cooperative study (CLASSICS). Circulation 2000;102:624–629.

5. Bhatt DL, Bertrand ME, Berger PB, et al. Meta-analysis of randomized and registry comparisons of ticlopidine with clopidogrel after stenting. J Am Coll Cardiol 2002;39:9–14.

6. Diener HC, Bogousslavsky J, Brass LM, et al. Aspirin and clopidogrel compared with clopidogrel alone after recent ischaemic stroke or transient ischaemic attack in high-risk patients (MATCH): randomised, double-blind, placebo-controlled trial. Lancet 2004;364:331–337.

7. Bhatt DL, Fox KA, Hacke W, et al. Clopidogrel and aspirin versus aspirin alone for the prevention of atherothrombotic events. N Engl J Med 2006;354:1706–1717.

8. Saw J, Exaire J, Lee D, et al. Statins reduce early death or stroke events following carotid artery stenting. Circulation 2004;110:III–646.

INDEX